TUBERCULOSIS IN THE WORKPLACE

Marilyn J. Field, *Editor*

Committee on Regulating Occupational Exposure to Tuberculosis
Division of Health Promotion and Disease Prevention

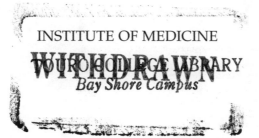

INSTITUTE OF MEDICINE

NATIONAL ACADEMY PRESS
Washington, D.C.

NATIONAL ACADEMY PRESS • 2101 Constitution Avenue, NW • Washington, D.C. 20418

NOTICE: The project that is the subject of this report was approved by the Governing Board of the National Research Council, whose members are drawn from the councils of the National Academy of Sciences, the National Academy of Engineering, and the Institute of Medicine. The members of the committee responsible for the report were chosen for their special competences and with regard for appropriate balance.

Support for this project was provided by the U.S. Department of Health and Human Services (Contract HHS-100-00-0008). The views presented are those of the Institute of Medicine Committee on Regulating Occupational Exposure to Tuberculosis and are not necessarily those of the funding organization.

Library of Congress Cataloging-in-Publication Data

Tuberculosis in the workplace / Marilyn J. Field, editor ; Committee on Regulating Occupational Exposure to Tuberculosis, Division of Health Promotion and Disease Prevention, Institute of Medicine.

p. cm.
Includes bibliographical references.
ISBN 0-309-07330-8
1. Tuberculosis—United States. 2. Medical personnel—Health risk assessment—United States. 3. Tuberculosis—Prevention—Government policy—United States. I. Field, Marilyn J, (Marilyn Jane) II. Institute of Medicine (U.S.). Committee on Regulating Occupational Exposure to Tuberculosis.

RC313.A2 .T83 2001
614.5′42′0973—dc21

2001030369

Additional copies of this report are available from:

National Academy Press
2101 Constitution Avenue, N.W.
Box 285
Washington, DC 20055
Call (800) 624-6242 or (202) 334-3313
(in the Washington metropolitan area)
Internet: www.nap.edu

Cover image: Mycobacterium tuberculosis. Copyright Dennis Kunkel Microscopy, Inc.

3/19/03

*"Knowing is not enough; we must apply.
Willing is not enough; we must do."*
—Goethe

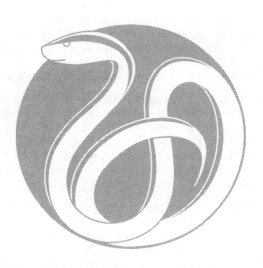

INSTITUTE OF MEDICINE

Shaping the Future for Health

THE NATIONAL ACADEMIES

National Academy of Sciences
National Academy of Engineering
Institute of Medicine
National Research Council

The **National Academy of Sciences** is a private, nonprofit, self-perpetuating society of distinguished scholars engaged in scientific and engineering research, dedicated to the furtherance of science and technology and to their use for the general welfare. Upon the authority of the charter granted to it by the Congress in 1863, the Academy has a mandate that requires it to advise the federal government on scientific and technical matters. Dr. Bruce M. Alberts is president of the National Academy of Sciences.

The **National Academy of Engineering** was established in 1964, under the charter of the National Academy of Sciences, as a parallel organization of outstanding engineers. It is autonomous in its administration and in the selection of its members, sharing with the National Academy of Sciences the responsibility for advising the federal government. The National Academy of Engineering also sponsors engineering programs aimed at meeting national needs, encourages education and research, and recognizes the superior achievements of engineers. Dr. William A. Wulf is president of the National Academy of Engineering.

The **Institute of Medicine** was established in 1970 by the National Academy of Sciences to secure the services of eminent members of appropriate professions in the examination of policy matters pertaining to the health of the public. The Institute acts under the responsibility given to the National Academy of Sciences by its congressional charter to be an adviser to the federal government and, upon its own initiative, to identify issues of medical care, research, and education. Dr. Kenneth I. Shine is president of the Institute of Medicine.

The **National Research Council** was organized by the National Academy of Sciences in 1916 to associate the broad community of science and technology with the Academy's purposes of furthering knowledge and advising the federal government. Functioning in accordance with general policies determined by the Academy, the Council has become the principal operating agency of both the National Academy of Sciences and the National Academy of Engineering in providing services to the government, the public, and the scientific and engineering communities. The Council is administered jointly by both Academies and the Institute of Medicine. Dr. Bruce M. Alberts and Dr. William A. Wulf are chairman and vice chairman, respectively, of the National Research Council.

COMMITTEE ON REGULATING OCCUPATIONAL EXPOSURE TO TUBERCULOSIS

Walter Hierholzer (*Chair*), Professor Emeritus of Internal Medicine, Infectious Diseases and Epidemiology, Yale University

Scott Barnhart, Medical Director, Harborview Medical Center, and Associate Dean, School of Medicine, University of Washington

Henry M. Blumberg, Associate Professor, Department of Medicine, Division of Infectious Diseases, Emory University and Hospital Epidemiologist, Grady Memorial Hospital

Scott Burris, Professor of Law, Temple University School of Law

Robyn Gershon, Assistant Professor, Division of Sociomedical Sciences, Mailman School of Public Health at Columbia University

Douglas Hornick, Associate Professor, Division of Pulmonary Diseases and Critical Care Medicine, Department of Internal Medicine, University of Iowa

Pamela Kellner, Director, Program Development Unit, Bureau of Tuberculosis Control, New York City Department of Health

James Melius, Executive Director, New York State Laborers' Health and Safety Trust Fund

Stephen G. Pauker, Sara Murray Jordan Professor of Medicine and Vice Chair, Clinical Affairs, Department of Medicine, Tufts/New England Medical Center

Robert C. Spear, Professor, Environmental Health Sciences, University of California, Berkeley

Lester N. Wright, Deputy Commissioner and Chief Medical Officer, New York Department of Correctional Services

Committee Consultants and Liaison

John J. Bass, Jr., Chair, Department of Medicine, University of South Alabama

Thomas M. Daniel, Professor Emeritus of Medicine and International Health, Case Western Reserve University

Lawrence Geiter, Director of Clinical Programs, Sequella Foundation, Maryland

Phillip Harber, Professor of Family Medicine and Chief, Occupational and Environmental Medicine, University of California, Los Angeles

Michael L. Tapper, Hospital Epidemiologist, Lennox Hill Hospital, New York City

Keith F. Woeltje, Assistant Professor of Medicine, Section of Infectious Diseases, Medical College of Georgia

M. Donald Whorton, Liaison, Board on Health Promotion and Disease Prevention, Institute of Medicine

v

Acknowledgments

In developing this report, the committee and staff benefited from the expertise and experience of many individuals. In particular, we learned much from the presenters and participants in the workshop and public hearing held in August, 2000. At the committee's request following the workshop, Ronald Bayer further developed his presentation about ethical issues, and Lisa Brousseau, Rachel Stricof, and Barry Farr also provided additional information or other assistance. Appendix A lists the workshop participants, presenters, and agendas.

The authors of the commissioned background papers presented in Appendixes B (John J. Bass, Jr.), C (Thomas M. Daniel), D (Keith F. Woeltje), E (Scott Burris and Jamie Crabtree), and F (Phillip Harber, Scott Barnhart, Douglas Hornick, and Robert Spear) made essential contributions to this report through their evidence reviews, and their extensive discussions with committee members and staff. Their ability to develop the evidence reviews on a tight schedule for discussion at the workshop was especially appreciated. Dr. Daniel also patiently allowed us to draw on his deep expertise and decades of experience in research on tuberculosis. Consultants Michael Tapper and Lawrence Geiter provided expert advice and information about many issues. M. Donald Whorton, the liaison to the committee from the IOM's Board on Health Promotion and Disease Prevention, likewise provided useful insights about the committee's deliberations and analyses.

The project officer at the National Institute for Occupational Safety and Health (NIOSH), Greg Wagner, always responded promptly to questions. Others at the agency who provided information and explanations about NIOSH research and statements included Paul Jensen and Christopher Coffey. At the Division of Tuberculosis Elimination (which is also part of the Centers for Disease Control and Prevention [CDC]), Renee Ridzon and Amy Curtis patiently answered many questions about CDC data, guidelines, and procedures. The weekly summary of news about tuberculosis developed by John Seggerson was an invaluable resource.

At the Occupational Safety and Health Administration (OSHA), Amanda Edens was unfailingly helpful in answering questions about the proposed rule. She and Claudia Thurber helped clarify aspects of OSHA's legislative, administrative, and judicial framework and differences between the language of the 1997 proposed rule and the 1994 CDC guidelines. Others at OSHA who provided useful information or explanations included Susan Sherman for her review of legal matters, Steven Bayard, Marthe Kent, and John Rainwater.

At the Institute of Medicine, study staff appreciate the assistance of Sue Barron, Claudia Carl, Mike Edington, Pat Spaulding, Rita Gaskins, Karen Autrey, and Melissa Goodwin among others. Michael Hayes helped in copy editing the report.

REVIEWERS

This report has been reviewed in draft form by individuals chosen for their diverse perspectives and technical expertise, in accordance with procedures approved by the NRC's Report Review Committee. The purpose of this independent review is to provide candid and critical comments that will assist the institution in making its published report as sound as possible and to ensure that the report meets institutional standards for objectivity, evidence, and responsiveness to the study charge. The review comments and draft manuscript remain confidential to protect the integrity of the deliberative process. We wish to thank the following individuals for their review of this report:

James August, American Federation of Labor and Congress of Industrial Organizations

Alfred Franzblau, M.D., School of Public Health, University of Michigan

Victoria Fraser, M.D., Washington University School of Medicine

Alan Hinman, M.D., M.P.H., Task Force for Child Survival and Development

Richard Menzies, M.D., Respiratory Epidemiology Unit, McGill University, Montreal Chest Institute

Mary L. Powell, Ph.D., University of Kentucky, Lexington

Although the reviewers listed above have provided many constructive comments and suggestions, they were not asked to endorse the conclusions or recommendations nor did they see the final draft of the report before its release. The review of this report was overseen by **Robert Lawrence**, M.D., School of Hygiene and Public Health, Johns Hopkins University, appointed by the Institute of Medicine and **Elaine L. Larson**, R.N., Ph.D., Columbia University School of Nursing, appointed by the NRC's Report Review Committee, who were responsible for making certain that an independent examination of this report was carried out in accordance with institutional procedures and that all review comments were carefully considered. Responsibility for the final content of this report rests entirely with the authoring committee and the institution.

Contents

BOXES, FIGURES AND TABLES

Boxes

Figures

Tables

TUBERCULOSIS
IN THE
WORKPLACE

Summary

Tuberculosis is a treatable, communicable disease that has two general states: latent infection and active disease. With few exceptions, only those who develop active tuberculosis in the lungs or larynx can infect others, usually by coughing, sneezing, or otherwise expelling tiny infectious particles that someone else inhales.

Although tuberculosis is still a major killer in poor countries, 50 years of effective drug treatment has greatly reduced the toll that the disease takes in developed countries. Nonetheless, after more than 30 years of declines in reported tuberculosis cases and deaths, the mid-1980s and early 1990s saw a reversal of that trend in the United States. This resurgence of tuberculosis, which included several outbreaks of the disease among hospital patients and workers, prompted considerable concern among health care workers, administrators, public health professionals, and policymakers. Renewed public and private efforts to control the disease followed. These efforts included the initiation of a rulemaking process by the federal Occupational Safety and Health Administration (OSHA) that led, in 1997, to the publication of proposed regulations on occupational tuberculosis.

In November 1999, the U.S. Congress requested that the National Academy of Sciences undertake a short-term study to examine the risk of tuberculosis among health care workers and the possible effects of federal guidelines and regulations intended to protect workers from this risk. Between April and September 2000, a committee of the Institute of Medicine (IOM), the health policy arm of the Academy, investigated three questions:

1

1. Are health care and selected other categories of workers at a greater risk of infection, disease, or mortality due to tuberculosis than others in the communities in which they reside?

2. What is known about the implementation and effects of the 1994 Centers for Disease Control and Prevention (CDC) guidelines for the prevention of tuberculosis in health care facilities?

3. What will be the likely effects on rates of tuberculosis infection, disease, and mortality of an anticipated OSHA standard to protect workers from occupational exposure to tuberculosis?

The committee's charge from Congress for this limited study did not include the development of recommendations for regulatory policy. It also did not include an evaluation of the costs or cost-effectiveness of implementing a standard.

Overall, the committee concludes that tuberculosis remains a threat to some health care, correctional facility, and other workers in the United States. Although the risk has been decreasing in recent years, vigilance is still needed within hospitals, prisons, and similar workplaces, as well as in the community at large. Fortunately, tuberculosis control measures recommended by the CDC in response to tuberculosis outbreaks in health care facilities appear to have been effective. Available evidence suggests that where tuberculosis is uncommon or where basic infection control measures are in place, the occupational risk to health care workers of tuberculosis now approaches community levels, which have been declining. The primary risk to workers today comes from patients, inmates, or others with unsuspected and undiagnosed infectious tuberculosis.

The committee also concludes that an OSHA standard on occupational tuberculosis can have a positive effect if it meets three basic conditions: (1) it is consistent with tuberculosis control measures that appear to be effective, (2) it increases or sustains the level of compliance with those measures, and (3) it allows appropriate flexibility for organizations to adopt tuberculosis control measures appropriate to the level of risk facing workers. The committee expects that a standard will meet the first two conditions by sustaining or increasing the use of effective tuberculosis control measures. The committee is, however, concerned that if a final OSHA standard follows the 1997 proposed rule, it may not meet the third condition of allowing reasonable flexibility to adopt measures appropriate to the level of risk.

CDC GUIDELINES AND THE PROPOSED OSHA RULE

1994 CDC Guidelines

In 1994, CDC published its most extensive guidelines for preventing the transmission of tuberculosis in health care facilities (including health care units in prisons, jails, and certain other settings). The guidelines present a three-level hierarchy of tuberculosis control recommendations comprising

1. administrative controls (in particular, protocols for early identification, isolation, and treatment of individuals with infectious tuberculosis),
2. engineering controls (in particular, negative-pressure ventilation of isolation rooms for patients with infectious tuberculosis), and
3. personal respiratory protection (primarily use of specially designed facemasks to prevent inhalation of infectious particles).

The CDC guidelines, which followed statements issued in 1982 and 1990, also set forth a risk assessment process that defines five categories of facilities (or areas of facilities) based on the risk of tuberculosis transmission. The guidelines recommend fewer tuberculosis control measures for the facilities in the "minimal" and "very low" risk categories. The risk assessment process for a facility covers the profile of tuberculosis in the community, the numbers of tuberculosis patients examined or treated in different areas of the facility, and the tuberculin skin test conversion rates for workers in different areas of the facility or in different job categories. The process also takes into account evidence of person-to-person transmission of tuberculosis resulting in active disease as well as information from medical record reviews or workplace observations that suggests possible problems in tuberculosis control measures. In the summer of 2000, CDC began a reassessment of its guidelines for health care facilities, and the results are expected in mid-2002.

1997 Proposed OSHA Rule

When the committee began work in April 2000, OSHA expected to publish the final standard on occupational tuberculosis in July. Subsequently, OSHA indicated that publication would likely occur by the end of the year 2000, which would follow the committee's final meeting in September 2000. Thus, the committee had to undertake its analyses without knowing the content of the final regulations. It is possible that the new Administration will not issue any final standard.

By law, OSHA can directly regulate only private employers and, with certain restrictions, federal agencies. Through agreements with states that choose to participate, OSHA regulations may also be applied to employees of state and local governments. About half the states have entered into such agreements.

In its 1997 proposed rule on occupational tuberculosis, OSHA followed the 1994 CDC guidelines in most respects. Also, OSHA concluded that the CDC guidelines in their original form were not specific and directive enough to be adopted directly as a regulatory standard. The proposed rule, therefore, differs from the CDC guidelines in certain ways. First, the proposed rule is written to be enforced and, therefore, tends to be more specific and directive than the CDC guidelines. Second, it would cover a broader group of employers and employees. Third, it is intended to protect employees and not, for example, patients, prisoners, or visitors. Fourth, it sets forth very restrictive criteria for defining "low-risk" employers that would not be expected to implement all the rule's requirements.

The 1997 proposed OSHA rule defines a category of employers that would be exempt from some of its requirements, but the qualifying criteria are narrower than those set forth in the 1994 CDC guidelines. Specifically, a facility must neither admit nor provide medical services to individuals with suspected or confirmed tuberculosis, it must have had no confirmed cases of infectious tuberculosis during the previous 12 months, *and* it must be located in a county that has had no confirmed cases of infectious tuberculosis during 1 of the previous 2 years and less than six cases during the other year. Even if a facility had admitted no tuberculosis patients in the preceding 12 months, had no tuberculosis cases in its service area, and had a policy of referring those with diagnosed or suspected tuberculosis, that facility could not qualify for this "lower risk" category if the surrounding county had reported one case of tuberculosis in each of the preceding 2 years.

ASSESSMENT AND CONCLUSIONS

Context: Changing Tuberculosis Case Rates and Community and Workplace Responses

The committee's conclusions need to be understood in context. This context includes the changing epidemiology of the disease over the past two decades, the evolution of community and institutional responses to the perceived threat of tuberculosis, and the persistence of geographic variations in community levels of tuberculosis.

Resurgent Tuberculosis, 1985–1992

Between 1985 and 1992, reported cases of tuberculosis increased by 20 percent, from 22,201 in 1985 to 26,673 in 1992. The case rate per 100,000 population increased by more than 12 percent, from 9.3 in 1985 to 10.5 in 1992. The number of deaths rose from 1,752 in 1985 to 1,970 in 1989. In the early 1980s, about 0.5 percent of new tuberculosis cases were resistant to the two major antituberculosis drugs, isoniazid and rifampin. By 1991, that figure had risen to 3.5 percent.

In addition, during the late 1980s and early 1990s, several U.S. hospitals experienced outbreaks of tuberculosis that affected both patients and employees. Some outbreaks involved a particularly lethal combination of multidrug-resistant disease and people with suppressed immune systems, most often related to HIV infection. Outbreaks also occurred in prisons and other workplaces serving people at increased risk of tuberculosis.

Lack of Preparation

In general, public health departments, health care facilities, prisons, and similar organizations were not prepared to cope with the resurgence of tuberculosis in the mid-1980s. After years of effective treatment and declining case rates, tuberculosis control measures were not a priority in either the community or the workplace. The HIV/AIDS epidemic and its interaction with tuberculosis were not well documented or understood. Similarly, the threat of multidrug-resistant tuberculosis resulting from incomplete treatment of the disease had yet to be clearly appreciated. Workplace outbreaks of tuberculosis were often associated with lapses in infection control measures.

Rebuilding Capacity

The resurgence of tuberculosis in communities and the outbreaks of the disease in workplaces prompted a range of public and private responses. Congress revived federal funding for tuberculosis control programs, which had virtually disappeared in the 1970s. States and some cities and counties also began to rebuild programs that had been neglected or dismantled. These programs focused on groups at increased risk of tuberculosis such as people with HIV infection or AIDS, and they emphasized directly observed therapy for individuals with active tuberculosis. Hospitals, prisons, and perhaps other institutions, especially those affected by outbreaks and those located in high-risk areas, improved their infection control programs.

Guidelines and Regulations

In 1990, CDC issued new guidelines for tuberculosis control measures in health care facilities. In 1993, in response to calls from health care and other workers, OSHA began to enforce some tuberculosis control measures under its general powers to protect worker safety and under other regulations related to airborne hazards. In 1994, the agency began a formal rulemaking process to develop specific regulations on occupational tuberculosis. Also in 1994, CDC issued a major revision of its 1990 guidelines for the prevention of transmission of tuberculosis in health care facilities. OSHA published a proposed rule on occupational tuberculosis in 1997 and solicited comments on the rule in 1998 and again in 1999. In addition, some state licensure agencies and private accrediting organizations required tuberculosis control measures.

Decreasing Rates of Disease

The epidemiology of tuberculosis has changed substantially since the early 1990s. In 1993, the trend of increasing tuberculosis case rates began to reverse, and declines have now been recorded for 7 successive years. Tuberculosis case rates reached new lows in 1999, when CDC reported a rate of 6.4 per 100,000 population, a 35 percent drop since 1992. Cases of multidrug-resistant disease have also decreased; in 1999, they accounted for just 1.2 percent of cases. In general, fewer cases of tuberculosis and less multidrug-resistant disease mean less risk for nurses, doctors, correctional officers, and others who work for organizations that serve people who have tuberculosis or who are at increased risk of the disease.

Continuing Geographic Variation

Despite the general decline in tuberculosis rates in recent years, a marked geographic variation in tuberculosis case rates persists, which means that workers in different areas face different potential risks. Among metropolitan statistical areas, 1999 case rates varied from 1.3 per 100,000 population in Omaha to 17.7 per 100,000 in New York City and 18.2 per 100,000 in San Francisco. Between 1994 and 1998, six states—California, Florida, Illinois, New Jersey, New York, and Texas—accounted for 57 percent of tuberculosis cases but had just under 40 percent of the U.S. population. These states also account for a large proportion of people with risk factors for the disease, notably, HIV infection and immigration from countries with a high prevalence of tuberculosis. More than 40 percent of tuberculosis cases reported in the United States in 1999 involved people born in other countries, primarily Mexico, the Philippines, and Vietnam.

Conclusions

One problem facing the IOM committee as well as CDC and OSHA was the lack of prospective, controlled studies documenting the effectiveness of specific protective measures in preventing the transmission of tuberculosis in the workplace. Most studies of these protective measures are retrospective or observational, and they are inconsistent in their methods and reporting. The studies typically involve organizations—mainly hospitals—that experienced tuberculosis outbreaks and then implemented multiple control measures in a fairly short period of time.

No national data on occupational risk of tuberculosis infection are available, and data from surveys, outbreak studies, and other sources are subject to various biases. Data are especially sparse for workplaces other than hospitals. This lack of information is troubling because many of these facilities serve people at increased risk of active tuberculosis—including people who are unemployed, homeless, or poor; people with human immunodeficiency virus (HIV) infection or AIDS or substance abuse problems; and recent immigrants from countries with high rates of tuberculosis. These other workplaces may lack the resources and expertise available to hospitals to assess the risk to workers and undertake appropriate precautions. External oversight may also be more limited.

After reviewing scientific and other literature, considering discussions held during the committee's public meetings, and drawing on its members' experience and judgment, the committee reached several conclusions in response to the questions posed to it. Again, the committee's charge and resources did not provide for consideration of policy options and recommendations.

> *Question 1:* Are health care and selected other categories of workers at greater risk of infection, disease, or mortality due to tuberculosis than others in the community in which they reside?

Through at least the 1950s, health care workers were at higher risk from tuberculosis than others in the community. Currently available data suggest where tuberculosis is uncommon or where basic infection control measures are in place, the occupational risk to health care workers of tuberculosis infection now approaches the level in their community of residence. Tuberculosis risk in communities has been declining since 1993. Overall, rates of active tuberculosis among health care workers are similar overall to those reported for other employed workers. Data do not allow comparisons of mortality risk, but health care workers and others with compromised immune function are at high risk of death if they contract multidrug-resistant disease.

The primary risk to health care, correctional, and other workers now comes from patients, inmates, or clients with unsuspected, undiagnosed infectious tuberculosis. Risk is influenced by the prevalence of tuberculosis in the community that the workplace serves and by the extent and type of worker's contact with people who have infectious tuberculosis. The available data do not allow precise quantification of the risk to health care workers or conclusions about the historical or current risk to other categories of workers covered by the 1997 proposed OSHA rule.

Question 2: What is known about the implementation and effects of the 1994 CDC guidelines for the prevention of tuberculosis in health care facilities?

Conclusions about the implementation and effect of the CDC guidelines must be read within the larger context of the social response to resurgent tuberculosis. The actions recommended in the CDC guidelines are consistent with general standards of good infection control, and the 1994 guidelines were built on a series of earlier government and professional recommendations. In addition, by the mid-1990s, OSHA and some state agencies were also requiring many of the same basic measures.

Implementation

Data from surveys, facility inspections, and other sources indicate that institutional departures from recommended tuberculosis control policies and procedures were common, if not the norm, in the late 1980s and the early 1990s. By the mid-1990s, hospitals, and, less clearly, other health care organizations and correctional facilities began to take tuberculosis control measures more seriously. The adoption of written tuberculosis control policies does not, however, always translate into consistent day-to-day practice.

Implementation is probably most complete for administrative controls including procedures for promptly identifying, isolating, diagnosing, and adequately treating people with active tuberculosis. For engineering controls, available data suggest that the rate of installation of negative-pressure isolation rooms has increased, but not all in-use rooms are assessed on a daily basis to ensure that they remain under negative pressure. Information about personal respiratory protection programs is very limited. It suggests that most hospitals have been providing some kind of protection and have been updating the equipment provided as new options, such as the N95 respirator, have been developed and certified by the National Institute for Occupational Safety and Health.

Effects

Overall, the measures recommended by CDC in 1994 and earlier to prevent the transmission of tuberculosis in health care facilities have contributed to ending hospital outbreaks of tuberculosis and preventing new ones. Studies of outbreaks as well as logic and biologic plausibility support CDC's stress on administrative controls, particularly the rigorous application of protocols for the prompt identification and isolation of people with signs and symptoms suspicious for infectious tuberculosis. Studies of outbreaks and modeling exercises suggest that engineering controls also make a contribution in limiting the transmission of tuberculosis. Available information suggests that most of the benefit of control measures comes from administrative and engineering controls. Modeling studies support the tailoring of personal respiratory protections to the level of risk faced by workers—that is, more stringent protection for those in high-risk situations and less stringent measures for others.

Although control measures have helped to end workplace outbreaks of tuberculosis and prevent transmission of the disease, these measures cannot prevent all types of worker exposure to tuberculosis. In areas with moderate to high levels of tuberculosis, some worker exposure to patients with unsuspected infectious tuberculosis can be expected. Not all infectious individuals have easily recognized symptoms or signs of the disease, so workers may be exposed to them for a period before tuberculosis is suspected, a diagnosis is made, and precautions are initiated. Conscientious implementation of tuberculosis control measures does not guarantee that transmission will never occur, but it appears to reduce risk significantly, especially in high-prevalence areas.

Question 3: What will be the likely effects on rates of tuberculosis infection, disease, and mortality of an anticipated OSHA standard to protect workers from occupational exposure to tuberculosis?

Because the committee had to work without access to the final OSHA regulations on occupational tuberculosis, it could not be certain of whether or how the final standard would differ from the 1997 proposed rule or from the 1994 CDC guidelines. Therefore, rather than concentrate narrowly on individual features of the proposed rule, the committee decided to consider more generally the conditions that would need to be met for a standard to have positive effects on tuberculosis infection, disease, or mortality. It identified three such conditions.

First, implementation of workplace tuberculosis control measures as recommended by CDC and proposed by OSHA must contribute meaningfully to the prevention of transmission of *Mycobacterium tuberculosis* in hospitals and other covered workplaces. Second, an OSHA standard must sustain or increase the level of adherence to workplace tuberculosis control measures, especially in high-risk institutions and communities. Third, an OSHA standard must allow reasonable adaptation of tuberculosis control measures to fit differences in the levels of risk facing workers.

Overall, the committee expects that the first of the conditions outlined above—that tuberculosis control measures are effective—will be met for hospitals and possibly correctional facilities. Insufficient information is available to assess the effectiveness of control measures in other workplaces.

The committee expects that the second condition will also be met; that is, an OSHA standard will sustain or increase the level of compliance with mandated tuberculosis control measures. A standard is likely to motivate more organizational adherence to control measures than can be achieved by voluntary guidelines. A standard is also likely to be clearer, more hazard specific, and easier to use than the other legal strategies available to OSHA. In addition, by providing a firmer basis for OSHA enforcement actions, a standard should put workers on stronger ground in identifying and challenging an employer's inadequate implementation of mandated tuberculosis control measures.

The committee is concerned, however, that if an OSHA standard follows the 1997 proposed rule, it may not meet the third condition of allowing organizations reasonable flexibility to adopt tuberculosis control measures appropriate to the level of risk facing workers. The 1997 proposed rule defines a category of employers that would be excused from some of the rule's requirements, but the criteria defined are very narrow and would likely subject too many low-risk organizations to the rule's full scope. In addition, as an indicator of tuberculosis risk in the community, the proposed rule would require use of county-level data to assess community risk, even though a facility's service area might be quite different and have a much different incidence of tuberculosis. To the extent that an OSHA standard inflexibly extends requirements to institutions that are at negligible risk of occupational transmission of *M. tuberculosis*, the standard is unlikely to benefit workers at the same time that it would impose significant costs and administrative burdens on covered organizations and absorb institutional resources that could be applied to other, potentially more beneficial uses.

The committee also concludes that OSHA's 1997 estimates overstated the number of infections, cases of disease, and deaths due to tuberculosis that would be averted by adoption of the 1997 proposed rule. (The committee did not have access to OSHA's recently revised estimates.) Tuberculosis case rates are down substantially from 1994 and the earlier years used for the estimates, and implementation of community and workplace tuberculosis control measures appears to be considerably improved. Recent data on tuberculosis infection are limited but indicate low levels of tuberculosis infection in health care facilities and suggest that exposure in the community is a significant factor in health care worker infections. In addition, the agency's estimates relied on assumptions about the progression of tuberculosis from infection to active disease and from disease to death that are widely used but inconsistent with available data and are unlikely to fit employed workers with reasonably good access to health care.

PUBLIC POLICY AND THE
CHANGING EPIDEMIOLOGY OF TUBERCULOSIS

Unlike typical workplace health problems such as those involving exposure to hazardous chemicals or dust, the likelihood of occupational exposure to tuberculosis has a close connection to the risk of tuberculosis in the surrounding community. Those responsible for occupational health programs cooperate with those responsible for public health programs to track and prevent the transmission of tuberculosis.

The committee draws a parallel between the circumstances facing workplace tuberculosis control programs and the circumstances described in the recent IOM report *Ending Neglect: The Elimination of Tuberculosis in the United States* (IOM, [2000]). That report attributed the resurgence in tuberculosis in the mid-1980s to the complacency that followed the introduction and spread of effective treatment beginning around 1950. Complacency led to neglect of basic public health measures including surveillance, contact tracing, outbreak investigations, and case management services to ensure that individuals completed treatments for latent infection and active disease. This neglect helped set the stage for the resurgence of tuberculosis when new circumstances emerged—including the HIV/AIDS epidemic, the increase in multidrug-resistant disease (largely due to incomplete treatment), and expanded immigration from regions of the world with high rates of tuberculosis.

For health care facilities, prisons, and other organizations that serve people at high risk of tuberculosis, a similar pattern of workplace complacency in the late 1980s and early 1990s—combined with an increasing incidence of tuberculosis in the community—contributed to workplace outbreaks of tuberculosis. Surveys, investigations of outbreaks, and facility inspections all pointed to institutional lapses in tuberculosis control measures including inattention to the signs and symptoms of infectious tuberculosis, delays in the initiation of appropriate evaluation and treatment, and improper ventilation of isolation rooms.

Just as community neglect interacted with workplace neglect to set the stage for workplace outbreaks of tuberculosis, it now appears that community control measures have interacted with workplace control measures to help end outbreaks of tuberculosis and reduce the potential for new ones. For example, increased government funding and public health efforts to ensure that individuals complete their treatments for active tuberculosis can be credited with reducing the number and proportion of infectious people—including those with multidrug-resistant disease—who appear in hospitals and other workplaces. At the same time, the implementation of tuberculosis control measures as recommended by CDC has almost certainly reduced the rate of transmission of drug-sensitive and multidrug-resistant tuberculosis in hospitals and in the broader community into which patients are discharged.

The challenge now is for policymakers, managers, and health professionals to understand and adapt to the decreasing incidence of tuberculosis without re-creating the conditions that would make institutions and workers vulnerable to new and possibly more deadly outbreaks of the disease. If tuberculosis case rates continue to decline, the maintenance of expertise and vigilance will not be easy.

Ending Neglect laid out a strategy for maintaining long-term vigilance and moving toward the elimination of tuberculosis in the United States. This strategy stresses (1) better methods for identifying people with recently acquired tuberculosis infection, (2) stronger efforts to effectively treat people who could benefit from treatment of infection, (3) research to develop effective vaccines, (4) more active product development initiatives focused on diagnostic and treatment technologies, and (5) research to tackle the problem of patient and provider failure to follow treatment recommendations.

If implemented, many of the recommendations from that IOM report—especially those related to better diagnostic tests and treatments for latent infection—would benefit workplace as well as community-based tuberculosis control programs. *Ending Neglect* also calls for the United States to increase its support for global tuberculosis control. With more than 40 percent of the tuberculosis cases in the United States (and in health care facilities in particular) involving people born in other countries, policymakers and public health authorities cannot ignore the international aspect of tuberculosis.

In summary, just as the risk of tuberculosis in the workplace is linked to the risk of tuberculosis in the surrounding community, the risk in American communities is affected by that elsewhere in the world and by the migration of infected persons within and across U.S. borders. Effective tuberculosis control measures in the workplace are one element of much broader national and international strategies to prevent and eventually eliminate the disease. The resurgence of the disease in the United States in the mid-1980s and early 1990s and the rise of multidrug-resistant disease demonstrate that tuberculosis remains a threat that public health programs cannot afford to ignore.

1

Introduction

Tuberculosis is a treatable, communicable disease that has two general states: latent infection and active disease.[1] With few exceptions, only those who develop active tuberculosis in the lungs or larynx can infect others, usually by coughing, sneezing, or otherwise expelling tiny infectious particles that someone else inhales.

After more than 30 years of declines in reported tuberculosis cases and deaths, the mid-1980s and early 1990s saw a reversal of that trend in the United States. Between 1985 and 1992, reported cases of tuberculosis increased by 20 percent, from 22,201 in 1985 to 26,673 in 1992 (CDC, 2000b).[2] The case rate per 100,000 population increased by more than 12 percent, from 9.3 in 1985 to 10.5 in 1992. The number of deaths rose from 1,752 in 1985 to 1,970 in 1989. Especially alarming was the increase in the number of more lethal multidrug-resistant strains of *Mycobacterium tuberculosis*, the organism that causes the disease. In the early 1980s, about 0.5 percent of new tuberculosis cases were resistant to the two major drug treatments (isoniazid and rifampin). By 1991, the figure stood at 3.5 percent (Edlin, 1992).

---

[1]Consistent with most recent literature, this report treats "infection with *Mycobacterium tuberculosis*," "latent tuberculosis infection," and "tuberculous infection" as synonyms. The first two terms are used, for example, in the recent statement from the American Thoracic Society and the Centers for Disease Control and Prevention on the classification of tuberculosis in adults and children (ATS/CDC, 2000a).

[2]Unless otherwise indicated, statistics reported in this chapter come from CDC (2000b).

Reasons cited for the increasing rates of tuberculosis and drug-resistant disease include the deterioration of public health programs aimed at preventing tuberculosis and encouraging completion of therapy for the disease (IOM, 2000). Incomplete treatment is a major cause of drug resistance. Increasing rates of HIV infection, homelessness, imprisonment, and immigration also contributed to the resurgence of tuberculosis. Depending on region and age group, up to 35 percent of those with tuberculosis were also infected with HIV.

The rise in tuberculosis, particularly multidrug-resistant disease, created considerable public alarm. For example, a 1992 opinion piece in the *Washington Post* on the combined threat of AIDS, substance abuse, and tuberculosis (headlined as the "three-headed dog from hell") described tuberculosis as a deadly and highly contagious disease "that you could catch from the person next to you in a movie theater or classroom" (Califano cited in OTA, 1993, p. 28). Transmission of the disease under such conditions is not very likely, but the description illustrates the level of concern being voiced by some commentators at the time.

Figure 1-1 shows both the increase in the number of tuberculosis cases beginning in the mid-1980s and the subsequent decrease in the number of cases starting in 1993. By 1999, the number of cases nationwide had dropped to 17,528 (an all-time low), and the case rate stood at 6.4 per 100,000 population (also the lowest ever). The rate of multidrug-resistant tuberculosis stood at 1.2 percent of reported cases, approximately one-third the level in 1991. In addition, the death rate had dropped to 0.4 per 100,000 population in 1998 (the latest year for which data are available), down from 0.8 per 100,000 population in 1988.

National case rates mask considerable geographic variation in the incidence of tuberculosis. In 1999, case rates varied from less than 1.0 per

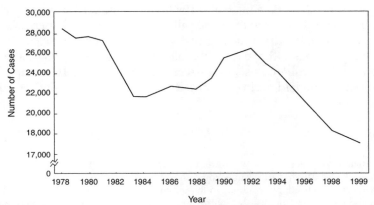

FIGURE 1-1. Reported cases of tuberculosis, 1978–1999. Source: IOM (2000) and CDC (2000b).

100,000 population in Vermont and Wyoming to more than 10 per 100,000 population in California (10.9), New York (11.0), and Hawaii (15.5) (CDC, 2000b). Some metropolitan statistical areas have even higher rates. For example, in 1999, case rates per 100,000 population were 17.7 for New York City and 18.2 for San Francisco. In 1998, the case rate in central Harlem was 63.7 per 100,000 population, which is similar to rates seen in developing countries such as Brazil (75 per 100,000 population) although it is far lower than the rates in the most severely affected countries, such as Zimbabwe (540 per 100,000) (Dye et al., 1999).

More than 40 percent of the tuberculosis cases reported in the United States in 1999 involved people born in other countries (IOM, 2000; CDC, 2000b). Individuals from Mexico, the Philippines, and Vietnam accounted for nearly half (45 percent) of these cases, with 151 other countries accounting for the remainder.

RISKS TO HEALTH CARE AND OTHER WORKERS

The resurgence of tuberculosis in the mid-1980s and early 1990s also affected health care workers and others employed in settings that served patients, inmates, or clients with tuberculosis. A number of high-profile outbreaks of tuberculosis—including cases of multidrug-resistant disease—were documented in hospitals, nursing homes, prisons, homeless shelters, and other settings (see, e.g., CDC [1994a], Dooley and Tapper [1997], and Garrett et al. [1999]). Most such outbreaks have been linked to lapses in infection control practices, delays in diagnosis and treatment of infectious individuals, and the presence of high-risk populations including people with HIV infection or AIDS and recent immigrants from countries with high rates of tuberculosis.

In 1999, of the 16,223 cases of tuberculosis for which occupational data were reported (92.5 percent of all reported cases), unemployed individuals accounted for nearly 60 percent of reported tuberculosis cases (CDC, 2000b). Such individuals accounted for less than 5 percent of the total workforce (BLS 2000a, 2000b). Health care workers accounted for about 2.6 percent or 422 of the cases in 1999. In 1998, health care workers accounted for about 9 percent of employed persons and 8 percent of tuberculosis cases among employed persons (Amy Curtis, CDC, 2000, personal communication) and about 5 percent of the total workforce. As discussed in Chapter 5, it can be difficult to determine whether tuberculosis in health care and other employed workers is due to workplace or community exposure.

Several health care and correctional workers have died of tuberculosis following documented work-related exposure to the disease (Dooley and Tapper, 1997), but no comprehensive mortality figures are available. Most of these workers as well as patients or inmates who died suffered from poorly functioning immune systems related to medical conditions such as HIV infection or AIDS or to medical treatments such as cancer chemotherapy.

Newly reported outbreaks of tuberculosis in health care facilities have dropped off since the mid-1990s, but recent outbreaks have been reported in correctional facilities (see Chapter 5). Reports on facilities that experienced tuberculosis outbreaks in the late 1980s and early 1990s describe lapses in tuberculosis control measures followed by the implementation of new protective measures, and the subsequent reduction of worker exposures and new infections.

OVERVIEW OF REPORT

In 1999, the U.S. Congress requested that the National Academy of Sciences undertake a short-term study of occupational tuberculosis (P.L. 106-113, Conference Report 196-749). A committee of the Institute of Medicine (IOM), which is the health policy arm of the Academy, prepared this report. Consistent with legislative conference language, the committee focused on three questions:

1. Are health care and selected other categories of workers at a greater risk of infection, disease, and mortality due to tuberculosis than others in the community within which they reside? If so, what is the excess risk due to occupational exposure? Can the risk of occupational exposure be quantified for different work environments and different job classifications?

2. What is known about the implementation and effects of the 1994 Centers for Disease Control and Prevention (CDC) guidelines for the prevention of tuberculosis in health care facilities?

3. What will be the likely effects on tuberculosis infection, disease, or mortality of an anticipated Occupational Safety and Health Administration (OSHA) standard to protect workers from occupational exposure to tuberculosis?

The committee's charge from Congress from this limited study did *not* include the development of recommendations for regulatory policy. It also did not include an evaluation of the costs or cost-effectiveness of the implementation of a standard.

According to the congressional request, work on this report was not to delay the issuing of the final rule, nor was the IOM study to be delayed pending the rule's publication. When the study committee officially began work on April 1, 2000, publication of the rule was expected in July 2000. When the committee met for the final time in September 2000, the final standard had not been issued, and its status was uncertain following the change in control of the Executive Branch in January 2001. As explained in Chapter 7, in the absence of the final standard, the committee focused on the conditions that a standard would need to meet to be effective.

The rest of this chapter briefly reviews responses to resurgent tuberculosis and proposed strategies for the elimination of tuberculosis in the United States and worldwide. Chapter 2 provides a basic review of tuberculosis transmission, infection, and disease. Chapter 3 discusses the proposed OSHA rule in the larger context of regulatory and other strategies used to protect worker health and safety. It also examines the statutory, judicial, and administrative frameworks within which the rule was developed. Chapter 4 summarizes the 1994 CDC guidelines and describes how the 1997 proposed OSHA rule differs from the guidelines. Chapter 5, 6, and 7 are organized around the three questions posed to the committee: the extent of occupational exposure to tuberculosis, the effects of the CDC guidelines, and the likely effects of an OSHA rule, respectively.

Appendix A describes the committee's activities in more detail. Appendix B discusses the strengths and limitations of the tuberculin skin test, Appendix C reviews the literature on the occupational risk of tuberculosis, and Appendix D reviews the literature on the effects of workplace tuberculosis control measures. Appendix E discusses OSHA from a legal perspective. Appendix F reviews issues related to the use of personal respiratory protection devices and programs in health care and other settings. Appendix G lists the recommendations of another recent IOM report on strategies for the elimination of tuberculosis in the United States, and Appendix H includes brief biographies for members of the committee.

RESPONSES TO RESURGENT TUBERCULOSIS

Responses to Tuberculosis in the Community

The increase in tuberculosis case rates in the mid-1980s and early 1990s prompted public health authorities to revive and adapt traditional strategies to prevent and control tuberculosis in the community. Specific federal funding for tuberculosis control programs, which had virtually disappeared in the 1970s, resumed in the 1980s and increased substantially in the 1990s, as shown in Figure 1-2 (IOM, 2000). States and some cities and counties began to rebuild programs that had been neglected or dismantled in the 1970s and early 1980s.

A particular focus of federal, state, and community efforts was drug-resistant disease, particularly that related to inappropriate or incomplete treatment. One measure, directly observed therapy, targeted the failure of many with active tuberculosis to complete their full, several-month treatment regimen (Addington, 1979; Chaulk et al., 1995; ATS/CDC, 2000a). Physician failure to prescribe the appropriate drugs at the appropriate level and frequency for the appropriate period of time is another problem (Rao

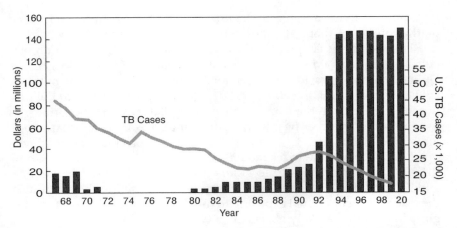

FIGURE 1-2. Trends in tuberculosis funding (CDC, fiscal years 1967–2000) and numbers of tuberculosis cases in the United States (in thousands). SOURCE: IOM (2000), p. 36 and CDC (2000b).

et al., 2000; Iseman, 1999a, 1999b). The development of practice guidelines and physician education programs are partial responses to such treatment errors (see Chapter 4), but physician awareness of and adherence to tuberculosis treatment guidelines remain concerns (DeRiemer et al., 1999; Evans et al., 1999). Other elements of the attack on drug resistant disease have included faster laboratory identification of drug-resistant strains of the disease (Tenover et al., 1993), surgical treatment of resistant disease, and the development of alternative drug regimens (Iseman, 1999a, 1999b).

Responses to Outbreaks in the Workplace

Outbreaks of tuberculosis in several health care and correctional facilities prompted additional actions by public health officials, health care and other managers, and those representing workers in these institutions (see Box 1-1 for a selective chronology). Federal and state investigations of these outbreaks often pointed to lapses in basic infection control protocols including failure to promptly identify and isolate suspected cases and failure to provide, maintain, and properly use negative-pressure isolation rooms designed for patients with infectious tuberculosis.

Beginning in 1990, CDC and other public and private health groups issued guidelines for the prevention and control of workplace transmission of tuberculosis in health care facilities, correctional facilities, and settings that serve homeless people (CDC, 1990a,b, 1992a, 1994b, 1996b). The 1990 CDC guidelines for health care facilities were adapted from earlier infection control guidelines. They did not reflect the changing epidemiology of the disease or the occupational safety and health perspec-

Box 1-1
Regulating Occupational Exposure to Tuberculosis:
Selective Chronology of Events

1950s	Health care workers' risk of tuberculosis accepted by most experts
1953	National reporting of tuberculosis cases initiated
1953–1984	Consistent declines in tuberculosis cases and deaths reported
1982	CDC issues guidelines on preventing tuberculosis transmission in health care facilities
1985/1986	First increase in numbers of tuberculosis deaths (1985) and cases (1986) since national data reporting began
1990	CDC issues new tuberculosis prevention guidelines for health care settings with specific focus on those with HIV infection and AIDS
1991	Outbreak of multidrug-resistant tuberculosis in a New York State prison results in the deaths of seven inmates and one correctional officer
1992	CDC advisory committee presents recommendations to prevent and control tuberculosis among homeless persons
1992	National Institute for Occupational Safety and Health recommends that health care workers in contact with tuberculosis patients wear industrial-type powered air purifying respirators
1992	Labor Coalition to Fight TB in the Workplace requests OSHA enforcement actions
1993	OSHA issues nationwide enforcement procedures related to occupational exposure to tuberculosis
1993	CDC issues draft revised guidelines on preventing tuberculosis transmission in health care facilities
1993	Decline in tuberculosis cases recorded, reversing 1986–1992 trend
1994	OSHA announces initiation of rulemaking process but declines request for an emergency temporary standard
1994	CDC issues revised and expanded guidelines for health care facilities
1995	OSHA meets with "stakeholder groups" to discuss workplace tuberculosis standard; seeks peer review of its risk assessment; publishes tuberculosis training and resource guide for field inspectors
1995	NIOSH issues revised certification procedures for nonpowered air-purifying personal respirators
1995	CDC initiates demonstration project to improve skin test surveillance for health care workers
1996	CDC advisory committee presents recommendations for correctional facilities
1997	OSHA issues proposed standard on workplace tuberculosis and provides for comment period and hearings
1998	OSHA conducts public hearings in Washington, New York, Chicago, and Los Angeles
1999	OSHA reopens comment period on the proposed rule with focus on issues related to homeless shelters, risk assessment, and other matters
1999	Continued decrease in tuberculosis cases and case rates
2000	CDC begins reexamination of 1994 guidelines

tives evident in later guidelines (Nardell, 1997). The 1994 revision of the guidelines was a specific response to disease outbreaks in health care facilities and the contributing factors identified during investigations of the outbreaks. In 1995, the National Institute for Occupational Safety and Health, which is part of the CDC, certified a new class of respirator for use in preventing transmission of tuberculosis.

One problem faced by CDC in 1990 and then again in 1994 was the lack of rigorous, prospective, controlled studies documenting the effectiveness of individual protective measures in preventing workplace transmission of tuberculosis. Both the lack of research and the expected cost of tuberculosis control measures contributed to the controversy over the revised guidelines for health care facilities that CDC issued in draft form in 1993 and final form in 1994 (Sepkowitz, 1995).

In 1993, the Congressional Office of Technology Assessment observed that none of the measures described in CDC's 1990 guidelines for health care facilities were thought to have been widely adopted (OTA, 1993, p. 6). Survey data supported these suspicions (see Chapter 6).

Groups representing health care and other workers created the Labor Coalition to Fight TB in the Workplace. In 1992, the coalition petitioned OSHA to issue an "advisory notice" with enforcement guidelines designed to protect workers from occupational exposure to tuberculosis. In 1993, it asked OSHA to issue a permanent standard (Labor Coalition, 1993).[3] In addition to citing the 1990 CDC guidelines, the coalition cited enforcement guidelines issued by Region II of the Occupational Safety and Health Administration and by the state of California's occupational safety and health agency. The Secretary of Labor announced in 1994 that OSHA would initiate a rulemaking process to establish formal standards to prevent workplace transmission of the disease. The U.S. Department of Labor, however, declined to issue the emergency temporary standard sought by labor groups, which had argued that the 1990 CDC guidelines were not being adequately implemented.

In 1993 and 1996, OSHA issued statements that emphasized the statutory obligations of employers to provide a safe workplace, described the applicability of certain existing regulations, and outlined procedures for investigating worker complaints and inspecting workplaces identified by CDC as having a higher incidence of tuberculosis than the general population (OSHA, Fact Sheet No. OSHA 93-43, 1993; OSHA directive CPL 2.106, February 9, 1996). Consistent with those statements, OSHA has cited or fined employers for failure to protect

---

[3]Unions signing the petition included the Service Employees International Union, the American Federation of State, County, and Municipal Employees, and the American Federation of Teachers.

workers from known hazardous conditions that put workers at risk of exposure to tuberculosis (ACCP/ATS, 1995). Recently, OSHA cited a federal agency, the Immigration and Naturalization Service, for such conditions (OSHA Region 6, 2000). Federal agencies cannot be fined by OSHA (see Chapter 3); the fines for an equivalent private-sector violator would have been $390,000.

In 1997, OSHA published a proposed rule (62 FR 201, October 17, 1997). It requested comments and information from affected groups. The proposed rule generated both support and opposition including lobbying by some groups for Congress to delay or block issuing of a final rule. In 1998, the agency conducted four public hearings. The agency reopened the public comment period in the summer of 1999, specifically requesting information and comments on homeless shelters and the agency's preliminary risk assessment. Altogether, the agency received approximately 1,500 comments on the proposed rule including testimony at the four hearings and comments submitted when the record was reopened in 1999 (Amanda Edens, OSHA, personal communication, December 6, 2000).

THE BROADER PUBLIC HEALTH CONTEXT: ELIMINATING TUBERCULOSIS IN THE UNITED STATES AND WORLDWIDE

Today, tuberculosis is a largely preventable and curable disease. Nonetheless, it continues to cause disability and death, especially in poor and disadvantaged communities around the world. The combination of HIV infection or AIDS and tuberculosis and the rise of multidrug-resistant disease have refocused policymakers and public health authorities on the goal of eliminating tuberculosis in the United States and worldwide. Workplace programs to prevent the transmission of tuberculosis operate within these broader national and international contexts.

Eliminating Tuberculosis in the United States

In the recently released Institute of Medicine report *Ending Neglect: The Elimination of Tuberculosis in the United States*, another IOM committee set forth a broad strategy for the elimination of the disease in this country (IOM, 2000). The report argues that the resurgence of tuberculosis in the 1980s was the price exacted from disregard of earlier calls for a drive to eliminate the disease and from neglect of the public health infrastructure needed to control tuberculosis. It then goes on to propose a strategy to prevent a return to complacency and, eventually, to eliminate the disease in this country. The strategy includes five broad tasks:

1. maintaining control in an environment of declining disease incidence and a changing health care system;

2. speeding the decline in disease incidence and moving toward elimination of the disease by focusing on targeted skin testing and treatment of latent infection;

3. developing additional diagnostic, treatment, and vaccination tools;

4. increasing U.S. involvement in efforts to eliminate tuberculosis worldwide; and

5. mobilizing public support and measuring progress toward the goal of tuberculosis elimination.

The strategy emphasizes the importance of early diagnosis of latent tuberculosis infection and active tuberculosis, especially among immigrants from countries with a high-prevalence of the disease. It also stresses appropriate treatment of latent tuberculosis infection with the use of directly observed therapy, when indicated, to ensure the completion of treatment.

Although workers' risk of tuberculosis is not explicitly discussed in the earlier IOM report, the success of a national tuberculosis elimination strategy would clearly benefit health care and other workers. Eliminating a hazard is much more effective than trying to control exposure to it a known or suspected danger.

Eliminating Tuberculosis Worldwide

With more than 40 percent of the tuberculosis cases in the United States involving people born in other countries, policymakers and public health authorities cannot ignore the global problem of tuberculosis. As noted above, a key recommendation of the recent IOM report on tuberculosis elimination in the United States was that this country should "expand and strengthen its role in global tuberculosis control efforts" (IOM, 2000, p. 11). Another recommendation was that those applying for immigration visas from countries with high rates of tuberculosis be tested for tuberculosis and that those with positive tests be evaluated and, if indicated, treated before being issued a permanent residency card.

Eliminating tuberculosis in the United States is a challenge that pales beside the challenge of eliminating tuberculosis worldwide. According to the World Health Organization (WHO), approximately one-third of the world's population is infected with M. tuberculosis (WHO, 1996, 2000b). Each year about 8 million people are newly diagnosed with the disease, and about 95 percent of these people live in developing countries (WHO, 1996, 2000b). Worldwide, tuberculosis kills about 2 million people yearly. It accounts for more deaths among adults than AIDS, malaria, and all other infectious diseases combined.

In 1993, the WHO declared a global tuberculosis emergency, and it has stated that "poorly managed TB programmes are threatening to make

TB incurable" (WHO, 2000a, p. 2). Twenty-two countries[4] account for nearly three-quarters of all new cases of the disease, and WHO has targeted them for special attention and assistance (WHO, 2000a).

WHO recently issued guidelines for the prevention of tuberculosis in health care facilities in resource-limited settings (WHO, 1999). The measures emphasize relatively inexpensive control measures involving natural ventilation (e.g., opening windows and providing special open-air areas for people waiting for care or visiting infectious patients). The focus is on first-line district health care facilities that lack the resources to support more expensive measures such as negative-pressure isolation rooms and personal respirators, which are advised only for referral facilities. Tuberculin skin testing is recommended only in research settings and at sites that offer preventive therapy for latent infection. Although these recommendations are aimed at resource-poor countries, they may also, under some circumstances, be relevant for some settings in this country. For example, crowded, underfunded homeless shelters may, when weather permits, have people with suspected tuberculosis wait outside in fresh air until transportation and treatment can be arranged.

CONCLUSION

Although tuberculosis is still a major killer in poor countries, 50 years of effective drug treatment has greatly reduced the toll that the disease takes in the United States. Nonetheless, the resurgence of the disease in the mid-1980s and early 1990s and the rise of multidrug-resistant disease demonstrate that tuberculosis remains a threat that public health programs cannot afford to ignore. Likewise, outbreaks of the disease in hospitals, prisons, and other facilities have underscored the potential for harm to nurses, doctors, guards, and others who work with people at increased risk of tuberculosis.

Will government mandates be effective in protecting health care and other workers from tuberculosis? The final chapter of this report considers this question. The next five chapters provide the foundation for that assessment by reviewing the basic features of the disease and its treatment, describing the legal context for OSHA regulations, comparing the regulations proposed by OSHA in 1997 with the voluntary guidelines published by CDC in 1994, examining the historical and recent occupational risk of tuberculosis, and evaluating the implementation and effects of the 1994 CDC guidelines.

---

[4]Afghanistan, Bangladesh, Brazil, Cambodia, China, Democratic Republic of Congo, Ethiopia, India, Indonesia, Kenya, Myanmar, Nigeria, Pakistan, Peru, Philippines, Russia, South Africa, Tanzania, Thailand, Uganda, Vietnam, and Zimbabwe.

2

Basics of Tuberculosis

Although tuberculosis has two general states, latent infection and active disease,[1] only those who develop active tuberculosis can transmit the disease. Table 2-1 summarizes the basic differences between latent tuberculosis infection[2] and active pulmonary tuberculosis, which is the most common form of the disease.

An understanding of both latent tuberculosis infection and active tuberculosis is needed to develop effective policies and programs to prevent and control transmission of tuberculosis in communities generally and in workplaces specifically. Detection and treatment of active, transmissible disease is the highest priority for both clinicians and public health officials. Detection and, in certain cases, treatment of latent tuberculosis infection is also important. For an infected individual, treatment helps prevent progression to active disease. For the broader community, detection and treatment of infection contribute to the broader public goal of tracking and eliminating tuberculosis. This chapter briefly reviews how latent tuberculosis infection and active tuberculosis develop and are diagnosed and managed.

---

[1]This chapter's discussion of infection, disease, and transmission draws on the works of Haas and Des Prez (1995), Daniel (1997), Gangadharam and Jenkins (1998), Reichman and Hershfield (2000), ATS/CDC (2000a,b), and CDC (2000a).

[2]As noted in Chapter 1, this report treats "infection with *Mycobacterium tuberculosis*," "latent tuberculosis infection," and "tuberculous infection" as synonyms.

TABLE 2-1. Differences Between Latent Tuberculosis Infection and
Active Pulmonary Tuberculosis

Latent Tuberculosis Infection	Active Tuberculosis (in the lungs)
Few tuberculosis bacteria in the body	Many tuberculosis bacteria in the body
Tuberculin skin test reaction usually but not always positive	Tuberculin skin test reaction usually but not always positive
Chest radiograph normal	Chest radiograph usually abnormal
Sputum smears and cultures negative	Sputum smears and cultures usually positive
No symptoms	
Not infectious	Symptoms (e.g., cough) often present
	Potentially infectious before treatment

SOURCE: Adapted from CDC (1999c, Module 1, p. 7).

TRANSMISSION AND DEVELOPMENT OF LATENT TUBERCULOSIS INFECTION AND ACTIVE TUBERCULOSIS

Tuberculosis is primarily caused by *Mycobacterium tuberculosis* (also called the tubercle bacillus). Humans can also develop bovine tuberculosis, a less serious disease that is primarily caused by drinking milk from cattle infected with *Mycobacterium bovis*.[3] Other mycobacteria can cause tuberculosis in various animals, but they rarely cause disease in humans.[4] As discussed later in this chapter, bovine and other mycobacteria may produce positive reactions to the tests used to screen people for tuberculosis.

Although *M. tuberculosis* was first identified in 1882, its behavior remains poorly understood in some important respects. In particular, much remains to be learned about the mechanisms of latent tuberculosis infection and disease activation and reactivation.

Transmission of *M. tuberculosis*

M. tuberculosis typically spreads through the air when people who have infectious tuberculosis in their respiratory tract cough, sneeze, speak, sing, or otherwise expel tiny particles containing the bacteria. A fine mist (an aerosol) of infectious particles can also be created in other ways, for

---

[3]In developed countries, bovine tuberculosis has largely been eliminated by programs of tuberculin testing in cattle followed by slaughter of infected animals. Infected cattle, deer, and other animals are still occasionally found in the United States, and human cases continue to be reported (Dankner and Davis, 2000; Hernandez and Baca, 1998; Palmer et al., 2000; Pillai et al., 2000; Schmitt et al., 1997). Aside from testing and destruction of infected animals, public health programs rely on compulsory pasteurization and certification of milk to prevent transmission of the disease to humans.

[4]For patients with AIDS, *Mycobacterium avium* complex disease can be life-threatening, but information about its epidemiology and effective management is limited (Gangadharam and Jenkins, 1998).

example, during a procedure to irrigate a tuberculosis-infected abscess, during laboratory processing of infected tissue, or during an autopsy or embalming.[5]

Whether produced by coughing or other actions, most of the largest, heaviest bacterium-bearing particles will settle fairly quickly and harmlessly on surfaces such as walls, furniture, and clothing. Some airborne particles will reach another person's nose and throat but will be trapped and then removed when the person swallows or spits. The smallest, lightest particles (called droplet nuclei) may reach the lung's alveoli, which are the tiny, endmost parts of the respiratory tract and the starting point for most tuberculosis infections. In poorly ventilated spaces, droplet nuclei may stay in the air for hours or even days. The bacteria are very sensitive to sunshine and other ultraviolet light.

Extended, close, indoor contact is usually required for tuberculosis to be transmitted from one person to another. At least one report has, however, documented transmission after workplace exposure limited to a few minutes (Templeton et al., 1995).

Tuberculosis is considered moderately infectious, with infection developing in perhaps 30 to 50 percent of those who have extended, close, indoor contact with people with active disease. Measles, by contrast, is considered highly infectious, with infection developing in an estimated 80 percent of susceptible people who come in contact with an infected individual (Haas and Des Prez, 1995).

The likelihood that *M. tuberculosis* will be transmitted from one person to another depends on several factors. These factors include

- the infectiousness of a person with infectious tuberculosis, which is related to the number of bacteria he or she expels and, possibly, the virulence (disease-causing potential) of the bacteria;
- the length of exposure to an infectious person or to air contaminated with tuberculosis bacteria;
- the environment surrounding an infectious person, for example, the size of a room and how well it is ventilated; and
- the functioning of an exposed person's immune system.

Infection with *M. tuberculosis*

Typically, when tuberculosis bacteria reach the alveoli in the lungs, they attract and are engulfed by white blood cells called macrophages.[6] The bacteria multiply within the macrophages, and some may escape and

---

[5]Transmission by other routes has also been reported (e.g., from inadequately sterilized bronchoscopes, accidental self-inoculation, and a kidney transplant) (Dooley and Tapper, 1997).

[6]This is a greatly simplified description of a very complex pathological process, aspects of which are still not fully understood.

eral population screening is not recommended in areas where active tuberculosis is uncommon, testing at the start of employment and sometimes periodically thereafter has been advised for otherwise low-risk individuals who work in health care facilities, prisons, or other settings that serve or house higher-risk populations. As discussed in Chapter 4, the 1994 CDC guidelines for health care facilities and the rule proposed by OSHA in 1997 provide for slightly different workplace programs for skin testing. A CDC advisory committee has recommended a reexamination of the 1994 recommendations, and a CDC working group recently began that process. The following discussion identifies some of the limitations of tuberculin skin testing (see also Appendix B).

Administering and Interpreting the Tuberculin Skin Test

To conduct a tuberculin skin test, a specified amount of tuberculin (a preparation made from killed tuberculosis bacteria) is injected into the skin of the forearm by a health care worker trained in the procedure. The only skin testing procedure recommended by CDC is the tuberculin skin test with PPD (a purified protein derivative of tuberculin).

After the injection, a reaction to the tuberculin skin test in an infected individual will generally occur and should be examined within 48 to 72 hours. A reaction should be interpreted by a physician or other trained health care worker who should follow a specific protocol to measure the raised, hardened area (induration) around the injection site. (Redness may also develop around the test site but is not considered in interpreting the test.)

Interpretation is based on the size of the reaction site and certain characteristics of the tested individual. For example, a 5- or 10-millimeter (mm) reaction may be classified as a negative response in an individual with no risk factors for disease but as a positive result in someone who does have risk factors. Absence of a reaction is recorded as 00 mm. Table 2-2 shows CDC recommendations for interpreting skin test reactions.

For groups being tested periodically as part of a tuberculosis surveillance program, both the number and rate of reactions and the rate of conversions from negative to positive test results are of interest. A conversion is generally defined as an increase of 10 mm or more in the reaction size within a 2-year period from the last test. Such a conversion is generally interpreted as indicating recent infection with *M. tuberculosis*. (As described below, high rates of false-positive test results are a concern in some environments.) Conversions are typically investigated to assess the possibility of workplace-related exposure to tuberculosis. To assess the possibility of community exposure, workers whose tests have converted may be questioned about possible contacts with family members or friends outside work who have active tuberculosis.

TABLE 2-2. CDC Recommendations for Interpreting Reactions to the Tuberculin Skin Test

I. Classify induration of ≥5 mm as positive for
- HIV-positive persons
- Recent contacts of individuals with tuberculosis
- Persons with fibrotic changes on chest radiograph consistent with prior tuberculosis
- Organ transplant recipients and others with conditions or treatments that suppress their immune systems

II. Classify induration of ≥10 mm as positive for
- Recent immigrants (within 5 years) from high-prevalence countries
- Injection drug users
- Residents and employees of high-risk congregate settings: prisons and jails, nursing homes and other long-term care facilities for elderly, individuals, hospitals and other health care facilities; residential facilities for AIDS patients, homeless shelters*
- Mycobacteriology laboratory personnel
- Persons with diabetes and other clinical conditions (other than those identified in category I) that place them at high risk
- Children under 4 years of age or children and adolescents exposed to adults in high-risk categories

III. Classify induration of ≥15 mm as positive for
- Persons with no known risk factors for tuberculosis

*For employees who are otherwise at low risk and who are tested upon hiring, an induration of ≥15 is considered positive. SOURCE: Adapted from ATS/CDC (2000a).

Measures of Test Accuracy

Several measures have been developed to help in assessing the accuracy and utility of screening tests (Daniel and Daniel, 1993; USPSTF, 1996). *Sensitivity* is defined as the proportion of people with a condition (e.g., infection with *M. tuberculosis*) who have positive test results.[9] The lower the sensitivity of a test, the more likely a test will miss people who actually have the disease or condition but show *false-negative* test results. The sensitivity of the tuberculin skin test has been estimated at 95 percent except for those with active tuberculosis or very recent infection (ATS/CDC, 1999a, Appendix B).

The *specificity* of a test is defined as the proportion of people without the condition who have negative test results. The lower the specificity of a test, the more people who do not have the condition will show *false-positive* results and be told that they do have it. Specificity for the tuberculin skin

---

[9]Calculation of sensitivity and specificity requires some way of identifying those with the condition who have negative results. (For the tuberculin skin test, the condition is latent tuberculosis infection.) This requires a "gold standard" reference test, which does not exist for many common screening tools, including the tuberculin skin test.

TABLE 2-3. Positive Predictive Value of a Positive Tuberculin Skin Test Assuming 95 Percent Sensitivity

Prevalence of Infection (%)	Predictive Value (%) at the Following Specificity		
	95%	99%	99.5%
90.0	99.4	99.9	99.9
50.0	95.0	99.0	99.5
25.0	86.4	96.9	98.4
10.0	67.9	91.3	95.5
5.0	50.0	83.3	90.9
2.0	27.9	66.0	79.5
1.0	16.1	49.0	65.7
0.1	1.9	8.7	16.0
0.05	0.9	4.5	8.7
0.01	0.2	0.9	1.9

SOURCE: ATS/CDC (2000a), with recalculation to correct predictive values for 0.01 percent prevalence.

test has been estimated at 99 percent or better in areas where exposure to other mycobacteria is uncommon and at 95 percent in areas where such exposure is relatively common (ATS/CDC, 1999a, Appendix B).

A third measure helpful in assessing the usefulness of a screening test is its *positive predictive value*, which is defined as the probability of a disease or condition in a tested person given a positive test result. A test's positive predictive value is affected by the prevalence of the disease or condition in the community of those being tested.[10] Table 2-3 illustrates how prevalence affects calculations of positive predictive value for the tuberculin skin test.

Another way of understanding the effect of disease or condition prevalence relies on Bayesian analysis, as shown in Table 2-4. Given the sensitivity and specificity levels assumed in the table, the positive predictive value—the probability of infection given a positive test result—drops from 49 to 8.7 percent when the prevalence of infection in the community drops from 1 to 0.1 percent.

Thus, even for a reasonably sensitive and specific test, the lower the prevalence of a disease or condition, the higher the proportion of false-positive results. In very low-prevalence areas, a majority of positive test results will be false positives.

---

[10]Prevalence is a measure of the probability of infection or disease in a population at a particular point in time. Incidence is the probability of new infection or disease in a specified time period, usually a year. In the context of workplace surveillance programs, results for baseline skin tests are analogous to prevalence data and results for repeated tests correspond to incidence data.

TABLE 2-4. Importance of Disease or Condition Prevalence, Bayesian
Probability Analysis

Test conditions:
  sensitivity of test, 95 percent
  specificity of test, 99 percent

Patient Status	Prior Probability (%)	Probability of a Positive Skin Test (%)	Product of Probabilities (col 1 * col 2) (%)	Revised Probability (col 3$_I$ * 100/ sum col 3) (%)
If prevalence is 1%				
TB infection	1	95	95	49.0
No TB infection	99	1	99	51.0
			Sum = 194	
If prevalence is 0.1%				
TB infection	0.1	95	9.5	8.7
No TB infection	99.9	1	99.9	91.3
			Sum = 109.4	

NOTE: TB = tuberculosis.

For individuals, false-negative results are a concern because of the
lost opportunity for treatment to reduce their likelihood of developing
active tuberculosis. False-positive results are a concern because they may
lead to unneeded and potentially harmful treatment for someone who
does not actually have latent tuberculosis infection. They can also provoke considerable anxiety. In some situations, a positive test result may
be socially stigmatizing. For public and occupational health personnel,
false-negative test results may lead to missed opportunities to control the
transmission of tuberculosis and identify weaknesses in community or
workplace control measures. False-positive results may lead to unnecessary use of limited resources for investigations and medical follow-up.

Other Limitations of the Tuberculin Skin Test

A number of factors can lead to false-positive or false-negative readings for a tuberculin skin test. They include

• *The inadequate conduct or management of the skin test or the skin testing
program.* With good training and careful practice, the tuberculin skin test
is not difficult to administer correctly and to interpret accurately and
consistently. A lack of resources and inadequate training and oversight
can, however, jeopardize the proper storage of the test material, the quality of testing procedures, and the appropriate recording and use of test
results (Chaparas et al., 1985; Ozuah, 1999; see also Perez-Stable and
Slutkin [1985]). In addition, differences in the products (reagents) used in

the test and in different batches of the same product may produce variable results (Villarino et al., 1999; Blumberg et al., 2000).

• *The possibility that repeated skin tests may stimulate a reaction in those with long-standing latent tuberculosis infection (a response called boosting).* If people infected many years ago have not been tested recently, some will incorrectly test negative on a tuberculin skin test (a false-negative result). The test itself may then stimulate—boost—their sensitivity to tuberculin. If given a second test a few weeks or months later, these individuals may correctly test positive. This boosted reaction can be mistaken for evidence of exposure to tuberculosis and new infection. To control for this phenomenon, workplace surveillance programs may provide two-step baseline testing (two skin tests given 1 to 4 weeks apart). In this context, a positive result for the second test following a negative result for the first test is interpreted as a boosted result rather than as a true conversion. A worker with a boosted test result would not be included in a periodic retesting program.

• *The difficulty of interpreting test reactions in people who have been vaccinated against tuberculosis with BCG.* Bacille Calmette and Guérin (BCG) vaccination is uncommon in the United States but fairly common in Europe and elsewhere.[11] Thus, many immigrants to the United States have been vaccinated and may show false-positive reactions to the tuberculin skin test.

• *The geographic prevalence of other mycobacteria that produce reactions to tuberculin.* In the southeastern United States (especially coastal areas) and other similar locales around the world, common exposure to mycobacteria other than *M. tuberculosis* can produce false-positive tuberculin skin test results.

• *The existence of anergy (failure of a person with tuberculosis infection to react to a tuberculin skin test).* Approximately 10 to 25 percent of those with active untreated tuberculosis may have no reaction to the tuberculin skin test (CDC, 2000a). Anergy can be caused by immunosuppression related to HIV infection and certain other infections, poor nutrition, certain drugs and vaccinations, and a number of other factors. Although procedures that can be used to test for anergy exist, the interpretation and accuracy of these tests are uncertain, and CDC and others do not recommend their routine use (CDC, 1997; Slovis et al., 2000).

---

[11]As described by CDC, "BCG vaccines are live vaccines derived from a strain of Mycobacterium bovis that was attenuated by Calmette and Guérin at the Pasteur Institute in Lille, France (29). BCG was first administered to humans in 1921. Many different BCG vaccines are available worldwide. Although all currently used vaccines were derived from the original M. bovis strain, they differ in their characteristics when grown in culture and in their ability to induce an immune response to tuberculin" (CDC, 1996c, p. 5). Although it is common in many European and other countries, the CDC does not recommend BCG vaccination except in rare circumstances.

  • *The lag between the earliest stages of infection and the ability of the tuberculin skin test to detect infection.* The tuberculin skin test depends on what is called a delayed-type hypersensitivity reaction that generally does not develop for 2 to 10 weeks after initial infection.

These additional limitations of the tuberculin skin test need to be recognized in implementing skin testing programs and developing policy recommendations and requirements for community and workplace programs for tuberculosis surveillance. As recommended in the recent Institute of Medicine report on the elimination of tuberculosis in the United States (IOM, 2000) and discussed further in Chapter 7, better screening tests are needed to detect latent tuberculosis infection more quickly and more accurately.

Treatment of Latent Tuberculosis Infection

Treatment of latent tuberculosis infection helps reduce the likelihood that the infection, especially recent infection, will progress to active disease. Treatment of latent tuberculosis infection is also a major element in public health strategies for the elimination of tuberculosis in the United States because it reduces the proportion of people who will develop active, transmissible disease (IOM, 2000). Thus, treatment benefits both the infected individual and the broader community, including workplaces. Completion of a recommended treatment regimen is estimated to cut the rate of progression from infection to disease by about 80 to 90 percent (ATS/CDC, 2000b).

Recommendations for Treatment of Latent Infection

The drugs used to treat latent tuberculosis infection are a subset of the drugs used to treat active disease, although specific treatment regimens vary. Because treatment of latent tuberculosis infection is not risk- or inconvenience-free, it is usually aimed at individuals at higher risk of developing active disease including those with recent infection and those with AIDS or other conditions that place them at higher risk of progression.

Selection of a treatment regimen depends on the characteristics of the person being treated, for example, whether the person has HIV infection or whether he or she is at high risk for failing to complete the full course of treatment. Alternative regimens vary in their potential risk, and burdens. Therefore, patients should be carefully advised of the options and their possible consequences. Patient preferences need to be considered in selecting a regimen.

The regimen most highly recommended by ATS and CDC (based on nonrandomized clinical trials) involves 9 months of daily or twice-weekly doses of isoniazid. The twice-weekly regimen is recommended only if the taking of the medication is directly observed (ATS/CDC, 2000b). An "acceptable," shorter isoniazid regimen for those without other risk factors involves 6 months of daily or twice-weekly doses of the drug (the latter only with direct observation). The shortest, currently acceptable regimen involves two drugs, rifampin and pyrazinamide, taken daily for 2 months.

Side Effects of Treatment

The major concern about treatment of latent tuberculosis infection has been the potential for liver damage. A recent analysis of 7 years of experience at a Seattle public tuberculosis clinic suggests that the risk of liver damage form the most widely used drug (isoniazid) is lower than previously thought—less than 0.2 percent, compared with the 0.5 to 2.0 percent reported from earlier studies (Nolan et al., 1999). Other analyses (Salpeter, 1993; Garcia Rodriguez et al., 1997) have also suggested risks of adverse treatment effects that are lower than assessed earlier. Those at possible increased risk of liver damage include those who use alcohol daily, those with preexisting liver disease, older people, and pregnant or postpartum women (ATS/CDC, 2000b). Liver damage is also a concern with the rifampin-pyrazinamide treatment regimen, which is being closely monitored as more experience with the regimen accumulates (CDC, 2000c).

Careful screening, patient education about signs and symptoms of hepatitis, and prompt discontinuation of drugs when symptoms occur can reduce or eliminate the potential for adverse effects (ATS/CDC, 2000b). Baseline testing of liver function is recommended for patients at risk for liver disorders and for patients who have a history of liver disease, are infected with HIV, use alcohol regularly, or are pregnant or within 3 months of having given birth. In addition, monthly laboratory monitoring of liver function is advised for patients who have abnormal results on baseline liver function tests or who are otherwise at risk for hepatic disease. Nonetheless, for people with an infection that produces no symptoms and that usually has a fairly small chance of progressing to active disease (which usually can be successfully treated), even a very small possibility of liver damage or death may dissuade them from treatment of latent infection. Depending on the drug, less serious adverse reactions include rashes, gastrointestinal upsets, fever, and joint pain (ATS/CDC, 2000b). Some of these reactions may be bothersome enough to prompt a switch to another drug—or abandonment of therapy altogether. As with other treatments, careful communication of risks and benefits is important, perhaps more so when much of the expected benefit will accrue to the broader community, not just the individual. [12]

Adherence to Treatment for Latent Infection

One consideration in the choice among alternative drug regimens is the trade-off between the higher degree of efficacy of a longer duration of treatment and the lower levels of individual adherence to such regimens. A number of studies suggest that rates of initiation and completion of treatment of latent tuberculosis infection are sometimes quite low. One study of an indigent urban population found that only 55 of 466 people with tuberculosis infection were prescribed drug therapy and only 20 of those completed it (Schluger et al., 1999). Another study involving high-risk inner-city residents identified 809 people with a positive skin test result of whom 409 fit ATS/CDC criteria for therapy for latent tuberculosis infection; only 84 (20 percent) actually completed treatment (Bock et al., 1999). Although the rate of treatment adherence might be expected to be high among health care workers, studies suggest otherwise. For example, one study found that only 8 to 10 percent of physicians whose skin tests had converted from negative to positive had been treated for latent tuberculosis infection (Ramphal-Naley et al., 1996). In another study, of 40 health care workers who were identified as having been eligible for isoniazid treatment following a skin test conversion, only 15 (38 percent) had completed at least 6 months of therapy (Fraser et al., 1994).

The highest rates of completion of treatment among health care workers were reported in a study of a hospital in a city with relatively high rates of active tuberculosis (Blumberg et al., 1996). Of 125 workers with a recent positive tuberculin skin test result, all got a chest radiograph and almost all (98 percent) saw a physician. Although 84 percent started therapy for latent tuberculosis infection, only 66 percent of those who started therapy completed at least 6 months of treatment. Almost three-quarters of the 34 physicians in the group completed therapy whereas not quite half (44 of 91) of other workers completed therapy. Of all those who started but did not complete treatment, one-third stopped because of side effects.

---

[12]Studies suggest that people often misunderstand numerical explanations of risks and benefits provided by health professionals (Schwartz et al., 1997). How information is provided is important (Ransohoff and Harris, 1997). For example, people may find it easier to understand frequency information (e.g., a 4 in 1,000 chance of some outcome) than probability information (e.g., a 0.4 percent chance of the outcome) (Gigerenzer, 1996). They may also better understand comparisons of absolute risk to a baseline (e.g., reduction in risk to 4 in 1,000 with treatment compared to 12 in 1,000 without treatment) than they understand presentation of relative risk information with no baseline (Schwartz et al., 1997). Treatment may appear more attractive when described in terms of gain (e.g., 99 percent of patients will not develop the disease) rather than loss (e.g., 1 percent will develop the disease) (Mazur and Hickam, 1990; Hux and Naylor, 1995).

DIAGNOSIS AND TREATMENT OF
ACTIVE TUBERCULOSIS

Diagnosis

Both the 1994 CDC guidelines on tuberculosis control for health care facilities and the 1997 proposed OSHA rule on tuberculosis control emphasize the fact that prompt identification, isolation, and treatment of people with infectious tuberculosis is critical to an effective tuberculosis control program. Following several outbreaks of tuberculosis in hospitals and other settings, CDC, OSHA, state health departments, and others initiated educational programs to make physicians, nurses, and others more aware of the symptoms of infectious tuberculosis. Nonetheless, as described below, prompt identification of infectious tuberculosis is complicated because symptoms are not highly specific to the disease.

Symptoms and Diagnostic Steps

According to CDC's case reporting requirements (CDC, 1999b), a laboratory definition of a case of tuberculosis requires either the isolation of *M. tuberculosis* from a clinical specimen or demonstration of acid-fast bacilli in a clinical specimen when a culture was not or could not be obtained. (The processing of laboratory smears of sputum or some other specimen uses a dye that leaves only mycobacteria colored after processing with an acid-alcohol solution. The bacteria are thus often described as acid-fast bacilli [AFB] and the smears as AFB positive or negative.) The clinical case definition of tuberculosis requires all of the following: a positive tuberculin skin test result, other signs and symptoms compatible with active tuberculosis (e.g., abnormal and unstable radiologic findings and persistent cough), treatment with two or more antituberculous medications, and a completed diagnostic evaluation. This clinical definition is for reporting purposes. Physicians may begin treatment of individuals with suspected infectious tuberculosis on the basis of symptoms and risk factors while awaiting test results.

Common symptoms of pulmonary tuberculosis include chronic cough, a cough that produces sputum, chest pain associated with coughing, and less commonly, coughing up of blood. Other symptoms, which also appear in nonpulmonary tuberculosis, include fever, weight loss, night sweats, and fatigue. Some people with infectious tuberculosis report less specific symptoms or, rarely, no symptoms. The higher the prevalence of active tuberculosis in the community, the higher "the index of suspicion" should be that those with symptoms warrant further evaluation.

Diagnostic evaluation of someone suspected of having active tuberculosis involves

- a medical history that includes questions about symptoms, possible exposure to someone with infectious tuberculosis, past history of the disease, country of origin, age, place of work, and other medical conditions such as HIV infection associated with higher risk of tuberculosis;
- a physical examination;
- a chest radiograph to look for abnormalities suggestive of active pulmonary tuberculosis (or signs of infection or past tuberculosis that might warrant treatment); and
- laboratory tests for evaluation of sputum samples.[13]

Laboratory samples are usually first assessed with a smear that can be quickly processed to provide a report within 24 hours. Smears allow the identification of mycobacteria but not the identification of *M. tuberculosis* specifically. A follow-up culture will produce more accurate and specific information, but even with the latest technology, reports will generally not be available for several days. Tests to evaluate drug susceptibility may be done sequentially after culture confirmation of disease, thus adding further to delays in starting appropriate treatment.

Molecular analysis (DNA fingerprinting) compares isolates of *M. tuberculosis* recovered from different individuals. Such analysis can help establish a chain of transmission that links new cases of active disease to source cases. It sometimes allows cases of active tuberculosis among workers to be more accurately linked to previously identified cases in the community or the workplace than was previously possible. The establishment of such links can help guide tuberculosis control efforts. As discussed in Chapter 5, uncertainty about the origins of tuberculosis infection and disease among health care and other workers contributes to uncertainty about the value of regulations in the control of occupational exposure. Some health care worker groups with the high rates of positive skin test results come from populations with high rates of active tuberculosis in the community (Appendix C). Current tests cannot identify the source of tuberculosis infection.

Improving Diagnostic Timeliness and Accuracy

Failures to promptly identify, isolate, and treat those with diagnosed or suspected infectious tuberculosis are major weak points in programs to prevent occupational exposure to the disease. Unfortunately, community- and workplace-based efforts to improve timely and accurate diagnosis of

---

[13]A tuberculin skin test is optional. Even if it is negative, it does not rule out the disease, especially in someone with symptoms or risk factors such as HIV infection or recent (less than 10 weeks) exposure to a person with infectious tuberculosis. For those with possible nonpulmonary tuberculosis, testing may involve blood, bone marrow, and other tissue.

infectious tuberculosis face a significant obstacle: the common symptoms of active tuberculosis are not highly specific to the disease. Particularly in areas where the disease has been rare for a considerable period, physicians are more likely to think of other, more common conditions—for example, bronchitis or lung cancer—when they see someone with symptoms such as a persistent cough. Clinicians likewise may not initially link radiologic signs of active tuberculosis to the disease. Moreover, some individuals with active tuberculosis, especially those with HIV infection, may show radiologic signs that are not typical of the disease, and a few may experience no symptoms. In addition, as tuberculosis has become less common and clinicians and laboratory personnel see fewer instances of the disease, it becomes more difficult for them to maintain proficiency in obtaining, processing, and accurately interpreting specimens.

Two recent reviews of episodes of tuberculosis transmission in health care facilities found that nearly all instances involved source cases with undiagnosed and untreated disease (Dooley and Tapper, 1997; Garrett et al., 1999). Many also involved lapses in infection control processes. In several instances, the patient identified as the source case had atypical radiologic signs and negative smears. Thus, the failures were not just the result of inattention to obvious signs and symptoms.

Unfortunately, because the symptoms of active tuberculosis are nonspecific, early identification protocols are likely to identify a sizeable percentage of people who do not actually have the disease. Isolation of these people results in an expensive, unnecessary use of isolation rooms. For example, one study in a high-prevalence hospital found that for every eight patients isolated, only one had confirmed tuberculosis (Bock et al., 1996). Later, as tuberculosis case rates dropped, this ratio increased to 10 to 1 (Blumberg, 1999). In low-prevalence areas, the ratio may be as high as 100 to 1 (Scott et al., 1994).

Researchers and clinicians have attempted to develop more precise diagnostic criteria and decision-support tools to allow quicker and more accurate identification of people with tuberculosis (Scott et al., 1994; Bock et al., 1996; Knirsch et al., 1998). This would promote earlier isolation and treatment. It would also help conserve resources by reducing the number of people incorrectly identified and isolated (false positives). Typically, however, such adjustments in prediction rules or decision criteria will result in more missed cases of active, potentially infectious disease (false negatives). For example, in one study, the use of prediction rules that were developed to reduce overisolation of nontuberculosis patients would have reduced the number of such patients with false-positive results from 253 to 95, but it would have missed 8 of 42 patients with (those with true disease) false negative results (Bock et al., 1996).

In addition to increasing the costs of care, overisolation may be emotionally stressful for patients. It typically reduces an individual's contact with family and friends and often limits contacts with health care work-ers. People may also feel stigmatized by the apparatus of isolation includ-ing the warning signs outside rooms and the requirement that patients be masked during transport outside the isolation room.[14]

Treatment of Active Tuberculosis

Treatment Regimens

The discovery in 1946 that streptomycin was effective against active tuberculosis began the transformation of the disease from an often lethal illness to one that could almost always be effectively treated (Daniel, 1997). Six years later, a much more effective drug, isoniazid, came on the market, and in 1970, rifampin, another very effective drug, became available. The use of these two drugs in combination made short-course therapy possible, reducing the length of treatment from 18 months to 6 to 9 months for drug-sensitive strains. As noted earlier, treatment of active tuberculosis cuts death rates from 50 percent or more to near zero for immunocompetent people who have drug-sensitive disease and who receive timely, appropriate care.

Unfortunately, multidrug-resistant strains of tuberculosis are much more difficult to treat, especially for patients with poorly functioning immune systems. Treatment of multidrug-resistant disease may require major surgery (e.g., removal of all or part of a lung) and long hospital stays. Patients may also undergo trials of treatment with second-line drug combinations that often must be used for long periods. These drugs also tend to produce more side effects than first-line drugs. Even with treat-ment, death rates among those with multidrug-resistant tuberculosis and immunosuppression may range from 40 to over 90 percent (CDC, 1994a).

Drug therapy regimens differ depending on the type of tuberculosis, the likelihood or identification of multidrug-resistant disease, the pres-ence of other medical conditions such as HIV infection or AIDS, patient age, risk of patient nonaderence to the regimen, and treatment side ef-fects. For drug-sensitive disease, the most common treatment regimen first uses a combination of four drugs (izoniazid, rifampin, pyrazinamide, and ethambutol) for 2 months followed by treatment with two drugs (izoniazid and rifampin) for 4 months (Fujiwara et al., 2000). Some drug schedules call for daily doses of medication; others call for twice-weekly

---

[14]Isolation for infectious tuberculosis does not require hospitalization if the person is not otherwise in need of inpatient care. Those isolated at home are instructed to stay at home without visitors. Home isolation may require that children and other high-risk individuals live elsewhere until the person with tuberculosis is no longer infectious. For those living in congregate settings such as nursing homes or prisons, however, protection of others may require use of properly functioning negative-pressure isolation rooms.

doses. Directly observed treatment is uniformly recommended for those on the latter schedule, which is often prescribed for those at high-risk of nonadherence.

Although the full course of treatment must be completed to cure the disease and limit the development of drug resistance, most individuals with active, drug-susceptible tuberculosis usually become noninfectious within 1 or 2 months of the start of treatment. Those with drug-resistant disease may remain infectious for much longer. People are considered no longer infectious when they meet three conditions: (1) they are receiving adequate therapy, (2) they have a significant clinical response to therapy, and (3) they have three consecutive negative sputum smear results for sputum collected on different days.

Directly Observed Therapy

As noted in Chapter 1, the strategy of short-course, directly observed therapy is targeted at the prevention of drug-resistant tuberculosis arising from incomplete treatment. The earliest use of directly observed therapy in the United States dates to the 1970s, but concerns about civil rights slowed its acceptance and use (Mangura and Galanowsky, 2000). CDC recommended the strategy in 1992 (CDC, 1992c), and it is a central component of the tuberculosis control initiatives of the World Health Organization (WHO, 2000a). The recent IOM report on the elimination of tuberculosis in the United States recommended that "all states have health regulations that mandate completion of therapy (treatment to cure) for all patients with active tuberculosis" (IOM, 2000, p. 6).

For individuals not living in prisons, nursing homes, or similar settings, directly observed treatment may involve scheduled appointments that bring a patient to a physician's office, clinic, or other site so that a nurse or other trained individual can watch the person take the required medications. In some cases, outreach workers may travel to an individual's residence. For health care and other workers, therapy may be observed in the employee health clinic.

Even when directly observed therapy is prescribed, it does not guarantee full and complete therapy. Enhancements to the basic strategy (such as multidisciplinary case management teams or the addition of economic and other incentives) can significantly improve the results of therapy (IOM, 2000).

CONCLUSION

Today, tuberculosis is a disease that can almost always be cured if it is diagnosed promptly and treated fully in people who have well-functioning immune systems and drug-sensitive disease. Recently, treatment priorities in community and workplace tuberculosis control programs have expanded to include latent tuberculosis infection. Faster, more accurate tests for both latent infection and active disease would benefit efforts to prevent and control tuberculosis in both the workplace and the community.

The next chapter reviews the statutory basis for the 1997 proposed OSHA rule on occupational tuberculosis. Chapter 4 compares the proposed rule with the 1994 CDC guidelines to prevent transmission of tuberculosis in health care facilities.

3

Occupational Safety and Health Regulation in Context

The creation of safer workplaces and the reduction in the number of occupational injuries, diseases, and deaths have been counted among the 10 leading public health achievements of the last century (CDC, 1999a,d). Safer workplaces are the cumulative result of many changes involving social attitudes and expectations, economic development, class and power relationships, science and technology, information resources and analytic capacities, government policies, and more.

This chapter focuses on government regulatory policy and the legal context within which the Occupational Safety and Health Administration (OSHA) has operated in developing the 1997 proposed rule on occupational tuberculosis. (See also Appendix E.) Understanding this context helps in understanding some of the differences between the proposed rule and the 1994 guidelines of the Centers for Disease Control and Prevention (CDC). First, however, it is useful to consider briefly the strategies available to workers seeking safer workplaces.

STRATEGIES FOR REDUCING WORKPLACE HAZARDS

Governmental regulation of workplace hazards is one of several possible strategies for workers seeking protection from unsafe working conditions. One way of categorizing these strategies is shown in Table 3-1, which distinguishes public versus private strategies and individual versus collective options. Each strategy has its strengths and limitations. These may vary depending on the kinds of workers and workplace hazards involved and on the economic environment, including the level of unemployment (Mendeloff, 1978, 1988; Robinson, 1991).

TABLE 3-1. Worker Strategies to Control Workplace Hazards

Strategy Type	Individual	Collective
Private	I. Quitting hazardous jobs; searching for jobs in safe workplaces	III. Joining labor unions; bargaining with employers for safe working conditions
Public	II. Suing in court for individual rights to information about hazards, to refuse hazardous assignments, and to report hazards without reprisal	IV. Organizing to secure government action to prevent or reduce health and safety hazards in the workplace

SOURCE: Adapted from Robinson (1991).

People quit jobs (Option I) for many reasons under many different circumstances. In theory, if employers perceive that employee departures are motivated by safety concerns and if they find hiring new workers troublesome, they may be motivated to improve working conditions. As a workplace-change strategy, the quitting option has serious limitations. In particular, workers with low levels of education and skills, who are often found in the most hazardous jobs, may lack better alternatives and, possibly, a real understanding of the risks that they face. Such individual workers are also not well prepared to challenge employers' unsafe working conditions in court (Option II).[1]

Unions and collective bargaining (Option III) have given workers a more powerful voice to influence employers and improve working conditions. The priorities in collective bargaining, however, generally involve wages, benefits, and job security. These objectives are relatively easy to understand, measure, and assess if achieved. They also generally affect union members across a wide range of job circumstances.

In contrast, unsafe working conditions may be less visible and may affect a smaller proportion of a union's members. Unions do negotiate with employers over issues such as hazard pay, provision of protective equipment, safety training, and reduction or elimination of workplace hazards. They have, however, cited lack of technical capacity to analyze health and safety problems and evaluate possible remedies for these problems as a barrier to the use of collective bargaining to negotiate workplace safety issues (Mendeloff, 1978). Lack of technical capacity and other resources may also constrain union use of litigation as a strategy to improve workplace conditions.

---

[1]Workers' compensation laws also constrain workers' ability to use litigation as a strategy to improve workplace safety because they bar suits based on an employer's alleged negligence.

Furthermore, the winning of worker protections on a company-by-company or industry-by-industry basis is a formidable challenge. Therefore, workers have often sought government—especially federal government—protections (Option IV), including protection for the very right to organize workers and bargain collectively. Regulatory strategies usually put the main burden of identifying and analyzing hazards and remedies on government officials rather than on workers.

Regulatory strategies to improve workplace safety and health have their own limitations. Some regulations face little resistance from those who are regulated; others are highly unpopular and provoke years of litigation. Policymakers are frequently challenged for not adequately weighing the expected benefits of regulation against the expected costs. Some regulations are relatively inexpensive and technically easy to implement, monitor, and enforce, but others are not. In any case, implementation of regulations as intended cannot be assumed.

The above discussion emphasizes strategies available to workers. Even when they are not actively sought by workers, employers, government officials, and others may take steps on their own initiative to identify and correct workplace hazards. For example, employers may easily become aware of real or potential hazards before workers recognize them and may take steps to reduce the hazard (and the liability that might result). Public health and other researchers may likewise identify hazards that affect both workers and members of the general community. They may then seek to publicize the hazards and find ways to eliminate or reduce them through voluntary action, scientific discovery, or technological innovation.

THE OCCUPATIONAL SAFETY AND HEALTH ACT OF 1970 AND ITS ADMINISTRATION

The first federal agency that focused on workplace safety was the U.S. Bureau of Mines, established in 1910 (CDC, 1999d). Its creation followed increasing attention to deaths in the workplace. For example, in 1906–1907, the first systematic survey of workplace accidents was undertaken in Allegheny County, Pennsylvania. It counted 526 deaths from such accidents in the county, including 195 among steelworkers.

Until 1970, states had the primary responsibility for regulating workplace conditions. The first state laws on worker safety date to 1837, and a few states had created inspection programs and started collecting injury and illness data before 1900 (OSHSPA, 1999). As they developed, state programs tended to rely more on education and consultation with employers rather than on formal enforcement of regulations backed by fines for employer violations (Mendeloff, 1978).

Not surprisingly, state laws and activities that regulate workplace health and safety were—and are—highly variable. Today, for example, states can choose to develop and adopt their own plans under the Occupational Safety and Health Act, and about half have chosen to do so (see below). If states choose not to develop such plans, federal occupational safety and health rules—including rules intended to protect workers from tuberculosis—will not apply to state and local government employees.

Whether or not they choose to develop state plans, states may innovate in areas not covered by federal regulations. For example, some states adopted so-called worker right-to-know laws before federal regulators first adopted a hazard communication standard in 1983 that applied to those working with hazardous chemicals (OSHSPA, 1999).

Creation of OSHA

The 1960s saw a broad expansion of the powers of the federal government in many areas such as civil rights, education, health, social welfare, and knowledge development. Toward the end of the decade, serious efforts began to secure federal regulation of workplace health and safety. In 1969, the U.S. Congress passed the Federal Coal Mine Health and Safety Act, which set health and safety standards for all mines and expanded the powers of federal mine inspectors (CDC, 1999d). The next year, Congress passed the Occupational Safety and Health Act (P.L. 91-596). As summarized at the beginning of the statute, the purpose of the legislation was to assure safe and healthful working conditions for working men and women

- by authorizing enforcement of the standards developed under the Act;
- by assisting and encouraging the States in their efforts to assure safe and healthful working conditions;
- by providing for research, information, education, and training in the field of occupational safety and health; and for other purposes.

The 1970 legislation created OSHA and assigned it responsibility for standard setting and enforcement. The statute also created the National Institute for Occupational Safety and Health (NIOSH), which undertakes training activities, makes recommendations to OSHA relating to health and safety standards, and supports epidemiologic, toxicologic, and other research on workplace hazards. NIOSH certifies personal respiratory protection devices for a wide range of workplace uses. OSHA is part of the U.S. Department of Labor (DOL), whereas NIOSH is part of CDC in the U.S. Department of Health and Human Services (DHHS).

The statute created two additional bodies. One is the National Advisory Committee on Occupational Safety and Health, which advises both DOL and DHHS on the feasibility of and alternatives to new standards.

The second is the quasijudicial Occupational Safety and Health Review Commission, which adjudicates citations and penalties. Decisions by this commission may be appealed to the federal courts. Rules may also be challenged in federal court on a "preenforcement basis" within 59 days of their publication in final form. A third body, the Federal Advisory Council on Occupational Safety and Health, which advises the Secretary of Labor on occupational safety and health issues involving federal agencies, was created by the Executive Order 11612 in 1974.

OSHA standards are predictably challenged in court both before and after enforcement. As discussed below and in Appendix E, several U.S. Supreme Court decisions have shaped how the agency does its work and justifies its proposals and policies.

For most of its 30 years, OSHA has survived amidst continued discussion about its basic premises (see, e.g., Page and O'Brien [1973], Mendeloff [1978, 1988], McCaffrey [1982], Mintz [1984], Robinson [1991], and Reich [1994]). Proposals are periodically introduced in Congress to curb or abolish the agency. In the 1980s, the Reagan administration trimmed federal regulation in many areas by means of executive orders and cuts in agency budgets including those of OSHA and NIOSH (Mendeloff, 1988; Robinson, 1991). In the 1990s, the Clinton administration issued Executive Order 12866, which requires more agency analyses of the costs relative to the benefits of regulations. Appendix E describes in more detail the key provisions of the OSHA statute and relevant executive orders and judicial decisions. The rest of this section provides a brief overview of OSHA's goals, the criteria that it uses in devising health and safety regulations, and the scope of its rules.

Goals and Criteria for OSHA Standards

The fundamental goal of the Occupational Safety and Health Act is "to assure so far as possible every working man and woman in the Nation safe and healthful working conditions" (29 USC 651 2[a]). The statute's general-duty clause provides that employers are to (1) furnish their employees work and a workplace that is free from recognized hazards that are likely to cause serious physical harm or death and (2) comply with safety and health standards set forth under the act.

The statute also provides that *employees* are to comply with applicable safety and health standards. In practice, this provision has little meaning. OSHA may not fine employees or otherwise punish them for failure to adhere to standards.[2]

---

[2]The agency may require employers to ensure certain actions by employees (e.g., use of personal respirators under certain circumstances). It cannot, however, hold an employer strictly liable for employee noncompliance if the employer has taken reasonable measures to train, monitor, and otherwise supervise employees. (984 F.2d 823).

OSHA's current regulations and enforcement actions to prevent the spread of tuberculosis are based on the statute's general-duty clause and on general standards involving respiratory protection (29 CFR 1910.134) and warnings of biological hazards (29 CFR 1910.145).[3] The 1997 proposed rule is based on separate provisions of the 1970 statute that authorize OSHA to issue mandatory occupational safety and health standards applicable to specific industries or hazards.

When OSHA creates a health standard, it must set the standard to "most adequately" ensure "to the extent feasible, on the basis of the best available evidence, that no employee will suffer material impairment of health or functional capacity even if such employee has regular exposure to the hazard dealt with by such standard for the period of his working life" (29 U.S.C. 655). The same paragraph of the statute also calls for "the attainment of the highest degree of health and safety protection for the employee." It provides, however, for "other considerations" to be taken into account, including the "latest available scientific data in the field, the feasibility of the standards, and experience under this and other health and safety laws." Whenever practicable, standards are to be stated in terms of objective criteria.

Reflecting its interpretation of its statute, case law, and executive orders, OSHA has described a workplace standard as "reasonably necessary or appropriate if it substantially reduces or eliminates significant risk and if it is economically feasible, technologically feasible, cost effective, consistent with prior Agency action . . . supported by substantial evidence." (62 FR 201 at 54169, October 17, 1997). Box 3-1 lists OSHA's interpretation of several of these phrases.

Significant Health Risk

In discussing what constitutes a significant health risk, OSHA has described such a risk as one that exposes a worker to a risk of death of 1/1,000 over a 45-year working lifetime. This criterion derives from the plurality statement of the U.S. Supreme Court that indicated that OSHA could regulate only a "significant risk" and that it is reasonable and acceptable for OSHA to regulate on the basis of odds of 1 in 1,000 that a practice or situation will prove fatal (448 U.S. 607 at 655). The ruling, which involved a standard on benzene, required that OSHA justify its rules with quantitative risk assessments. The decision, however, stated

---

[3]The most recent OSHA standard on personal respiratory protection, which was issued in 1998, does not apply to tuberculosis (29 CFR 1910.134). The agency, which had published the proposed rule on occupational tuberculosis in 1997, instead provided a separate interim regulation (29 CFR 1910.139). The interim regulation describes the provisions of the 1987 respiratory protection standard that apply until a tuberculosis standard is published.

> **Box 3-1**
> **Key Terms Relevant to Justification**
> **of OSHA Standards as Used by the Agency**
>
> *Significant risk:* "generally . . . at a minimum, a fatality risk of 1/1,000 over a 45-year working lifetime . . . [is] a significant health risk."
>
> *Substantially reduce risk:* No explicit definition found.
>
> *Material impairment:* No explicit definition found.
>
> *Economically feasible:* "A standard is economically feasible if industry can absorb or pass on the costs of compliance without threatening its long-term profitability or competitive structure."
>
> *Technologically feasible:* "A standard is technologically feasible if the protective measures it requires already exists, can be brought into existence with available technology, or can be created with technology that can reasonably be expected to be developed."
>
> *Cost-effective:* Within the context of the OSHA statute and applicable judicial decisions, the cost-effectiveness of required protective measures is narrowly defined in terms of "the least costly of the available alternatives that achieve the same level of protection."
>
> *Substantial evidence:* No explicit definition found. "Scientific certainty" is not required; rather, actions need only be supported by a "body of reputable scientific thought."
>
> SOURCE: 62 FR 201 at 54169 (1997)

that the risk determination was not to be a "mathematical straightjacket" nor did it require "anything approaching scientific certainty" (448 U.S. 607 at 655). The ruling also noted that "safe" was not the equivalent of "risk-free." In the 1997 proposed rule on tuberculosis, OSHA defines infection with *M. tuberculosis* as a material impairment of health and applies the 1/1,000 risk criterion to the risk of infection rather than the risk of death.

Substantially Reduce Risk

The committee found no quantitative guidance in case law or elsewhere about what constitutes a substantial reduction in a significant risk. In the benzene case, the court stated that evidence should indicate that it is "more likely than not" that a rule will eliminate or reduce the risk being regulated. The court further concluded "that Congress intended, at a bare minimum, that [OSHA] find a significant risk of harm and therefore a probability of significant benefits before establishing a new standard" (448 U.S. 607 at 642, 645). Chapter 7 discusses OSHA's estimate of the reductions in the numbers of cases of tuberculosis infection, disease, and death that would result from implementation of the 1997 proposed rule.

Material Impairment

In its 1997 proposed rule, OSHA concluded that tuberculosis infection was a material impairment of health because it poses some risk of progression to active disease and because treatment of infection involves some risk of adverse effects. (See Chapter 7 for commentary on this assessment.) The term "material impairment" is not defined explicitly in the proposed rule or the statute, nor has it apparently been defined in case law.

Other OSHA standards have also defined infections and subclinical conditions as material impairments. For example, in the rule on blood-borne pathogens, the agency declared that hepatitis B virus infection as well as the disease itself constituted a material impairment of health (56 FR 64004, December 6, 1991). Before that, in its standard on lead (43 FR 52952, November 14, 1978), OSHA designated not only death and overt symptoms of lead poisoning but also certain subclinical pathophysiological changes as material impairments.

Feasibility

The OSHA statute refers to standards that ensure "to the extent feasible" that workers' health and functional capacity will not be impaired. OSHA has interpreted technical feasibility to mean that a standard can be implemented with existing technology, adaptations of available technology, or reasonably foreseeable technological developments. Consistent with a 1981 U.S. Supreme Court decision on cotton dust regulations, OSHA has interpreted economic feasibility basically to mean that the cost of complying with a standard is not so high that it will cause a substantial number of businesses to fail (452 U.S. 490).

Cost-Effectiveness

For OSHA, a standard is cost-effective if the measures required are the least costly of the available alternatives that achieve the same high level of worker protection required by its statute. This is consistent with the Unfunded Mandates Reform Act of 1995, which requires the use of the most cost-effective means of accomplishing a regulatory objective. It is also consistent with the 1993 Executive Order 12866, which requires a regulatory flexibility analysis to determine—"to the extent permitted by law"—whether the costs of a regulation are justified by its benefits.[4]

The 1981 U.S. Supreme Court decision on cotton dust regulations held that "a cost-benefit analysis by OSHA is not required by the statute" (452 U.S. 490 at 500). In a 1993 appellate court decision that generally upheld 1991 OSHA regulations on bloodborne pathogens (29 CFR 1910.1030), the Seventh Circuit Court of Appeals noted that

> OSHA did not (indeed is not authorized to) compare the benefits with the costs and impose the restrictions on finding that the former exceeded the latter. Instead it asked whether the restrictions would materially reduce a significant workplace risk to human health without imperiling the existence of, or threatening massive dislocation to, the health care industry . . . this is the applicable legal standard (984 F.2d 823 at 825).

The same court also suggested some boundaries of reasonable costs for a life saved by a regulation. It noted that the bloodborne pathogen rule's "implicit valuation of a life is high—about $4 million—but not so astronomical, certainly by regulatory standards, . . . as to call the rationality of the rule seriously into question" (984 F.2d 823 at 825).[5] It also noted that the diseases targeted—infection with Hepatitis B or AIDS—were diseases that killed people "in their prime" (984 F.2d 823 at 826). The court goes on to note the benefits of avoiding serious consequences other than death.

In sum, OSHA's application of cost-effectiveness analysis is fairly circumscribed. It is similar to the kinds of analyses occasionally used by the Health Care Financing Administration program to limit Medicare payments to the level of the less expensive of two treatments that achieve equivalent outcomes for a health problem (HCFA, 1999 [Carriers Manual section 2100.2]).

---

[4]Cost-effectiveness analyses examine the costs associated with achieving a desired outcome such as saving a life or preventing a case of disease. Cost-benefit analyses use monetary measures of benefits as well as costs. Notwithstanding this distinction, cost-effectiveness analyses frequently use the term "benefit" more generally to describe a desired effect or outcome (e.g., a life saved) without an explicit monetary valuing. A valuing may be implicit; for example, if a rule is estimated to save up to 200 lives yearly at a total estimated direct cost of $200,000,000 yearly, it implies that a life saved is worth at least $1,000,000.

[5]In the rule on bloodborne pathogens, OSHA estimated that implementing the rule would cost employers $813 million per year and would avert 187–197 deaths per year among workers and their sexual contacts. Dividing yearly costs by yearly deaths approximates the $4 million figure cited by the appellate court. In the 1997 proposed rule on tuberculosis, OSHA estimated that implementing the rule cost employers $245 million per year in direct costs and would avert an estimated 138–190 deaths per year among workers and their families and other contacts. It estimated $89 million to $116 million in cost savings related to avoided costs for medical care and absenteeism.

Role of Evidence

The statute provides that OSHA can regulate on the basis of the "best available evidence" [(29 USC 655(f), 6(b)(5)]. The U.S. Supreme Court has said that "scientific certainty" is not required; rather, actions need only be supported by a "body of reputable scientific thought" (448 U.S. 607 at 655). The court also said that OSHA could also use assumptions that risked error on the side of overprotection. The court explicitly acknowledged the relevance of epidemiologic evidence.

OSHA Standards and Communicable Diseases

The agency has traditionally focused on materials used in industrial processes to which exposure was relatively predictable and measurable. A cotton dust standard in the cotton-textile industry, for example, could assume that workers in a cotton-textile mill would be exposed to cotton dust.

The 1997 proposed rule on occupational tuberculosis was only the second that OSHA has developed to deal with an infectious disease hazard. The other led to the 1992 standard on bloodborne pathogens. Regulation of the occupational risk of communicable disease introduces at least three additional complications for regulators that must be kept in mind in assessing the proposed rule on occupational tuberculosis.

First, exposure to *Mycobacterium tuberculosis* is not readily predictable and cannot reliably be measured, so exposure must be inferred from epidemiologic and other data. Because exposure depends upon numerous factors that vary considerably from workplace to workplace, it cannot be assumed that health care and other workers will actually be exposed to *M. tuberculosis*.

Second, the risk of exposure and negative health effects has the potential to change rapidly because of events outside the workplace, requiring unusual flexibility and coordination with other actors involved in preventing the transmission of tuberculosis. If community prevalence drops substantially or infection control measures change significantly, OSHA's risk assessment or regulatory response may cease to be relevant.

Third, the risk of communicable disease may not originate in the workplace. No one brings formaldehyde or other regulated toxins into the workplace, but workers, patients and others do bring communicable diseases into workplaces. Thus, OSHA must deal with the question of whether infections in a hospital or other covered workplace are to be attributed to a worker's occupational risk or community risk.

Application to Private and Public Employers and Employees

For the most part, OSHA's direct regulatory focus is on private employers. Separate provisions of the statute describe its application to federal workers and to state and local employees.

Under the statute, federal agencies are to develop safety standards consistent with those issued by OSHA, maintain occupational safety and health records, and report to the Secretary of Labor regarding their programs. As set forth in a 1980 executive order, federal agencies must (1) follow OSHA standards unless the Secretary of Labor approves an alternative safety plan, (2) comply with the act's general-duty clause by eliminating recognized hazards that cause or are likely to cause death, (3) permit unannounced inspections under certain conditions, and (4) allow employees to report safety problems without fear of discrimination or retaliation. OSHA may inspect and cite federal agencies, but it cannot fine them.

State and local employees are not covered by OSHA rules unless their states have adopted state occupational safety and health plans approved by OSHA. If states adopt plans that are "at least as effective as" the federal plan, the federal government pays up to 50 percent of the cost of enforcing the plans.

Almost half the states and territories have approved plans, and two of these states (New York and Connecticut) cover only public employees.[6] If OSHA adopts a final rule on tuberculosis, states with state plans would have to adopt a comparable standard within 6 months. States with approved plans must still require employers to submit reports to OSHA as though no plan were in place, and OSHA may also inspect workplaces in these states to monitor state performance. In states without approved plans, public hospitals, medical examiners' offices, most prisons and jails, and other facilities would not be subject to an OSHA tuberculosis standard. They might, however, be affected by general or tuberculosis-specific infection control provisions in state licensure laws, Medicare or Medicaid requirements, or private accreditation standards. Further, if a public facility such as a prison contracted with a private agency to operate the health unit in the facility, then that agency would have to comply with OSHA requirements even if the rest of the facility was exempt.

Multiple-Employer Workplaces

For hospitals and other employers covered by OSHA rules, outsourcing arrangements have become an increasingly popular way to cut costs and increase flexibility. Thus, some nurses may work for the hospital directly, whereas others may be supplied by one or more outside agencies. Food-service employees may be supplied by one contract and janitors by another. As a result, professional and nonprofessional workers at

---

[6]The other jurisdictions are Arizona, California, Hawaii, Iowa, Kentucky, Maryland, Michigan, Minnesota, Nevada, New Mexico, North Carolina, Oregon, Puerto Rico, South Carolina, Tennessee, Utah, Vermont, Virginia, Virgin Islands, Washington, and Wyoming.

hospitals and other workplaces may be employed by a number of different employers. These employers share responsibility for employee safety and health under OSHA.

For example, a hospital may operate a tuberculin skin testing program only for its employees, meaning that each contractor that supplies the hospital with workers may have to set up its own testing program. Alternatively, a hospital may agree—for a fee—to also test a contractor's employees.

Some responsibilities for tuberculosis control are not readily shared. In particular, hospitals typically must provide isolation rooms and ventilation equipment that protect both their employees and the employees of independent contractors. They may, however, contract for maintenance of the equipment.

Employees and Nonemployees

Federal law obligates employers to provide employees with safe working conditions and to comply with specific OSHA standards. In most situations, employers' obligations do not extend to volunteers. If volunteers receive some significant compensation in kind (e.g., room and board), OSHA claims that an employee-employer relationship exists. Medical or other residents and fellows who are compensated for their services qualify as employees for purposes of federal occupational safety and health regulations. Medical, nursing, and other students who are not compensated do not appear to be covered, although a health care facility may still choose to test them or require that they be tested by their schools.

The situation with respect to physicians can be complicated. Within a hospital, patients may be seen by physicians who are employed by the hospital, physicians who are employed by an affiliated medical school, physicians who are employed by a managed care plan or other corporation, physicians who have incorporated their own practices, and physicians who practice without having incorporated or created an equivalent legal entity. Physicians in all but the last category appear to be subject to OSHA's requirements for employee protection.

Resources and Enforcement Actions

The fiscal year (FY) 2000 budget authority for OSHA provided for $381 million in funding and for 2,262 full-time-equivalent employees (DOL, 2000). About $82 million of this total was designated for grants to state plan programs, and $141 million was designated for agency enforcement activities. Another $54 million was designated for federal compliance assistance, which involves various kinds of voluntary employer and employee technical assistance and training programs. In 1998, when OSHA's budget was $336.5 million, the agency reported that states and territories with state plans allocated another $111.3 million to their own programs (OSHSPA, 1999).

In its FY 2001 budget request, OSHA stated that it expected to issue seven standards in FY 2000 and five more FY 2001 (DOL, 2000). For FY 2000, the agency estimated that federal OSHA employees would conduct more than 34,500 inspections and 27,500 consultation visits. State plan personnel would conduct another 55,000 inspections in FY 2000.

OSHA's enforcement activities include responding to complaints made by employees covered by OSHA and periodically inspecting covered workplaces on a scheduled basis. OSHA's compliance officers inspect work sites and counsel employers regarding compliance concerns. The reports of these compliance officers provide the basis for regional office personnel to determine whether violations exist and citations should be issued. In 1999, OSHA began a targeted inspection program that focuses on the work sites with the highest injury and illness rates on the basis of the data reported to OSHA (Jeffress, 2000).

Penalties for violations range from zero in the case of *de minimus* technical violations that do not affect safety or health to $70,000 for the most serious repeated or willful violations. If violations are not corrected within a specified time, a "failure to abate" violation can result in fines of up to $7,000 per day. Appendix E describes enforcement activities and penalties in more detail.

CONCLUSION

OSHA operates within the boundaries provided by its statute, applicable executive orders, and relevant judicial decisions. The provisions of the 1997 proposed rule on tuberculosis reflect the directions and constraints set by each of these sources. The next chapter compares that rule and the 1994 CDC guidelines on tuberculosis in health care facilities.

4

Comparison of CDC Guidelines and Proposed OSHA Rule

As described in Chapter 1, both the Centers for Disease Control and Prevention (CDC) and the Occupational Safety and Health Administration (OSHA) responded to the resurgence of tuberculosis that began in the mid-1980s and continued into the early 1990s. Beginning in 1990, CDC issued a series of tuberculosis control guidelines aimed at different settings and populations. In 1993 and 1994, OSHA issued enforcement procedures based on existing respiratory protection regulations and on statutory requirements that employers provide safe workplaces. Also, in 1994, OSHA initiated a rule-making process that led to the 1997 proposed rule. As this report was being completed in Fall 2000, OSHA had not published the final standard.

This chapter summarizes the provisions of the 1994 CDC guidelines for health care facilities and describes points of difference between the guidelines and the 1997 proposed OSHA rule. The proposed rule "incorporated the basic elements" of the 1994 guidelines with some differences (62 FR 201 at 54170 [October 17, 1997]). For example, as described later in this chapter, the CDC guidelines set forth a more extensive process for assessing the risk facing workers in a health care facility and determining which control measures apply on the basis of the level of risk. More generally, OSHA drafted the proposed rule to be enforced, and it therefore tends to be more specific and directive than the CDC guidelines. It would cover a broader range of employers and employees than the guidelines but would not extend to patients, prisoners, or visitors.

Some of the differences between the two documents reflect differences in the basic missions of CDC and OSHA. For example, consistent with its broader public health mission, the CDC guidelines for health care facilities include recommendations related to patients, family members, and visitors as well as employees. Similarly, CDC's discussion of tuberculosis control measures is generally more detailed, clinically oriented, and educational than the discussion of such measures in the proposed OSHA rule. Consistent with OSHA's regulatory responsibilities, the proposed rule is often more specific and directive than the guidelines.

Both the CDC guidelines and the proposed OSHA rule were published during a period of change, and as discussed in Chapters 5, 6, and 7, circumstances continue to change. This chapter provides a descriptive overview and comparison of the guidelines as issued by CDC in 1994 and the rule as proposed by OSHA in 1997. Chapter 6 presents the committee's assessment of the impact of the CDC guidelines, and Chapter 7 examines the likely impact of an OSHA standard. Complicating this latter assessment was the lack of a final published standard.

CDC GUIDELINES ON PREVENTING TRANSMISSION OF TUBERCULOSIS IN HEALTH CARE FACILITIES

CDC has published guidelines and recommendations for controlling tuberculosis in health care facilities (CDC, 1990b, 1994b), correctional facilities (CDC, 1996b), and facilities serving homeless people (CDC, 1992a). It has also developed guidelines focusing on special populations including migrant workers (CDC, 1992b), at-risk minority groups (CDC, 1992c), foreign-born persons (CDC, 1998b), and those with human immunodeficiency virus (HIV) infection (most recently, CDC, 1998a, 2000c).[1]

CDC's 1994 guidelines for health care facilities, which replaced those issued in 1990, served as the foundation for the rule proposed by OSHA in 1997. In the fall of 2000, CDC began a reexamination of the guidelines, in particular, the recommendations on tuberculin skin testing. No new recommendations are expected before 2002.

The 1994 CDC guidelines present a three-level hierarchy of measures to prevent transmission of tuberculosis in health care facilities. As explained below, the hierarchy consists of (1) administrative controls, (2) engineering controls, and (3) personal respiratory protection.[2]

---

[1]Other organizations have also issued guidelines and recommendations on preventing the transmission of tuberculosis. The American College of Chest Physicians (ACCP) and the American Thoracic Society (ATS) issued a joint statement on institutional measures to control tuberculosis in 1995 (ACCP/ATS, 1995). The next year the ATS (1996) issued a statement on respiratory protections. (For a comparison of these and other guidelines, see Nardell, 1997.) Recent joint statements from ATS and CDC include recommendations on skin testing and treatment for latent tuberculosis infection (ATS/CDC, 2000a,b).

[2]In occupational health, the traditional hierarchy of strategies to control workplace hazards emphasizes engineering controls first (McDiarmid et al., 1996). For example, one text states that "Engineering controls are the most desirable and reliable means for reducing workplace exposures [to toxicants]" (Cohen, 1992, p. 1401).

The guidelines for health care facilities focus primarily on hospitals, with special sections on ambulatory care settings, emergency departments, autopsy rooms, and laboratories. They also include brief discussions of emergency medical services, hospices, long-term-care facilities, correctional facilities, dental settings, home health care settings, and medical offices. The guidelines define health care workers to cover paid and unpaid workers including contract employees, students, and volunteers.

In 1996, a CDC advisory group published recommendations for the prevention of tuberculosis in correctional facilities (CDC, 1996b). These recommendations are organized around the core activities of screening, containment, and assessment rather than around the hierarchy of controls listed above. Although the recommendations reflect differences between the purposes of correctional facilities and those of health care facilities, many elements are similar to the 1994 guidelines. For example, the discussion of tuberculin skin testing and follow-up for employees is consistent with the 1994 guidelines, except that no category of prison worker is singled out for retesting more often than once a year. Prisons that have medical units are advised to follow the 1994 CDC guidelines in those units. Facility personnel are also advised to be familiar with guidelines published by American Thoracic Society (ATS) and the National Commission on Correctional Health Care (NCCHC, 1992, 1996).

CDC's 1992 recommendations for those who work with homeless people only briefly discuss protections for homeless shelter workers (CDC, 1992a). These protections include (1) tuberculin skin testing of shelter staff upon hiring and every 6 to 12 months thereafter, (2) evaluation of those with positive tests results, and (3) provision of treatment for those with latent tuberculosis infection, as appropriate.

In contrast to government regulations, the CDC guidelines on tuberculosis are advisory, which allows more leeway for institutional interpretation and judgment. The guidelines are not enforced by a government agency responsible for monitoring compliance and proposing penalties for noncompliance. Other federal and state agencies as well as accrediting organizations may, however, require tuberculosis control measures based on or similar to those recommended by CDC.[3] In some circumstances, health care

---

[3]To receive Medicare payments, hospitals, nursing homes, and some other health care providers must meet requirements set by the Health Care Financing Administration (HCFA). Many hospitals qualify for Medicare payment through accreditation by the Joint Commission on the Accreditation of Healthcare Facilities (JCAHCO), which may specify additional criteria for certification. Both HCFA and JCAHCO require infection control programs in hospitals and nursing homes. For nursing homes, the HCFA guidelines used by state inspectors specifically require that facilities demonstrate procedures for early detection and management of residents with signs and symptoms of infectious tuberculosis, screening of residents and workers for tuberculosis infection and disease, and evaluation of workers exposed to tuberculosis in the workplace (AHCA, 2000).

facilities might also be subject to OSHA sanctions under enforcement procedures based on the general-duty-clause of the agency's statute (see Chapter 3 and Appendix E). In addition, health care facilities that fail to follow CDC guidance might be more vulnerable to lawsuits by patients or others who contract tuberculosis in a facility. Employees who acquire active tuberculosis (and sometimes tuberculosis infection) through occupational exposure are covered under workers' compensation laws that preclude litigation against an employer (see Chapter 3 and Appendix E).[4]

Unlike some guidelines directed at health care practitioners, the 1994 CDC guidelines do not have a "sunset" provision that specifies a date after which users should not rely on the guidelines. These and similar provisions acknowledge that scientific knowledge is always advancing and that those who develop clinical practice guidelines should have a process to review and update recommendations to reflect current scientific evidence and changing circumstances (IOM, 1992; CDC, 1996a). As noted earlier, the agency recently began a reexamination of the 1994 guidelines.

PROPOSED OSHA RULE ON OCCUPATIONAL EXPOSURE TO TUBERCULOSIS

OSHA's mission, described in Chapter 3, differs from that of CDC. In addition, its rules must meet statutory, judicial, and administrative criteria that do not apply to CDC guidelines. In developing rules, OSHA must, however, consider available guidelines, research, and other information. For example, the agency incorporated basic elements of the 1994 CDC guidelines in the 1997 proposed rule. OSHA also notes that in enforcing a final rule on tuberculosis, it would ordinarily defer to subsequently updated CDC guidelines that had provisions in conflict with the rule.

OSHA concluded that the CDC guidelines were not an enforceable alternative to the proposed rule. Nonetheless, in the commentary (preamble) on the proposed rule, the agency asks for comments on this alternative, including how "compliance and efficacy" could be determined (62 FR 201 at 54227 [October 17, 1997]).

The proposed OSHA rule also includes nonmandated guidance on certain topics. These include the writing of the required exposure control plan, the use of ultraviolet germicidal irradiation lighting systems, and

---

[4]As described in Chapter 2, laboratory tests that can "fingerprint" strains of tuberculosis may help in evaluating whether the workplace is the source of tuberculosis in a patient or health care worker. Nonetheless, such testing in not always feasible, and it may not rule out exposure from a source in the community. As described elsewhere in this chapter, the proposed OSHA rule would provide certain financial protections for workers diagnosed with tuberculosis without requiring proof of its origin in the workplace.

performance-monitoring procedures for high-efficiency particulate air (HEPA) filters used for contaminated air that may be recirculated into general-use areas.

The rest of this section briefly reviews differences in the settings and people covered by the CDC guidelines and the proposed OSHA rule. The remaining sections focus on differences between the exposure control measures described in the guidelines and those in the proposed rule.

Covered Settings and Employers

The proposed OSHA rule is not limited to health care workers, employers, and settings. It would cover a wide range of employers and employees including

- Hospitals
- Long-term-care facilities serving the elderly
- Hospices
- Substance abuse treatment centers
- Home health care providers
- Emergency medical service providers
- Research and clinical laboratories handling tuberculosis bacteria
- Medical examiners' offices
- Other facilities where certain high-hazard procedures are performed
- Homeless shelters
- Correctional facilities
- Immigration detainment facilities
- Law enforcement facilities
- Contractors working on ventilation systems or areas that might contain airborne tuberculosis bacteria
- Social service workers, attorneys, and teachers visiting those with suspected or confirmed tuberculosis
- Personnel agencies or other organizations providing temporary or contract workers to covered facilities

The list of workplaces and employees provided above does not cover all those in which higher rates of tuberculosis have been documented. For example, workers in certain mining industries often have workplace-related physical conditions (e.g., silicosis) that make them more susceptible to tuberculosis. Because these workers are not anticipated to have a high risk of workplace *exposure* to the disease, the proposed OSHA rule does not cover them. (Also, mine safety is covered by another U.S. Department of Labor agency, the Mine Safety and Health Administration.)

Some health care settings are unexpectedly omitted from the listing in the 1997 proposed rule. For example, tuberculosis clinics are not mentioned, nor are HIV-AIDS clinics, although the latter serve populations at high risk of having infectious tuberculosis. Tuberculosis and HIV-AIDS clinics could, however, be affected by the proposed rule's coverage of facilities where high-hazard procedures (e.g., cough induction or administration of aerosolized drugs) are performed. If a clinic did not perform such procedures, no provisions of the proposed rule would apparently apply. In a presentation to the committee, OSHA staff suggested that the final rule is likely to cover tuberculosis and HIV-AIDS clinics explicitly.

The proposed OSHA rule also does not cover physicians' offices unless high-hazard procedures are performed there. Thus, physicians serving recent immigrants, AIDS patients, and other high-risk populations in high-prevalence areas would not be covered unless they performed bronchoscopies or similar procedures. The 1994 CDC guidelines state that it is likely that tuberculosis will be encountered in medical offices. They advise a risk assessment and the use of precautions consistent with that assessment. In the commentary on the proposed rule, OSHA asks whether all or some medical and dental offices should be covered.

OSHA likewise asks whether it should cover long-term care facilities other than those serving the elderly population. It specifically mentions psychiatric facilities.

Funeral homes are not covered by the proposed rule, although medical examiners' offices would be covered. OSHA's preliminary analysis of risk in the funeral industry was inconclusive, but more recent information provided to the agency indicates that some funeral homes use procedures that can produce airborne particles containing tuberculosis bacteria. One study of funeral home workers in Maryland found that employees involved in embalming were twice as likely as other funeral home employees to have positive tuberculin skin test results (Gershon et al., 1995b). At least one case of cadaver-to-embalmer transmission of tuberculosis has been documented (Sterling et al., 2000a).

As discussed in Chapter 3, OSHA's statutory jurisdiction and regulations do not extend to state and local government employees unless a state has an occupational safety and health plan approved by OSHA. In states without such plans, state, county, or municipal governments would not be required to follow an OSHA rule for their hospital employees, correctional facility workers, paramedics, social workers, medical examiners, and other public employees who may be at risk of occupational exposure to tuberculosis.[5] Federal government agencies such as the Veterans Health Administration are covered by OSHA standards under statute and the executive orders described in Chapter 3.

---

[5]State and local health care workplaces could potentially be affected if HCFA, JCAHCO, or state regulators required adherence to elements of a tuberculosis standard for accreditation, licensure, or Medicare certification.

In its commentary on the proposed rule, OSHA recognizes that protective measures need to be tailored to different kinds of workplaces. To clarify the responsibilities of several kinds of employers, OSHA presents several charts outlining what the proposed rule would require. These charts cover (1) work settings where individuals with suspected or confirmed infectious tuberculosis are admitted or provided medical services; (2) work settings where early identification and transfer procedures are used for those with suspected or confirmed infectious tuberculosis; (3) employers that serve individuals who have been isolated due to suspected or confirmed tuberculosis or individuals who work in areas where air contaminated with tuberculosis likely exists; (4) home health care and home-based hospice care; (5) emergency medical services; (6) clinical and research laboratories; and (7) personnel agencies.

In facilities that rely on outside contractors to provide nursing, food service, and other kinds of workers, several different employers may share responsibilities for implementing certain protective measures. For example, a hospital may provide skin testing for its own employees while requiring each outside contractor to test contract workers. Alternatively, a contractor may be able to arrange for the hospital to provide required skin testing and other employee health services. Responsibility for some protective measures—such as the provision of isolation rooms—cannot be shared.

Covered Individuals

The specific objective of the 1997 proposed OSHA rule is to protect employees rather than patients, prisoners, visitors, or volunteers.[6] The rule does not cover independent, nonemployed, nonincorporated physicians (see Chapter 3). Facilities may, however, require these physicians to certify compliance with certain measures (e.g., up-to-date skin test or successful treatment for recent infection or active disease) before they grant them privileges to see patients in the facility. Likewise, although medical, nursing, and other students are apparently not covered by the rule, the health care facilities in which they train may require that their sponsoring schools take responsibility for skin testing and certain other measures. Residents are considered employees for purposes of occupational safety and health regulation. Chapter 3 and Appendix E discuss more generally the scope of OSHA regulations.

The proposed OSHA rule would provide certain job and financial protections for employees with suspected or confirmed infectious tuberculosis that are not provided for in the CDC guidelines. These are described below in the section on administrative controls.

---

[6]Depending on several factors, such as the receipt of significant in-kind compensation (e.g., free meals), a volunteer may sometimes be considered a worker for purposes of OSHA regulations (see Appendix E).

COMPARISON OF GUIDELINES AND PROPOSED RULE: ADMINISTRATIVE CONTROLS

This and the next two sections of this chapter summarize and discuss the administrative, engineering, and personal respiratory protection provisions of the 1994 CDC guidelines for health care facilities. Because OSHA relied heavily on the CDC guidelines, in drafting its proposed rule, the summaries are organized around the guidelines with points of difference between the two noted in italics. The descriptions of control measures and differences in the guidelines and proposed rule were reviewed by both OSHA and CDC staff and revised as appropriate.

In its commentary on the proposal, OSHA identified some differences between the guidelines and the proposed rule. Other differences were identified in comments submitted to OSHA by various organizations including the American Hospital Association (AHA) (AHA, 1998) and the Association of Professionals in Infection Control and Epidemiology (APIC) (APIC, 1998). The committee's own review of the CDC guidelines and the proposed OSHA rule found a few additional points of difference.

Some control measures are discussed in more detail elsewhere in this report. Tuberculin skin testing and diagnosis and treatment for latent tuberculosis infection and active disease are discussed in Chapter 3. Appendix B provides a more detailed examination of the skin test. Respiratory protections are discussed further in Appendix F.

The following discussion does not cover the 1992 CDC guidelines for those serving homeless people. The 1997 proposed OSHA rule would require homeless shelters to follow essentially the same procedures required for correctional facilities and hospitals that refer rather than treat people with suspected or confirmed tuberculosis. In 1999, acknowledging serious concerns about the practicality and cost of the requirements for homeless shelters, OSHA reopened the comment period and record on the proposed rule to solicit additional information and comments on requirements for homeless shelters. In a presentation to the committee, OSHA staff have suggested that the final rule may include fewer requirements for homeless shelters.

Administrative Controls Related to Risk Assessment, Surveillance, Worker Education, and Coordination

Table 4-1 summarizes most of the key elements of the administrative controls recommended in the 1994 CDC guidelines for health care facilities. (The elements related to patient management are summarized in the next section of this chapter.) The italicized comments in the table highlight the differences between the CDC guidelines and the proposed OSHA rule that might influence the effectiveness or the burdensomeness of a final rule. A discussion of some of the differences follows the table.

TABLE 4-1. Summary of Administrative Controls (other than diagnosis and treatment) Recommended by CDC for Health Care Facilities, with Notes (in italics) on How Proposed OSHA Rule Differs

Assigning Responsibility
1. Assigning responsibility for the control program to qualified person(s)
2. Ensuring that the program includes experts in infection control, occupational health, and engineering
   NOTE: Assignment of responsibility to qualified individuals is implicit in the proposed OSHA rule.

Assessing Risk and Developing Tuberculosis Control Plans
1. Analyzing tuberculosis in the community: incidence, prevalence, drug resistance
   NOTE: The proposed OSHA rule would require county-level information and assessment for facilities seeking exemption from certain of the rule's provisions.
2. Analyzing tuberculosis in the facility: laboratory results, discharge diagnosis including data on drug resistance, medical record review; by location(s) of treatment
3. Analyzing worker tuberculin skin test conversions by work area or category
   NOTE: The proposed OSHA rule would not require assessment of laboratory results, data on drug resistance, medical records, or data on skin test conversions.
4. Matching a facility or area within a facility to one of several risk categories based on skin test conversion data and other factors (see Figure 4-1)
   NOTE: The proposed OSHA rule does not explicitly rank facility risk levels and does not consider skin test conversion data in matching work area or job category characteristics to regulatory requirements
5. Periodically reassessing risk based on new community data, review of patient records, observation of work practices, etc.
6. Preparing and implementing written tuberculosis control plans consistent with level of risk identified in the assessment
   a. Writing plans for each area of a facility and each relevant worker category
   b. Selecting infection-control protocols for each relevant work area or job category
   c. Disseminating plans to relevant managers and workers
   d. Evaluating implementation of plans and revising it as appropriate
   NOTE: The proposed OSHA rule would require annual review of the written exposure control plan and updating of the plan when necessary to reflect changes in tasks, procedures, engineering controls, or job classifications.

Establishing a Screening and Surveillance Program Consistent with the Risk Assessment
1. Providing two-step baseline tuberculin skin testing for those without a documented positive test result or a documented negative test result within the past 12 months (exceptions: when results for such testing suggest that no boosting is occurring, the two-step approach can be foregone; baseline testing is optional for minimal-risk facilities)
2. Providing periodic retesting at 3-, 6-, or 12-month intervals consistent with the risk assessment, area of employment, and employee characteristics
   NOTE: The proposed OSHA rule differs slightly on requirements for baseline skin testing and different frequencies of testing for certain workers. Unlike the CDC guidelines, the proposed rule would require skin testing within 30 days of termination of employment.

3. Providing follow-up diagnostic evaluation and—when appropriate—treatment for workers with positive skin tests

   NOTE: *The proposed OSHA rule would, in addition, require employers to provide each employee with a written medical opinion following evaluation by a physician or other licensed health care professional.*

4. Evaluating workers with symptoms or signs of tuberculosis and excluding those with infectious tuberculosis from the workplace until they are noninfectious

   NOTE: *The medical removal provisions of the proposed OSHA rule would, in addition, require wage, benefit, and other protections for workers removed from work due to suspected or confirmed infectious tuberculosis. The proposed rule would require employers to pay for follow-up services for employees with converted skin tests or suspected or confirmed active disease.*

1. Evaluating possible workplace exposure to and transmission of tuberculosis
   a. Establishing procedures to identify exposure incidents, transmission of disease, and factors associated with exposure or transmission
   b. Investigating worker skin test conversions, diagnoses of tuberculosis in workers, and exposure incidents

Educating, Training, and Counseling Workers
1. Educating workers (as appropriate for their work responsibilities) about tuberculosis infection, disease, transmission, symptoms, treatment, and risks in their community and facility
2. Training workers in tuberculosis control measures applicable to their work responsibilities

   NOTE: *The proposed rule would also require that workers be informed about the OSHA rule. It would require annual retraining unless the employer could show that each employee had the skills and knowledge needed. The proposed rule would require that training be appropriate to employees' level of literacy, education, and language.*

1. Counseling workers as appropriate about positive skin tests, suspected or known personal exposure to active tuberculosis, diagnosis of active disease, treatment options, etc.
2. Offering assignments involving low risk of tuberculosis exposure to employees known to be immunocompromised

   NOTE: *The proposed OSHA rule would not require alternative assignment for immunocompromised workers but would require that workers be educated about tuberculosis risks for individuals with these and other conditions.*

Coordinating with Public Health Officials
1. Reporting cases of active tuberculosis
2. Assisting in investigations of tuberculosis exposure and transmission

   NOTE: *The proposed OSHA rule would require reporting of cases of occupational tuberculosis infection and disease to OSHA, but it does not explicitly require coordination with public health authorities.*

   NOTE: *The proposed OSHA rule includes a variety of additional recordkeeping requirements related to employee medical records, medical surveillance, employee training, engineering controls, confidentiality, record availability and transfer, and other matters.*

SOURCES: CDC (1994b) and 62 FR 201 (October 17, 1997).

Risk Assessment and Exposure Control Plan

CDC Assessment Provisions   The CDC guidelines recommend that all health care facilities perform a comprehensive risk assessment and then adopt tuberculosis control measures appropriate for the level of risk identified. The guidelines describe five levels of risk: minimal risk, very low risk, low risk, intermediate risk, and high risk (Figure 4-1). The minimal-risk and very-low-risk categories apply only to entire facilities; the other categories apply to areas or groups within a facility. The guidelines specify the control measures appropriate for each category. Many measures (e.g., written tuberculosis control plan, worker education, and protocols for identifying patients with active tuberculosis) are recommended for all categories.

The assignment of risk is based on an analysis of several variables including the community's "tuberculosis profile" (including cases and rates of multidrug-resistant disease); the number and types of patients with tuberculosis seen by the facility and by areas within the facility; the facility's policy on the treatment or referral of patients with tuberculosis; comparative levels and trends in employee tuberculin skin test conversions (by area and job category) including clusters of conversions; and evidence of person-to-person transmission of active tuberculosis within the facility. The risk assessment process also provides for review of medical records and observation of tuberculosis control practices to identify possible delays or deficiencies in identifying or treating individuals with infectious tuberculosis.

On the basis of the risk assessment, the CDC guidelines assign a facility or an area within a facility to one of five risk categories: minimal, very low, low, intermediate, and high risk. The minimal-risk category applies only to facilities with no tuberculosis patients in the facility or the community. (For this assessment, no time period—e.g., the past 2 years—is explicitly specified.) The very low risk category applies to facilities that plan to refer patients with suspected or confirmed tuberculosis, that have admitted no patients with tuberculosis during the past year, and that have not experienced comparatively high rates of tuberculin skin test conversions or conversion clusters or apparent person-to-person transmission of *Mycobacterium tuberculosis*. These facilities may, however, be located in communities that have had recent cases of tuberculosis.

The risk assessment recommended by CDC calls for a "profile of tuberculosis in the community served by the facility" (CDC, 1994b, p. 17). The risk assessment described in the 1997 proposed OSHA rule calls for the use of county-level tuberculosis cases without reference to a facility's service area. County-level data are more readily and uniformly available than subcounty data. However, facilities located in large counties may draw patients from a much smaller service area; facilities may also have

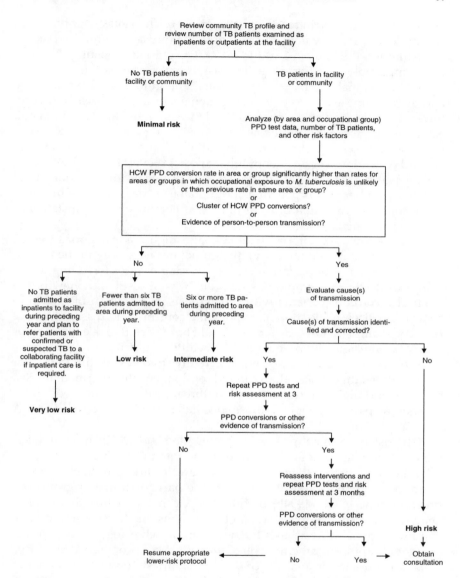

FIGURE 4-1. Protocol for conducting a tuberculosis risk assessment in a health care facility. PPD = purified protein derivative; HCW = health care worker; and TB = tuberculosis. SOURCE: CDC (1994b).

service areas that include all or part of more than one county. Thus, county-level data may not provide a good picture of community risk.

Although the Table 4-1 in the 1997 CDC guidelines listing the measures applicable to different facility risk categories uses the terms "required" "optional," and "not applicable," the guidelines are voluntary and do not impose enforceable requirements. For minimal-risk and very-low-risk facilities, the majority of control measures still apply to both risk categories (e.g., having protocols for investigating worker skin test conversions and contacts of patients not initially diagnosed with tuberculosis, and educating workers about tuberculosis). Several tuberculosis control measures are listed not applicable (e.g., protocols for initiation of the isolation of tuberculosis patients) or optional (e.g., evaluation of ultraviolet germicidal irradiation units or other engineering controls installed in triage or waiting areas).

For the low-risk, intermediate-risk, and high-risk categories (which applies to areas within a facility), the guidelines vary only in the recommended frequency of performance for several measures including tuberculin skin testing for employees (and analysis of results), review of the medical records of patients with tuberculosis, observation of infection-control practices, evaluation of engineering controls, and reassessment of risk. For example, a low-risk facility would be expected to take these steps yearly, whereas an intermediate-risk facility would have to undertake them every 6 to 12 months—which actually involves no difference for organizations that choose the 12 month option. For the intermediate-risk category and high-risk (tuberculosis outbreak) category, the frequencies for some steps are higher than those specified in the 1997 proposed OSHA rule.

The risk assessment process recommended by CDC includes a determination of whether a facility's conversion rate in "an area or group" is "significantly" higher than that (1) for an area or group unlikely to experience occupational exposure or (2) for the particular area or group at a previous time (CDC, 1994b, p. 10). OSHA concluded that this kind of analysis is unduly complicated and too burdensome to be required of all employers or used as a basis for determining what regulatory requirements will apply to an employer. Thus, the 1997 proposed OSHA rule does not provide for analysis of data on skin test conversions either in identifying low-risk settings or in developing or revising exposure control plans. However, in the list of issues on which it invites comments, OSHA does inquire about the benefits of requiring such analyses and the specific type of analysis that the agency might require. OSHA has not indicated whether such a requirement will appear in the final standard.

OSHA Provisions   Because some facilities are very unlikely to experience occupational exposures to tuberculosis, the proposed OSHA rule would—like the CDC guidelines—impose fewer requirements on facilities that meet certain requirements. To qualify, employers would need to document that they (or the places where their employees work):

1. neither admit nor provide medical services to individuals with suspected or confirmed tuberculosis,[7]

2. have had no confirmed cases of infectious tuberculosis during the previous 12 months, *and*

3. are located in counties that have had no confirmed cases of infectious tuberculosis during 1 of the previous 2 years and less than six cases during the other year.

These criteria do not include whether a facility has any evidence (e.g., clusters of tuberculin skin test conversions) of internal transmission of tuberculosis. No hospital in a county with one case of tuberculosis in each of the last two years could qualify for OSHA's "low-risk" category (a label not used by OSHA), even if the hospital had admited no patients with tuberculosis.

For facilities that meet all three criteria, regulatory requirements would be limited to a written plan for controlling exposure, provision of a medical history and two-step baseline skin testing without periodic retesting, medical management and investigation after an exposure incident, job protections for workers with active tuberculosis, employee training, and record keeping. Other than requirements for baseline skin testing, the requirements are similar to those that CDC recommends for minimal-risk and very-low-risk facilities. CDC, however, advises that two-step testing can be discontinued for the minimal-risk category if experience shows little or no boosting.

Except for the facilities that meet the three criteria listed above, the proposed OSHA rule would require facilities to identify employees whose duties could be reasonably anticipated to bring them into contact with people who have suspected or confirmed infectious tuberculosis or with *M. tuberculosis*-contaminated air. Individual protective measures (e.g., skin testing and respirator provision and fit testing) would apply to those with such anticipated contact, which OSHA terms "occupational exposure."

Program of Employee Tuberculin Skin Testing and Follow-up

During the course of the committee's work, CDC's ACET recommended that the agency examine the 1994 guidelines' provisions on tu-

---

[7]Facilities would still have to conform to federal and state laws that require specified categories of health care facilities (mainly hospitals) to provide certain kinds of treatment, for example, emergency evaluation and stabilization of an injured or ill person before transfer. These people are treated but not admitted.

berculin skin testing. In making the recommendation, ACET members noted declines in tuberculosis cases and rates in the United States since 1994, which increases concerns about false positive test results in low-prevalence areas (see Chapter 2 and Appendix B). CDC has accepted the recommendation and has begun the process of considering revisions to the testing and other recommendations of the 1994 guidelines.

Baseline Testing   The 1994 CDC guidelines describe baseline skin testing at hiring as optional for its category of minimal-risk facilities, but a footnote states that it "may be advisable so that if an unexpected exposure does occur, conversions can be distinguished from positive skin test results caused by previous exposures" (CDC, 1994b, p. 15). The 1997 proposed OSHA rule would require such testing for new employees with "occupational exposure" in all facilities, including those in its "low-risk" category. OSHA staff have indicated that the final standard may provide that employers follow CDC's recommendations on baseline testing. Thus, if the CDC recommendations change, so would OSHA's requirements.

Frequency of Testing   The 1994 CDC guidelines establish a testing scheme that recommends 3-month, "6 to 12"-month, and 12-month testing intervals based on the risk level for a work area or occupational category. The guidelines do not call for such periodic testing for the minimal risk and very-low-risk categories. The 1997 proposed OSHA rule would require 6-month testing for some categories of workers (e.g., those performing high-hazard procedures) and 12-month testing for all others. It would not require retesting after the baseline test for facilities in its "low-risk" category. The CDC guidelines for skin testing recommend that testing frequencies be based on, among other factors, analyses of a facility's past experience with skin test conversions. In contrast, the proposed OSHA rule reflects the agency's focus on an employee's type of work and its potential for creating occupational exposure.

Testing at Termination of Employment   The proposed OSHA rule would also require that employers offer skin testing within 30 days of termination of employment. The CDC guidelines include no such provision. AHA reported in 1998 that less than 6 percent of hospitals undertook such testing (AHA, 1998). OSHA staff have indicated that the final rule may clarify that employers would not be required to track down employees who, for example, quit with no or little notice.

Job and Financial Protections for Workers

The proposed rule provides various job and financial protections not included in the 1994 CDC recommendations. The rule would require what

OSHA terms "medical removal protections."[8] Such protections require continuation of wages and other benefits for workers who develop suspected or confirmed infectious tuberculosis and who must be excluded from the workplace until they are confirmed to be noninfectious.[9] The agency states that such protections encourage employees—especially low-income workers—who suspect that they have tuberculosis to seek early evaluation of symptoms for the good of themselves and those around them.

For workers who were unable to function adequately while wearing a properly fitted respirator, the 1997 proposed OSHA rule would require that they be assigned other tasks or have wages and other benefits continued for up to 18 months if no such tasks can be identified. Unlike the 1994 CDC guidelines, the proposed rule does not provide that immunocompromised workers be offered the voluntary opportunity of reassignment to work involving a low risk of exposure to tuberculosis.

The proposed OSHA rule would also require employers to cover the costs of skin tests, respirators, and similar services or equipment. If medical treatment for latent tuberculosis infection were advised after a skin test conversion, the employer would also have to bear the cost of such treatment. Furthermore, if an employee developed infectious tuberculosis after an exposure incident in a covered work setting, the employer would be required to cover the costs for medical evaluation and treatment.

Although the proposed rule calls for investigation of the circumstances surrounding a skin test conversion, the emphasis is on identifying possible lapses in infection control rather than on trying more definitively to determine the likelihood that the conversion resulted from occupational exposure. The CDC guidelines place more emphasis on such an investigation, in part, so that public health authorities can be informed and take steps to prevent further exposures if a likely community source of a worker's infection is identified.

Coordinating with Public Health Authorities

The CDC guidelines—reflecting the agency's public health orientation—highlight the importance of coordination and cooperation with public health authorities. The proposed OSHA rule is silent on such coordination. Employers would still be governed by state laws that require reporting of infectious diseases including active tuberculosis. OSHA's

---

[8]OSHA first included medical removal protections in its 1976 standard on lead.

[9]The proposed rule does not require proof that the disease was acquired through occupational exposure. Earnings and other protections may, however, be reduced to the extent that the worker is compensated for lost earnings by a public or employer-sponsored compensation program.

silence on requirements imposed by other federal or state laws does not alter employers' obligations to comply with these laws.

Record Keeping

The proposed OSHA rule includes a variety of record-keeping requirements related to employee medical records, medical surveillance, employee training, engineering controls, confidentiality, record availability and transfer, and other matters. Among other purposes, these records would assist OSHA inspectors with assessing employer compliance with regulations. Many of the record-keeping requirements are consistent with standard operating procedures in larger organizations but might require new procedures for smaller organizations.

Controls Related to Patient Management

Table 4-2 summarizes the provisions of the 1994 CDC guidelines that relate specifically to the development and application of procedures for identifying, diagnosing, and treating people with tuberculosis. Again, points of difference with the 1997 proposed OSHA rule are noted in italics.

Identification of Persons with Tuberculosis

The 1994 CDC guidelines stress the critical importance of early identification, isolation, and treatment of individuals who may have infectious tuberculosis. They recommend that institutions develop protocols for such identification based on the prevalence and characteristics of tuberculosis in the populations served by the institution (CDC, 1994b). The guidelines also list common symptoms of tuberculosis but note that the "index of suspicion" will vary depending on the characteristics of the population served.

The 1997 proposed OSHA rule would require employers to develop a written tuberculosis control plan that included procedures for the prompt identification of individuals with suspected or confirmed infectious tuberculosis. OSHA's commentary on the proposed rule notes that procedures will likely vary for different employers. It does not discuss the prevalence of tuberculosis in the population served as a factor to be considered in developing or applying these procedures.

The CDC guidelines recommend that hospitals receive laboratory analyses of sputum smears within 24 hours. The proposed OSHA rule has no parallel requirement, and the introduction to the proposed rule does not discuss the issue.

TABLE 4-2. Summary of Patient Management Recommendations by CDC, with Notes (in italics) on How Proposed OSHA Rule Differs

Identifying Individuals with Suspected or Confirmed Infectious Tuberculosis
NOTE: In general, the proposed OSHA rule provides less detailed specification of processes for identifying, diagnosing, and treating individuals with tuberculosis.
1. Establishing protocols to identify those with symptoms or signs of active disease
   a. At initial encounters in emergency department, admitting area, outpatient clinic
   b. Before scheduled admissions if possible
2. Assessing suspicious symptoms or test results after admission for patients not identified earlier
3. Initiating precautions (e.g., isolation) for suspected or confirmed cases of infectious tuberculosis
   NOTE: The proposed OSHA rule provides for either masking or segregation of patients before isolation or transfer to another facility. Facilities that transfer rather than admit suspected or confirmed infectious patients would be required to arrange appropriate isolation or transfer within 5 hours.
4. Evaluating patients with suspected cases of tuberculosis unless the institution's policy is to refer cases
   a. Performing appropriate laboratory tests (including tests for drug resistance)
   b. Providing results of smear analyses within 24 hours of collection
   c. Performing appropriate diagnostic radiologic procedures

Treating Patients with Suspected or Diagnosed Tuberculosis (unless the policy is to refer)
1. Selecting treatment regimen (including use of inpatient or outpatient care) based on patient characteristics, test results, and preferences
2. Monitoring response and making decisions about continued treatment, isolation, discharge, etc.
3. Performing diagnostic and treatment procedures for infectious patients in the isolation room when possible and, when not possible, scheduling procedures at times when they can be performed quickly and when waiting areas are less crowded
4. Delaying elective surgery and elective dental procedures until patient is confirmed to be noninfectious
5. Avoiding cough-inducing procedures on infectious patients unless absolutely necessary and performing these procedures using local exhaust ventilation devices when possible
   NOTE: The proposed OSHA rule refers more broadly to "high-hazard" procedures, which are defined as those that may produce aerosols that contain tuberculosis bacteria.

SOURCE: CDC (1994b), and 62 FR 201 (October 17, 1997).

Patient Evaluation and Management

The proposed OSHA rule would require facilities that do not treat patients with tuberculosis to either isolate those with suspected or confirmed tuberculosis or transfer them within 5 hours. The CDC guidelines do not have a specific recommendation about how quickly transfer or isolation should occur. In its discussion of the proposed rule, OSHA describes the 5-hour provision as a preliminary determination, and it asks for comments including suggestions about alternative means of protecting employees. The agency cites one study that showed that emergency departments—once a presumptive diagnosis of tuberculosis was made—"were able to initiate isolation in an average of 5 hours from the time of patient registration" (62 FR 201 at 54252 [October 17, 1997]). OSHA also notes statements by ATS (ATS, 1992, p. 1627) describing the use of surgical masks for longer periods (not defined) as "stigmatizing, uncomfortable, and probably ineffective." In the discussion of the proposed rule, OSHA states that if isolation or transfer cannot be accomplished within 5 hours, it must be done as soon as possible thereafter.

COMPARISON OF GUIDELINES AND PROPOSED RULE: ENGINEERING CONTROLS

The term "engineering controls" applies to an array of protective measures based on engineering principles and technologies. In the context of programs to prevent the transmission of tuberculosis, the controls apply primarily to the design, creation, and maintenance of isolation rooms or areas (e.g., booths used for cough-inducing procedures) and to ventilation or air purification procedures for general-use areas such as emergency departments and admitting areas.

Table 4-3 summarizes the engineering controls that the 1994 CDC guidelines recommend for health care institutions that serve people with tuberculosis. The italicized comments highlight differences between the CDC guidelines and the proposed OSHA rule that might affect the effectiveness or the burdensomeness of a final rule. The first category in the table—managing facility ventilation—is also an administrative control, but the topic is included here for convenience. Neither the CDC guidelines nor the proposed OSHA rule would require engineering controls for home-based services.

Warning Signs

The proposed OSHA rule describes the specific shape and text for signs outside isolation rooms. The CDC guidelines are silent on this issue.

The proposed OSHA rule also includes more extensive requirements for warning signs and labels for ultraviolet germicidal irradiation lighting systems and for ventilation systems. The proposed rule does not discuss whether signs should, under certain circumstances, provide warnings in languages in addition to English. A rule of reason would suggest that the warnings must be readable by the people whom they are intended to warn. The CDC guidelines mention the language issue in the discussion of warning signs for ultraviolet germicidal irradiation lighting systems.

TABLE 4-3. Summary of Engineering Controls Recommended by CDC for Facilities That Serve People with Tuberculosis, with Notes (in italics) on How Proposed OSHA Rule Differs

Managing Facility Ventilation
1. Ensuring that systems are regularly checked, maintained, and overseen by staff or consultants with appropriate engineering or other expertise
2. Ensuring that systems meet applicable federal, state, and local requirements
3. Providing appropriate warning signs for ventilation equipment and ultraviolet lighting systems
    NOTE: The proposed OSHA rule, in addition, sets forth shape and text requirements for warning signs in isolation areas and includes more precise requirements for labeling of vents than are provided for in the CDC guidelines.

Ventilating General-Use Areas (e.g., waiting rooms, and emergency departments)
1. Designing and operating systems to move air from cleaner to less clean areas
2. In high-prevalence communities, providing supplementary controls such as ultraviolet germicidal irradiation (UVGI) lighting or HEPA filtration system.
3. Providing local exhaust ventilation systems (e.g., booths, tents, and laboratory hoods) for areas where high-hazard procedures (e.g., bronchoscopy, administration of aerosolized medications, and sputum induction) are performed and ventilating them to achieve 99.9 percent removal of airborne contaminants
    NOTE: The proposed OSHA rule does not discuss ventilation requirements for general-use areas or for local exhaust ventilation systems. The proposed rule would not require supplementary UVGI systems for general-use areas in high-prevalence communities but does provide nonmandatory guidelines for their safe use.

Providing and Maintaining Isolation Rooms
1. Establishing air-change rates for in-use rooms of at least 6 per hour in existing facilities and 12 per hour in new or renovated facilities
    NOTE: The proposed OSHA rule would not require a specific number of air changes for isolation rooms. It would require ventilation to achieve 99.9 percent removal of airborne contaminants after an isolation room is vacated by a suspected or confirmed infectious patient.
2. Directing fresh air first to areas used by workers and then to patients (preferred strategy)
3. Maintaining negative pressure relative to hallways and other surrounding areas
4. Exhausting air to outside away from public areas and air intake vents (or if not possible, using HEPA filtration for exhausted or recirculated air)
5. Daily monitoring and periodic maintenance
6. Keeping the number of persons entering isolation room minimal
    NOTE: The proposed OSHA rule calls specifically for minimizing the number of employees entering isolation rooms and the time that they spend there.

SOURCES: CDC (1994b), and 62 FR 201 (October 17, 1997).

Ventilation Requirements

General-Use Areas

The CDC guidelines include recommendations regarding ventilation of general-use areas. The proposed OSHA rule does not include ventilation requirements for these areas.

Isolation Rooms or Areas

The CDC guidelines recommend 6 to 12 air changes per hour for an isolation room while it is in use for an infectious patient.[10] The proposed OSHA rule has no specific requirement for air changes. The commentary on the rule does not explain this departure from the CDC guidelines, nor does it ask for comments.

The proposed OSHA rule does discuss air changes in the context of a requirement for ventilation following the vacating of an isolation room by an infectious patient (see below). The proposed OSHA rule would require ventilation to achieve removal of 99.9 percent of airborne contaminants. An appendix to the proposed rule includes a CDC table on local exhaust ventilation that lists the air changes and minutes that are required to achieve different removal efficiencies (90, 99, and 99.9 percent).[11]

The CDC guidelines do not discuss ventilation requirements when an infectious patient has vacated an isolation room, but the guidelines do include a section on ventilation of isolation tents and booths (local exhaust devices). For these spaces, the CDC guidelines recommend at least 99 percent removal efficiency.

The CDC guidelines recommend that the number of persons entering isolation rooms be "minimal," but they do not specifically mention employees. The proposed OSHA rule would require provisions in an employer's exposure control plan to minimize the number of employees entering isolation rooms and the time that they spend there.

COMPARISON OF GUIDELINES AND PROPOSED RULE: PERSONAL RESPIRATORY PROTECTIONS

The term "personal respirator" applies generically to a range of devices that vary in complexity from flexible masks covering the nose and mouth to units that cover the wearer's head and have independently powered air supplies. Appendix F discusses the types and functions of personal respirators and the evidence of their effectiveness. As noted earlier, personal respiratory protection comes third in CDC's hierarchy of tuberculosis control measures.

In the sections on respiratory protections, the 1994 CDC guidelines mention the then-applicable 1987 OSHA regulations on respiratory pro-

---

[10]As defined by CDC, air changes refer to "the ratio of the volume of air flowing through a space in a certain period of time (i.e., the airflow rate) to the volume of that space (i.e., the room volume); this ratio is usually expressed as the number of air changes per hour (ACH)" (CDC, 1994b, p. 113).

[11]For example, according to the table, with 6 air changes per hour, it would take 46 minutes to achieve 99 percent removal efficiency and 69 minutes to achieve a 99.9 percent level. With 12 air changes per hour, the corresponding figures are 23 and 35 (62 FR 201 54299; CDC, 1994b, p. 72).

tection programs. Those standards were revised in 1998 (29 CFR 110.134). However, pending issuance of the standard on occupational tuberculosis, OSHA has specified provisions from earlier versions of the standard that apply pending publication of the tuberculosis standard (29 CFR 1910.139).

The National Institute for Occupational Safety and Health (NIOSH) has legal responsibility or authority for certifying personal respirators for use in a wide variety of hazardous work situations including different kinds of mining operations, construction activities, and health care services. When the 1994 CDC guidelines were issued, they specified criteria for respirators that were, at that time, met by only one type of NIOSH-certified respirator. Since then, NIOSH which is a part of CDC, has certified a new class of less expensive and simpler devices (N95 respirators) that meet the 1994 criteria in most situations.

CDC's recommendations related to personal respiratory protections are summarized in Table 4-4, which identifies in italics differences between the guidelines and the proposed OSHA rule. Again, the first category of recommendations relates to administrative measures, which are reviewed here for convenience.

Fit Testing and Fit Checking of Respirators

The 1994 CDC guidelines recommend that workers who wear respirators should undergo an initial fit test to identify an appropriately fitting respirator and that workers be taught to check the fit of the respirator before each use. The guidelines also state that facilities should have respirator protection programs that conform to the 1987 OSHA respiratory protection standard.

The 1987 OSHA respiratory protection standard did not require annual fit testing, but the 1998 revision of the standard added such a provision (29 CFR 1910.134). Pending publication of the final tuberculosis standard, the 1998 standard did not apply to the hazard of tuberculosis. OSHA's interim requirements for tuberculosis did not require annual fit testing (29 CFR 1910.139).

The 1997 proposed OSHA rule would require at least annual assessment of a worker's ability to wear a respirator. Unless this assessment determined that an annual fit test was not necessary, the rule would require at least an annual fit testing of respirators for most workers. OSHA asked for comments on whether an annual evaluation of the need for fit testing was adequate.

The 1997 *Federal Register* notice of the proposed OSHA rule takes over five pages (in small print) to describe the required fit testing procedures. These procedures are virtually identical to those described in the 1998 general respiratory protection standard.

The 1994 CDC guidelines do not describe the fit-testing process in detail but note that all facilities in which personal respirators are used

TABLE 4-4. Summary of Personal Respiratory Protections Recommended by CDC, with Notes (in italics) on How Proposed OSHA Rule Differs

Managing a Facility Respiratory Protection Program
1. Assigning responsibility to a person with appropriate expertise and experience to oversee worker training, device selection and maintenance, worker adherence to respirator use requirements, and other program provisions
   NOTE: Assignment of responsibility to qualified individuals is implicit in the proposed OSHA rule.
2. Ensuring that respirators meet criteria relating to such matters as
   a. Size of particles that respirator can filter under specific conditions
   b. Rate of leakage where the respirator seals to the face
   c. Ability to fit different sizes and kinds of faces (which usually means that some range of respirator sizes must be provided)
   d. Ability of respirator to be tested for fit to the face of a worker
3. Including all workers who use respirators in the respiratory protection program that facilities are required by OSHA to develop, implement, and maintain (as described in a supplement to the guidelines)

Identifying Workers Needing Respirators, Primarily
1. Personnel who enter patient rooms or residences to provide medical, nursing, and other services to people with suspected or confirmed infectious tuberculosis
2. Personnel who are present during procedures such as bronchoscopy during which patients are likely to expel *M. tuberculosis*-bearing particles into the air and who may require higher-performing devices
   NOTE: The proposed OSHA rule would not make provision of higher-performing respiratory devices a requirement for workers performing high-hazard procedures.
3. Personnel in other settings where administrative and engineering controls are not likely to be protective (e.g., personnel repairing ventilation equipment)
   NOTE: The proposed OSHA rule also would require either masking of patients or the use of personal respirators in two situations: (1) when personnel are transporting patients with suspected or confirmed tuberculosis and (2) when personnel are working in areas where patients with known or suspected tuberculosis are placed while awaiting transfer.

Providing Respirators and Ensuring Their Proper Use
1. Screening workers—at hiring and periodically thereafter (at least every 5 years)— to determine whether any medical condition precludes use of a respirator
   NOTE: The CDC guidelines make no explicit recommendation for periodic fit testing of personal respirators, although they briefly describe some elements of fit-testing procedures. They also note that all employers who use respiratory protection are covered by the then-applicable OSHA respiratory protection standard. The 1997 proposed OSHA rule includes explicit provisions for: (1) at least an annual assessment of worker's ability to wear a respirator, (2) at least an annual respirator fit test unless the preceding assessment determines that a fit test is not required, (3) an assessment whenever the size or make of a respirator used by a worker changes or the worker's facial characteristics change in ways that might affect respirator fit, and (4) use of both qualitative and quantitative fit-testing procedures.
2. Matching workers to appropriate respirators on the basis of physical characteristics, job requirements, etc.
   NOTE: The proposed OSHA rule would require that employers provide alternative work for personnel who cannot function adequately while using a respirator.
3. Training workers in a device's appropriate use (including checking the device's fit at each use), inspection, maintenance, and storage

4. Cleaning, repairing, and replacing respirators as appropriate
5. Providing respirators to those who are visiting patients with tuberculosis in isolation rooms and instructing visitors in their use

   NOTE: The proposed OSHA rule does not mention visitors.

SOURCES: CDC (1994b), and 62 FR 201 (October 17, 1997).

must have a respiratory protection program as required by OSHA. The guidelines include a supplement that discusses considerations in selecting a respirator and developing a personal respiratory protection program. In addition to referring to OSHA regulations, the 1994 guidelines also refer to a 1987 NIOSH guide. NIOSH issued a new users guide for respirators in 1998 (NIOSH, 1999; see also NIOSH, 1995, 1996).

Respirator Use Outside Isolation Rooms

The 1997 proposed OSHA rule requires respirator use when workers are either transporting unmasked individuals with suspected or confirmed infectious tuberculosis or when they are working outside isolation rooms in areas where such unmasked individuals are confined (e.g., while awaiting transport to another facility). The CDC guidelines call for masking of patients in these situations, but they also provide more generally for the use of respirators "where administrative and engineering controls are not likely to protect them" (CDC, 1994b, p. 33). The proposed rule states that OSHA cannot require masking of patients and notes that some combative individuals may not accept masking. If a known or suspected infectious person cannot be masked, then the worker transporting him or her must have personal respiratory protection.[12] In the latter situation (patients not masked), protection would not be provided to others who come near the patient (e.g., including workers, visitors, and other patients who share an elevator). The proposed rule has other provisions intended to protect such individuals, for example, the requirement that exposure control plans include policies to delay the moving of patients until they are no longer infectious unless a delay would compromise care.

Reflecting its broader perspective, the CDC guidelines stress that respiratory protections used by health care workers should protect both the worker and patients. For example, workers involved in surgical proce-

---

[12]Although OSHA arguably could require employers to make a practice of masking patients when necessary to create a safe workplace, it could not require patients or other nonregulated persons to comply with such requirements. If a patient refuses to wear a mask or otherwise comply with the institution's rules, the institution can (and, arguably under OSHA, must) take action to either secure compliance or eject the person from the facility. Such action would be based on the institution's proprietary authority or on public health law or some other body of law that gives it the power to act against a dangerous or unruly person.

dures should not use a respirator (e.g., one with an expiration valve) that might contaminate the surgical field.

Situations Requiring More Protective Respirators

The CDC guidelines note that facilities may identify certain situations (e.g., bronchoscopies on patients with diagnosed or suspected infectious tuberculosis) that warrant respiratory protections that exceed those recommended by standard criteria. The proposed OSHA rule would not require employers to identify such situations or supply more protective personal respiratory devices. OSHA, however, requested comments on whether the final rule should include such requirements.

CONCLUSION

Because OSHA relied substantially on the 1994 CDC guidelines in developing the its 1997 proposed rule, the two documents are generally similar in their basic provisions. Some differences, such as those related to record keeping, are mainly administrative. Others, particularly OSHA's proposed financial protections for workers temporarily removed from their position while undergoing treatment for active tuberculosis, reflect differences in organizational missions and responsibilities.

The final standard is likely to differ from the 1997 proposal but specific details were not available during the course of this study. In Chapter 7, the committee's assessment of the likely effects of a final OSHA standard examines three areas of difference that could affect its impact. These areas involve tuberculin skin testing, respiratory protections, and methods for assessing facility risk for occupational transmission of tuberculosis and requirements for control measures.

5

Occupational Risk of Tuberculosis

This chapter reviews what is known about the workplace risk of tuberculosis among employees covered by the proposed rule on occupational tuberculosis issued in 1997 by the Occupational Safety and Health Administration (OSHA). The specific questions addressed here include the following: Are health care and selected other categories of workers at a greater risk of infection, disease, and mortality due to tuberculosis than others in the community within which they reside? If so, what is the excess risk due to occupational exposure? Can the risk of occupational exposure be quantified for different work environments and different job classifications?

Most of the information relevant to these questions involves the occupational risk of tuberculosis in hospitals and, to a lesser extent, prisons. The committee found limited very information about the occupational risk of tuberculosis in other correctional settings, long-term-care facilities, home health and home care services, outpatient clinics of various kinds, and homeless shelters. The problem is not just that such information is unavailable to outsiders but that it may also be unavailable to support internal assessments of risk and then guide appropriate responses. This scarcity of surveillance information for settings such as homeless shelters and local jails is a concern because many of these facilities serve people at increased risk of active tuberculosis—including those who are unemployed, homeless, or poor; people with HIV infection or AIDS or substance abuse problems; and recent immigrants from countries with high rates of tuberculosis. Unlike hospitals, these organizations often lack strong institutional and professional traditions of infection control, and the extent of external oversight by government agencies, accrediting bodies, or other entities varies. In addition, many of these facilities do not operate in an environment in which an outbreak of tuberculosis might threaten their reputations, although they may be vulnerable to civil law suits (e.g., by inmates citing deficient health and safety measures).

An assessment of the occupational risk of tuberculosis needs to take historical context into account. As described in Chapter 1, during the late 1980s and early 1990s, outbreaks of tuberculosis in several large, urban hospitals helped focus attention on the risk of tuberculosis in health care settings. They also raised concern about lapses in infection control measures. These outbreaks occurred against a backdrop of resurgent tuberculosis that has been linked to underfunded public health programs, incomplete treatment of the disease, and increasing numbers of people at risk because of human immunodeficiency virus (HIV) infection, homelessness, imprisonment, and immigration from countries where tuberculosis is common. Although these problems have not disappeared, they have been mitigated by increased funding for community tuberculosis control, intensive programs of directly observed therapy, more effective treatments for HIV infection and AIDS, and increased attention to tuberculosis control measures in the workplace. Since 1993, national tuberculosis case rates have dropped for seven successive years.

The discussion in this chapter draws extensively on the background paper by Thomas M. Daniel in Appendix C. That paper provides a more detailed review of the relevant literature and its limitations.

CONCEPTS AND DEFINITIONS

In its simplest sense, *occupationally acquired disease* means disease acquired during the course of a person's work. The focus of those concerned about workplace transmission of tuberculosis is, however, on identifying workers whose duties could be reasonably anticipated to bring them into contact with (1) people who have infectious tuberculosis or (2) air that contains *Mycobacterium tuberculosis*. In OSHA's terminology, this anticipated contact—*not* actual exposure—constitutes *occupational exposure*. Thus, a respiratory therapist in a facility that treats patients with tuberculosis would normally be categorized as having occupational exposure, whereas a financial analyst in the facility's administrative offices normally would not.

Risk has a variety of technical and popular meanings, and the committee recognizes the technical, political, and ethical controversies and debates that surround the concept of risk, the characterization of risk, and public perceptions of risk (NRC, 1983, 1996). Used in a general sense, risk refers to the probability of adverse health effects of, for example, exposure to infectious tuberculosis.[1] The *occupational risk of tuberculosis* is the probability of acquiring tuberculosis infection or active tuberculosis as a result of workplace exposure. Occupational risk is usually described statistically. Depending on the purpose of an analysis and the available data, it can be described in absolute terms (for example, as the risk of acquiring active tuberculosis during a year or a working lifetime for a particular category of worker) or in comparative terms (for example, one group's risk compared with another's). Comparative data help in identifying possible causes of or contributors to a problem (e.g., by comparing skin test conversion rates in different areas of a facility). Comparisons also help in understanding or communicating the magnitude of a problem and in assessing priorities for spending public health funds or other resources.

CDC lists two options for defining a *case of active tuberculosis* (CDC, 2000b). The laboratory definition requires either the isolation of *M. tuberculosis* from a clinical specimen or the demonstration of acid-fast bacilli in a clinical specimen when a specimen for culture was not or could not be obtained. The clinical case definition requires all of the following: a positive tuberculin skin test result; other signs and symptoms compatible with tuberculosis (e.g., abnormal and unstable radiologic findings or persistent cough), treatment with two or more antituberculous medications, and a completed diagnostic evaluation. Physicians may begin treatment of suspected infectious tuberculosis based on symptoms and risk factors while awaiting test results.

The definition of *infection with M. tuberculosis* is based only on test results, specifically, the results of the tuberculin skin test. The foundation of workplace surveillance programs has been the finding and investigating of tuberculin skin test conversions. As discussed in Chapter 2 and Appendix B, the tuberculin skin test has serious limitations as a community or workplace surveillance tool, particularly in communities and workplaces where tuberculosis is uncommon. In very low-prevalence locales, most skin test conversions will be false positives.

In general, occupationally acquired tuberculosis infection or disease is easier to define than to document. Nationally reported data on the occupational status of reported tuberculosis cases do not distinguish between cases originating in the workplace and those originating in the

---

[1]The committee was not charged with undertaking a formal risk assessment. A formal risk assessment involves four basic steps (NRC, 1983). *Hazard identification* relies on epidemiologic studies, animal studies, and other tools to determine whether exposure to an agent can increase the incidence of a health condition. A *dose-response assessment* attempts to determine the relationship between the dose of an agent and the incidence of an adverse effect. An *exposure assessment* seeks to estimate the intensity, frequency, schedule, duration, and route of human exposures and the size and kinds of populations exposed. *Risk characterization* involves estimation of the incidence of a health effect under the exposure conditions described by the exposure assessment.

community. Direct evidence about the source of transmission typically comes from investigations of possible workplace outbreaks of tuberculosis. In this context, an "outbreak" may be defined as transmission of *M. tuberculosis* that results in infection or active disease among workers, patients, and others exposed in a health care facility, prison, or other setting in which people with tuberculosis are treated, served, or detained (Garrett et al., 1999).[2] Investigations of possible outbreaks include the careful questioning of affected workers not only about possible workplace exposures but also about possible community-related exposures involving family members and other close contacts outside of work.

Some outbreak investigations are supported by molecular epidemiology (*DNA fingerprinting*), which compares isolates of *M. tuberculosis* recovered from different individuals. Molecular analyses can help establish a chain of transmission that links workplace cases of active tuberculosis (but not infection) to source cases in the workplace or the community. As discussed further below, inferences about the source of infection or disease for a worker are still most often based on comparisons of occupational and demographic information for workers with and without occupational exposure to tuberculosis. In some cases, no clear source of infection or transmission—either work related or community based—is identified.

In analyses of tuberculosis risk in workplaces and communities, the term "community" or "community of residence" has no precise definition.[3] Although a facility's location may be identified as a particular city, county, or metropolitan area, the residences of workers in that facility may be widely spread across areas with very different rates of tuberculosis. For example, someone living in central Harlem can be expected to have a higher risk of community exposure to tuberculosis than someone from the Connecticut suburbs.

Few studies have matched detailed information on worker place of residence against equally detailed community data on tuberculosis cases. Information on a worker's home zip code may improve on city or county as an indicator of community of residence, but a single zip code may still encompass an area with quite variable resident characteristics (e.g., incidence of tuberculosis and income levels). Also, collection of zip code data

---

[2]For tuberculosis infection, investigators focus on excess rates or clusters of skin test conversions rather than on single conversions. If an investigation does not indicate workplace transmission, then the presence of skin test conversions or cases of active tuberculosis does not constitute a workplace outbreak.

[3]Sometimes community is described in social rather than geographic terms. An example might be a close-knit community of recent immigrants. Recently, CDC reported an outbreak of tuberculosis in a "social network of transgender persons (i.e., persons who identify with or express a gender and/or sex different from their biological sex)" (Sterling et al., 2000a, p. 1).

from workplace records can be very labor intensive, and address information may not be current or entered into computer databases. Because tuberculosis is negatively correlated with income, some studies have also investigated whether places of residence for workers with converted skin tests are clustered in low-income—and presumably higher-risk—areas. Others have simply used low income as a surrogate for higher risk of community exposure.

HISTORICAL PERSPECTIVES ON THE OCCUPATIONAL RISK OF TUBERCULOSIS

A review article by Sepkowitz (1994) summarizes studies from the 1920s through the 1950s that showed that nurses, physicians, and others working with tuberculosis patients had high rates of positive skin tests or skin test conversions compared to the rates expected in the broader community. For nursing students who were initially tuberculin skin test negative, conversion rates reported in studies in the United States and Europe ran as high as 95 to 100 percent by the time the students graduated. The reported yearly incidence of active tuberculosis ranged from 2 to 12 percent in nursing schools.[4] Comparative data on nonhealth care occupations or work settings is limited, but Sepkowitz cites studies in the 1930s that reported the incidence of active tuberculosis to be 1 percent for employees of a life insurance company and 2 percent for food handlers.

Other early studies reviewed by Sepkowitz focused on medical students. One survey of those who had been medical students between 1940 and 1950 reported a tuberculosis case rate of 334 per 100,000 medical students per year. In the general population during that period, the estimated tuberculosis case rates ranged between 32 and 100 per 100,000 population per year. Another study identified a particularly high risk to medical students of participation in autopsies on those who died with active tuberculosis.

---

[4]*Prevalence* is a measure of the probability of infection or disease in a population at a particular point in time. *Incidence* is the probability of new infection or disease in a specified period of time, usually a year. It is not always clear whether studies are reporting incidence rates or probabilities, which are based on different denominators (see, e.g., Kahn and Sempos [1989]). The denominator for a rate is based on the average population at risk of some event during a defined interval (reflecting reductions in the population due to the occurrence of the event, e.g., death or acquisition of disease). The denominator for a probability uses the population at risk at the beginning of the defined interval. Because the denominator of a rate reflects reductions in an at-risk population during an interval, a rate will be higher than a probability. The spread between the two increases as the level of risk increases. For example, if the annual probability of an event is 0.05 (and the event is experienced uniformly during the year), then the annual rate will be 0.051; if the probability is 0.12, the rate will be 0.128.

Sepkowitz cites a 1953 study (Mikol et al., 1953) that found that hospital workers with direct patient contact had an 8- to 10-fold higher incidence of tuberculosis compared with that for workers without direct contact. A review by Menzies and colleagues of studies conducted in the 1960s reported that health care workers exposed to patients with known tuberculosis had a four to six times greater incidence of infection with *M. tuberculosis* than unexposed workers (Menzies et al., 1995). The quality of the studies that they reviewed varied considerably.

In sum, a number of studies indicate that health care workers, especially those who cared for patients, have historically been at higher risk of infection and disease than the general population. By the 1960s, effective treatment of tuberculosis was becoming widely available and public health programs were mobilizing to control if not eliminate the disease. In addition, health care facilities were beginning to adopt some tuberculosis control measures such as screening patients with chest radiographs and isolating those with known or suspected infectious disease.

MORE RECENT INFORMATION ON THE COMMUNITY AND OCCUPATIONAL RISK OF TUBERCULOSIS

U.S. Government Surveys and Databases

General Population

Active Tuberculosis and Mortality from Tuberculosis CDC reports annually on cases of active tuberculosis nationwide and by state and selected cities (see, e.g., CDC [2000b]). It reports national mortality data but does not break deaths down by state or other category.

Chapter 1 described the resurgence in tuberculosis cases and case rates beginning in 1985, an increase that followed uninterrupted declines since national data were first reported in 1953. After reaching a high of 10.5 per 100,000 population in 1992 (13 percent higher than in 1985), rates began to decline again in 1993. Case rates and case numbers reached their lowest levels yet in 1999, when CDC reported a case rate of 6.4 per 100,000 population and 17,528 cases of tuberculosis (CDC, 2000b). Rates of death from tuberculosis, which also rose in the 1980s and early 1990s, have also declined in recent years from 0.8 per 100,000 in 1989 to 0.4 per 100,000 in 1998, and numbers of deaths declined from 1,970 to 1,110.

CDC data make it clear that tuberculosis is not evenly distributed within the United States. For example, the increase in case rates from 1985 to 1992 was largely concentrated in a few states. During this period, the seven states with case rate increases of 4 percent or more (1984 to 1991) showed a collective increase from 11.2 to 16.8 cases per 100,000 population (Comstock, 2000). In contrast, the overall case rate for the other states dropped from 8.5 to 7.4 cases per 100,000.

In 1999, case rates among states ranged from 0.5 per 100,000 population in Vermont to 15.5 per 100,000 population in Hawaii. Among metropolitan areas, rates varied from less than 1.3 per 100,000 population in Omaha to 17.7 per 100,000 population in New York City and 18.2 per 100,000 population in San Francisco. Data from government surveys and databases as well as other sources fairly consistently show that rates of active tuberculosis vary by race, ethnicity, age, and country of origin. Table 5-1 shows that such demographic variation persists despite the decline in case rates during recent years. As reported in Chapter 1, over 40 percent of tuberculosis cases reported in U.S. in 1999 involved people born in other countries with individuals from Mexico, the Philippines, and Vietnam accounting for nearly half of the cases among foreign-born persons.

TABLE 5-1. Tuberculosis Case Rates per 100,000 Population, United States, 1989–1999

Year	1989	1992	1993	1999
Race/ethnicity[a]				
White, non-Hispanic	4.0	4.0	3.6	2.2
Black, non-Hispanic	29.5	31.7	29.1	16.8
Hispanic[b]	19.3	22.4	20.6	12.4
American Indian/Alaska Native	19.8	16.2	14.6	11.8
Asian/Pacific Islander	39.8	46.3	44.5	35.3
Unknown/missing	0	0	1	0
Country of origin[c]				
U.S. born	NA[d]	8.2	7.4	4.0
Foreign born[e]	NA	34.2	33.6	29.2
Unknown	2	1	2	1
Age[a]				
0–14 years	2.5	3.1	3.0	1.8
15–24	4.8	5.5	5.1	4.0
25–44	10.6	12.7	11.6	7.3
45–64	12.4	13.4	12.5	8.2
65+	19.7	18.7	17.8	11.7
Not stated	0	0	0	0

[a]Denominators for computing these rates were based on official post-census estimates from the U.S. Census Bureau.
[b]Persons of Hispanic origin may be of any race.
[c]Denominators for computing these rates were obtained from Quarterly Estimates of the United States Foreign-born and Native Resident Populations: April 1, 1990 to July 1, 1999 (www.census.gov/population/estimates/nation/nativity/fbtab001.txt)
[d]NA equals data not available.
[e]Includes persons born outside the United States, American Samoa, the Federated States of Micronesia, Guam, the Republic of the Marshall Islands, Midway Island, the Commonwealth of the Northern Mariana Islands, Puerto Rico, the Republic of Palau, U.S. Minor Outlying Islands, U.S. Miscellaneous Pacific Islands, and the U.S. Virgin Islands.
SOURCE: CDC, 2000b (excerpted from Tables 2, 3, and 4).

Infection with *M. tuberculosis* In contrast to active tuberculosis, no routinely collected, national data document the prevalence or incidence of infection with *M. tuberculosis* in the U.S. population overall or in major population subgroups. The last effort to collect systematic information on the prevalence of tuberculosis infection nationwide dates back to the 1971–1972 National Health Survey. For that survey, trained personnel administered and read tuberculin skin tests for a national sample of American adults. Based on the results, analysts estimated the prevalence of skin test reactivity among adults aged 25 to 74 years to be 21.5 percent during the survey period (Engel and Roberts, 1977).

In the risk assessment section of its 1997 proposed rule on tuberculosis, OSHA presented an estimate of the prevalence of latent tuberculosis infection in the United States developed by Christopher Murray. Using a mathematical model of tuberculosis transmission, Murray estimated the prevalence of latent tuberculosis infection in 1994 to be about 6.5 percent for Americans over age 18 (62 FR 201 at 54199 [Table V-6] October 17, 1997).

Working from Murray's prevalence estimates, OSHA estimated the weighted annual risk of infection for the U.S. population to be approximately 0.146 percent. For individual states, the estimates ranged from 0.02 percent in New Hampshire to 0.30 percent in New York and 0.35 percent in Hawaii. OSHA used these prevalence and incidence estimates as the bases for comparing the occupational risk of tuberculosis with the background risk of the disease in the general population (see Chapter 7).

In Appendix C, Daniel uses a technique for estimating the annual risk of tuberculosis infection based on the empiric ratio between this risk and the incidence of active disease (Daniel and Debanne, 1997). Using data derived from white male naval recruits between 1958 and 1965, he estimated this ratio to be approximately 150. When that ratio is applied to the 1998 tuberculosis case rate for the United States, it yields an annual risk of infection of approximately 0.05 percent per year, which is about one-third of the 0.146 percent per year figure used by OSHA in its risk assessment. The higher OSHA figure may reflect differences in the reference year used, their inclusion of racial and ethnic minorities, and possibly other factors such as the impact of HIV infection and AIDS since 1980.

Health Care and Other Workers

Active Tuberculosis and Mortality from Tuberculosis Since 1994 (for the year 1993), the CDC has reported occupational information for people diagnosed with active tuberculosis. The CDC data do not allow one to draw conclusions about the source—workplace versus community—of workers' exposure to tuberculosis.

In 1999, those who had reported they were unemployed within the preceding 24 months accounted for nearly 60 percent of all cases of the disease (CDC, 2000b). Those who reported their occupation as health care workers within the preceding 24 months accounted for approximately 2.6 percent of the cases nationwide, down from 3.0 percent in 1998. In 1998, health care workers accounted for about 9 percent of employed persons and 8 percent of tuberculosis cases among employed persons (Amy Curtis, CDC, 2000, personal communication).[5] During the period from 1994 to 1998, six states—California, Florida, Illinois, New Jersey, New York, and Texas—accounted for 57 percent of the cases of tuberculosis among health care workers and about the same percentage of all tuberculosis cases. (The six states account for just under 40 percent of the U.S. population.)

As shown in Figure 5-1, for the period 1994 to 1998, the overall incidence of active tuberculosis among health care workers was similar to that for other employed workers—about 5.1 per 100,000 population for the former and 5.0 per 100,000 population for the latter (Curtis et al., 1999). Between 1994 and 1998, the tuberculosis case rate for health care workers dropped from 5.6 to 4.6 per 100,000 population, whereas the rates for other employed workers stayed relatively steady at 5.2 per 100,000 population in both 1994 and 1998.

Looking only at cases of drug-resistant tuberculosis among U.S.-born workers from 1994 to 1998, CDC analysts found significantly higher rates of drug-resistant disease for health care workers (3.2 percent of cases) than for other workers (1.5 percent of cases) (Panlilio and Curtis, 2000). For the 2 most recent years, the difference in rates for the two groups was not statistically significant.

Among foreign-born health care workers, those born in the Philippines account for the largest percentage of cases of active tuberculosis (about 33 percent) (Curtis et al., 1999). Among all foreign-born employed workers (and for the U.S. population generally), those born in Mexico accounted for the highest percentage (about 25 percent) of tuberculosis cases.

In 1999, CDC reported that workers in correctional facilities accounted for about 0.1 percent of cases of active tuberculosis (CDC, 2000b). Most information on correctional facilities focuses on inmates, who have much

---

[5]Health care and correctional workers account for about 95 percent of those covered by the proposed rule. The CDC data are based on reported occupation within the past 24 months (CDC, 2000b). Most of the progression from infection to active tuberculosis occurs within the first two years following infection. CDC first began collecting occupational data in 1993, but the initial reports are considered less reliable than subsequent ones. In recent years, approximately 500 to 600 cases of tuberculosis among health care workers have been reported yearly.

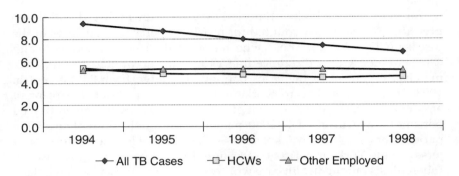

FIGURE 5-1. Tuberculosis incidence rates per 100,000 population by year and reported employment status within preceding 24 months. TB equals tuberculosis; HCW equals health care workers. SOURCE: Curtis et al. (1999).

higher rates of tuberculosis than the general population.[6] A 1999 U.S. Department of Justice report could not report national data on tuberculosis case rates for inmates, but it cited New York State data for inmates showing a decrease in case rates from approximately 175 per 100,000 population in 1991 to 30 per 100,000 population in 1997 (NIJ, 1999). Factors identified by CDC as contributing to increased tuberculosis risk in correctional facilities included increasing numbers of HIV-infected inmates, crowding, and poor ventilation. Many workers in correctional facilities are also likely to be affected (although less intensely so) by these conditions.

Occupational information is not routinely reported for tuberculosis deaths. It is, however, recorded on death certificates. The committee found one analysis of data for 1979 to 1990 from the National Occupational Mortality Surveillance database (CDC, 1995a). In that analysis, CDC researchers identified occupational groups that had both four or more deaths from pulmonary tuberculosis and a high proportionate risk of mortality from the disease. In the 21 occupational groups that met their criteria, two race- and sex-specific subgroups had potential workplace exposure to tuberculosis. They were white male funeral directors

---

[6]An analysis of 1985–1986 data from 29 states found that the rate of active tuberculosis was nearly four times higher for adult inmates of correctional facilities than for unincarcerated individuals of similar ages (Hutton et al., 1993). Data from the early 1990s showed that the rate of active tuberculosis for inmates was 6 times higher than the rate for the state population in New York, 8 times higher in New Jersey, and 10 times higher in California (CDC, 1996a). In 1994, CDC reported that inmates accounted for 4.8 percent of tuberculosis cases but only 0.6 percent of the U.S. population (CDC, 1996a). A 1997 New York State report showed that tuberculosis cases and case rates among inmates outside New York City closely tracked the increase and subsequent decrease in national case rates shown in CDC statistics (reported in NIJ [1999]).

and white male health and nursing aides, orderlies, and attendants. Of the other occupational subgroups identified, six were classified as having the potential for substantial exposure to silica and two were associated with low socioeconomic status.

Infection with *M. tuberculosis* In 1992, concerned about a number of hospital outbreaks of tuberculosis, CDC sent questionnaires all 632 public hospitals and a 20 percent sample (444 institutions) of private hospitals with 100 beds or more that were listed in the American Hospital Association database (Manangan et al., 1998). About 70 percent for each group responded (726 institutions in total). Ninety-six of 716 hospitals (13 percent) reported transmission of *M. tuberculosis* to health care workers. In 1996, CDC randomly selected and resurveyed half of the 272 hospitals that had reported six or more admissions of tuberculosis patients in the 1992 survey (Manangan et al., 1998, 2000). Seventy-five percent (103 facilities) responded. In that survey of higher-risk facilities, 7 percent of 103 respondents reported transmission of *M. tuberculosis* to workers.

In 1995, CDC began a demonstration project to develop better estimates of workplace-related skin test conversions among health care workers and to test software to support more systematic collection and analysis of skin test data (McCray, 1999a,b). The project recruited 32 participating facilities from nine jurisdictions including both high-prevalence areas (New York City and San Francisco) and low prevalence areas (Oregon and Colorado). Using data collected prospectively from the demonstration project sites, CDC analysts reported an overall tuberculin skin test conversion rate of 5.9 per 1,000 health care workers. Rates differed little among the types of participating organizations (nine hospitals, seven correctional facilities, five health departments, two nursing homes, and seven other types of facilities). After adjusting for race, foreign birth, New York City residence, and household exposure, analysts found no statistically significant associations between skin test conversions and the occupational categories used (administrative/clerical, nurse, outreach worker, physician/physician's assistant, and other). Data were not collected on the extent of workers' contact with patients or on their work location within facilities (e.g., medical ward). More than 20 percent of those participating had either a positive skin test history or a positive test result at the baseline.

Additional, older data analyzed in Appendix C by Daniel are mixed. He concludes that health care workers are at risk in the workplace of being infected with tuberculosis but that the risk has been declining in recent years and now approaches community levels. Where modern infection control measures have been implemented, occupational risk approaches the level of risk in the communities in which workers reside.

Overall, data for the mid-1990s do not show that health care workers as a group are at higher risk of active tuberculosis than other employed workers, but for some of the period they may have been at higher risk of multidrug-resistant disease. No national data report on the rate of tuberculosis infection among workers, but a small CDC demonstration project has suggested no association between job category and risk after demographic factors were taken into account. No recent occupation-specific mortality rates are available, but an analysis of older data suggests that some subgroups of health care workers may have been at higher risk of death than other workers.

Other Surveys and Reports Not Involving Outbreaks

Literature Reviews

In a 1995 review of data on tuberculosis among health care workers, Menzies and colleagues reviewed studies based on disease registries in several other countries. The studies reported "estimated risk ratios of 0.6 to 2.0, indicating at most only modest increased risk" of disease for health care workers compared with that for others in the community (Menzies et al., 1995, p. 92). Menzies and colleagues noted that such studies may underestimate risk because they do not standardize for age. This is important because the working population is younger and healthier than the general population. The authors also noted that cohort nor disease registry analyses are limited by "the inability to distinguish occupational from nonoccupational exposure" (Menzies et al., 1995, p. 92). The review also covered questionnaire studies from the 1950s through the 1980s that reported higher rates of disease for pathologists, certain laboratory technicians, and physicians. It noted concerns about modest response rates and possible recall biases for these studies. The authors identified no "recent" cohort studies comparing the risk of infection with *M. tuberculosis* among U.S. health care workers with the risk among individuals in the general community. Although they reviewed several studies reporting rates of tuberculosis infection among health care workers, the authors cited the limitations of the studies and did not present an overall assessment of infection risk in the postantibiotic era. They did not present mortality data.

Garrett and colleagues also reviewed U.S. surveys and surveillance reports for a variety of health care workers (e.g., physicians and house staff) and locales dating back to the 1960s (Garrett et al., 1999). They concluded that "available data suggest that the [annual] risk of [tuberculin skin test] conversions among hospital employees in general [i.e., for all categories of workers in nonoutbreak situations] is approximately 1 percent or less" (Garrett et al., 1999, p. 484). They did not present corresponding disease or mortality estimates. The authors noted that the data, which were sometimes inconsistent and subject to many methodologic limitations, also suggested that the risk of conversions varied considerably by type of hospital, geographic location, job category, and likelihood of contact with high-risk patients. (This review's discussion of outbreak reports is summarized later in this chapter.)

Another review by Dooley and Tapper (1997) similarly concluded that overall skin test conversion rates for facilities are typically 1 percent or less in nonoutbreak environments, but they emphasized that "overall rates in a facility can mask very high rates in some areas or occupational groups" (p. 368). In studies not specific to outbreak situations, the review authors found mixed results for comparisons of skin test conversion rates for different job categories and different assumed levels of patient contact. Some studies found higher skin test conversion rates for those in jobs with more patient contact (e.g., nursing and respiratory therapy); others did not. The work categorization and other methods and the detail reported in these studies varied considerably (e.g., whether categorizations by patient contact differentiated between contact with patients at high risk of tuberculosis and contact with other patients). The review authors noted that skin test conversion rates in health care workers probably represent a combination of community- and workplace-related transmission of *M. tuberculosis*. (This review's discussion of outbreak reports is summarized later in this chapter.)

Individual Studies and Reports

During the 1980s and 1990s, a number of published articles reported skin test conversion information from state databases, surveys, or studies in one or a few organizations. Most are limited to hospitals.

In a 1987 article entitled "Is the Tuberculosis Screening Program of Hospital Employees Still Required?," researchers at the University of Washington analyzed skin test conversion data for 1982 to 1984 for 114 hospitals in Washington (Aitken et al., 1987). They put the estimated overall conversion rate for these hospitals at 0.09 percent over the 3-year period (0.03 percent per year), with slightly higher rates for hospitals that admitted tuberculosis patients and slightly lower rates for those that did not. They concluded that the conversion rates in hospitals did not differ significantly from the estimated rate for the state population overall.

A study in a nonoutbreak environment found correlations between positive skin test conversions and the worker's age, the worker's race, and the poverty level in the worker's zip code of residence (Bailey et al., 1995). (Data on tuberculosis case rates were not reported by zip code.) For the period January 1989 through July 1991, the overall rate of skin test conversions was 0.93 percent (0.37 percent annually). After controlling for other variables, the analysts found an association between higher poverty levels and higher rates of positive skin tests and test conversions. Risk was not associated with patient contact or occupational category, so analysts concluded that community rather than occupational exposure was more likely.

In a national survey that focused on infection control measures, responding hospitals showed overall annual skin test conversion rates of 0.6 to 0.7 percent for 1989 through 1992 (Sinkowitz et al., 1996). Higher conversion rates were found among those involved in bronchoscopy (3.7 percent) and respiratory therapy (1.0 percent). No information was collected on employee demographic characteristics or on the details of the testing procedures used by the facilities.

Another study reporting higher rates of skin test conversions for respiratory therapists involved a military medical center in Maryland (Ball and Van Wey, 1997). Annual skin test conversion rates, which ranged between 0.4 and 2.6 percent across the occupational categories identified, did not differ significantly for patient-contact and non-patient-contact categories. Respiratory therapists, however, had an annual conversion rate of 15.6 percent.

In a study of 56 of 167 North Carolina hospitals reporting data on tuberculin skin test conversions, researchers reported a 5-year mean annual conversion rate for all employees of 1.14 percent (Price et al., 1987). Mean annual conversion rates varied by region of the state (1.80 percent in the east, 0.70 percent in the center, and 0.61 percent in the west). This was consistent with variations in rates for the general population in these sections of the state. The researchers concluded that this association pointed to community rather than workplace origins for new employee infections with *M. tuberculosis*. In its initial risk assessment for the proposed rule on tuberculosis, OSHA analysts also used these North Carolina data. After critics noted the high prevalence of atypical mycobacteria in the eastern part of North Carolina, the analysts used only the figures for hospitals in the western part of the state to estimate the risk of infection for workers in areas with a moderate prevalence of active tuberculosis. (Other criticisms of the data noted the high nonresponse rate, the limited use of two-step initial testing, and inconsistencies in testing practices. See Chapter 7 for further discussion.)

For its risk assessment, OSHA staff used 1994 Washington State data as a basis for estimating worker risk in low-prevalence areas (62 FR 201). Based on comparisons between hospitals "in zero-TB counties and with no known TB patients" and other hospitals, they estimated that the occupational risk of transmission of *M. tuberculosis* in Washington State hospitals was 1.5 times higher than the background rate of transmission. For other ways of comparing hospitals, the estimated risk was less. For employees of long-term-care facilities (including nursing homes) and home health care workers, OSAH estimated the risk to be 11 and 2 times the background rate respectively. As noted earlier, OSHA estimated the latter risk to be about 0.15 percent per year. (OSHA's risk assessment is reviewed in Chapter 7.)

A few reports focus on correctional facilities. A 1994–1995 survey of correctional facilities noted that many responding facilities could not report skin test conversions because skin testing for employees was done by private physicians and the results were not communicated and entered into employee records (NIJ, 1996). A later survey found that more than half of state and federal prison systems and more than a third of the jail systems failed to report conversion data (NIJ, 1999).

At the Cook County Jail in Chicago, the facility began offering tuberculin skin testing to health care workers (mandatory) and correctional officers (voluntary) in 1994 (McAuley, 2000). Health care staff at the jail have documented 24 known exposure episodes involving workers and have concluded that these were associated with 10 documented and 30 possible skin test conversions, none of which involved health care workers. The test results for correction officers did not differ by the area of the facility in which they worked.

Outbreak Reports

This section reviews information from published reports of workplace outbreaks of tuberculosis. Most reports of outbreaks have involved units of hospitals including inpatient medical wards (general medical, HIV, infectious disease, and renal transplant units), surgical suites, emergency departments, laboratories, intensive care units, an autopsy room, radiology suites, an inpatient hospice, outpatient clinics, and bronchoscopy rooms (see Dooley and Tapper [1997], Garrett et al. [1999], and Appendix D).

Probable cases of workplace transmission of tuberculosis have also been reported in prisons and jails (Campbell et al., 1993; Pelletier et al., 1993; Prendergast et al., 1999; Bergmire-Sweat et al., 1996; Jones et al., 1999), a freestanding primary care clinic (Howell et al., 1989), long-term-care facilities (Stead, 1981; Munger et al., 1983; Stead et al., 1985; Brennen et al., 1988 [and possibly Steimke et al., 1994]), a residential HIV infection treatment facility (Hoch and Wilcox, 1991), homeless shelters (Nolan et al., 1991; Curtis et al., 2000; Moss et al., 2000), public health laboratories (Kao et al., 1997), a medical examiner's office (Ussery et al., 1995), and a funeral home (Sterling et al., 2000a). In addition, outbreaks have been reported in settings where occupational exposure is not anticipated, including naval vessels and airplanes (DiStasio and Trump, 1990; Aguado et al., 1996).

Low-prevalence communities are not immune from outbreaks. For example, CDC investigators recently reported an outbreak in North Dakota. It involved a child from the Marshall Islands who transmitted *M.*

tuberculosis to 3 of 4 household members, 16 of 24 classmates, 10 of 32 school-bus riders, and 9 of 61 day-care contacts (Curtis et al., 1999). This case was also unusual because tuberculosis in children is not usually transmitted to others.

Although national CDC data show approximately 400 to 600 cases of tuberculosis in health care workers per year in recent years, case investigations of hospital or other outbreaks indicate that outbreaks reports account for only a small number of all cases of tuberculosis (Dooley and Tapper, 1997; Garrett et al., 1999, CDC, 2000b). For example, the 19 outbreak reports (1965 to 1995) summarized by Dooley and Tapper (1997) covering the period 1965 to 1995 account for fewer than 50 cases of active disease among health care workers. The 28 outbreak reports (one covering more than one institution) (1962 to 1996) reviewed by Garrett and colleagues (1999) account for fewer than 90 cases, of which 27 were associated with one 1962 to 1964 outbreak. The outbreak investigations have linked some cases of active disease to workplace exposure, but other cases were not explicitly linked to either a workplace or a community source. The reviews by Dooley and Tapper and Garrett and colleagues did not report on deaths associated with the outbreak studies they summarized, although Garrett and colleagues noted 9 deaths among at least 20 workers known to have contracted multidrug-resistant disease. Chapter 6 discusses what these investigations suggest about the association between outbreaks and the implementation of tuberculosis control measures.

Cautions

As a source of information on the occupational risk of tuberculosis, outbreak reports have a number of limitations. Most are retrospective or observational. Skin testing procedures are often poorly described, as are data about test skin conversions and cases of tuberculosis. Important information about the facilities and their employees is often missing, inadequately described, or inconsistently measured across outbreak studies. For example, many reports do not include information about variables such as employee age, length of employment, job category, work location within a facility, country of origin, race, and past vaccination with bacille Calmette-Guérin (BCG).

In addition to the limitations of individual reports, no comprehensive, systematic national system exists for the reporting and publishing of information on workplace outbreaks of tuberculosis. Published reports do not represent the universe of outbreaks (even those investigated by CDC staff), and they may appear years after the first investigation of an outbreak. Moreover, published reports on outbreaks probably over represent unusual circumstances (e.g., an unusual location). Indeed, as the very label suggests, outbreaks represent atypical rather than normal circumstances, at least in relatively low-prevalence regions such as the United States.

Thus, reports of outbreaks do not provide a solid basis for estimating the occupational risk of latent tuberculosis infection or active disease. Nonetheless, careful analyses of outbreaks can provide suggestive information about the potential risk of infection or disease among different types of workers. Particularly useful are studies that have compared workers with and without potential risk factors such as contact with patients at increased risk of tuberculosis (e.g., those on medical wards, HIV/AIDS units), work involving aerosol-generating procedures, and various demographic characteristics (e.g., income, race, place of birth, and place of residence). Although statistical analyses may find similar levels of risk in workplaces and workers' community of residence, workplace investigations, including DNA analyses, make clear that workers do face a real risk of acquiring tuberculosis from patients, inmates, or others who they encounter on the job.

Review Articles

Garrett and colleagues searched the literature for published reports of tuberculosis outbreaks in health care settings (Garrett et al., 1999). They located reports on 28 outbreaks occurring between 1960 and 1996, mostly in hospitals. The more recent outbreaks (late 1980s and 1990s) differed from earlier outbreaks in that they more often involved serious cases of multidrug-resistant disease, affected relatively large numbers of patients and workers, and spread rapidly enough to be picked up by hospital and public health surveillance systems. A high percentage of the cases involved patients or workers who were seriously immunocompromised due to HIV infection or AIDS and who were thus at high risk of progressing quickly from tuberculosis infection to active disease. This made it easier for clinicians and others to recognize possible links to earlier hospital stays. In these more recent outbreaks, at least 20 health care workers developed multidrug-resistant tuberculosis, and 9 of them died. Skin test information for workers was often incomplete but pointed to additional workers who had become infected with *M. tuberculosis* without developing active disease. Garrett and colleagues described the epidemiological evidence for transmission of tuberculosis in the health care setting as "compelling" (Garrett et al., 1999, p. 489).

A review by Dooley and Tapper (1997) of 21 outbreaks in adult inpatient settings (many also reviewed by Garrett and colleagues [1999]) reported that a single source of transmission was identified for 10 settings, whereas the others involved multiple sources. Some sources were discovered as a result of formal investigations, whereas others were discovered incidentally. The source cases often had HIV infection or AIDS and had atypical radiographs and negative sputum smears that made it easier for them to go undetected and untreated. A majority of the health care workers who developed active multidrug-resistant tuberculosis had HIV infection or AIDS, as did most of those who died. The estimated duration and consequences of reported exposures varied widely. In one outbreak involving an autopsy on a person with unsuspected tuberculosis, all five of those present for the 3-hour procedure—including one person present for only 10 minutes—subsequently had skin test conversions and two developed active tuberculosis (Templeton et al., 1995). Two developed active tuberculosis. Other reports also indicate that transmission of *M. tuberculosis* can occur during relatively short periods of exposure (e.g., 2 to 4 hours).

Individual Reports: Hospitals

Some studies of hospital outbreaks of tuberculosis have reported information useful in assessing the likelihood of occupational versus community transmission of tuberculosis. Most of these studies have also attempted to assess the effects of implementing tuberculosis control measures consistent with the 1990 or 1994 CDC guidelines. The discussion below focuses on evidence of workplace transmission of *M. tuberculosis*. Chapter 6 reviews evidence on the effects of tuberculosis control measures.

After an outbreak of multidrug-resistant tuberculosis at St. Clare's Hospital and Health Center (New York City) in the early 1990s, researchers compared tuberculin skin test conversion rates for different occupational categories (nurse, physician, laboratory, housekeeping, social service, and finance) (Louther et al., 1997). They found the highest rate of skin test conversions among housekeeping employees. A multivariate analysis showed that significant differences in conversion rates by job category remained after adjustment for differences in age, BCG vaccination status, country of birth, gender, and the tuberculosis incidence in the zip code area of residence. In the multivariate analysis, residence was not associated with risk of conversion. As discussed in Chapter 6 and Appendix D, that study also reported decreases in conversion rates following the implementation of tuberculosis control measures.

Following an outbreak at the Cabrini Medical Center (New York City), researchers compared rates of skin test conversion for workers on wards admitting patients with tuberculosis with rates for workers on wards that did not admit such patients (Maloney et al., 1995). For the 18-month period before tuberculosis control measures were implemented, conversion rates were 16.7 percent for the former group and 2.8 percent for the latter group, a statistically significant difference. Following the introduction of infection control measures from June through October 1991, rates fell on wards that admitted patients with tuberculosis but not on other wards.

For the 13-month period from June 1991 through August 1992, the difference in conversion rates for the more exposed and the less exposed groups of workers had narrowed to a nonsignificant 5.1 versus 4.0 percent respectively. The researchers did not find that conversion rates correlated with zip code of residence, race, or other demographic characteristics. Again, the investigators documented lapses in infection control measures.

At Grady Memorial Hospital in Atlanta, hospital staff tracked skin test conversion rates after an outbreak of tuberculosis and the implementation of infection control measures (Blumberg et al., 1995; Sotir et al., 1997).[7] In the first period studied, January through June 1992, 3.3 percent (annual rate, 6.49 percent) of workers with previous negative skin tests converted. For January through June 1994, the conversion rate had dropped to 0.4 percent (annual rate, 0.89 percent).

A later report focused on house staff, who served in hospitals affiliated with Emory University and typically spent about half their training at Grady Memorial Hospital (Blumberg et al., 1998). Over the study period, skin test conversion rates dropped from approximately 6.0 per 100 person-years to 1.1 after implementation of expanded tuberculosis control measures. Over the entire period studied, house officers in the medicine and obstetrics/gynecology departments had significantly higher skin test conversion rates than house officers in other departments, but the rates for the groups were not significantly different by the end of the study period. Graduates of foreign medical schools had much higher conversion rates than graduates of U.S. medical schools. Throughout the study period the house staff continued to care for large numbers of patients with active tuberculosis.

Some workplace investigations have used DNA fingerprinting in an effort to assess the likelihood of a workplace rather than community source of transmission. Some have concluded that transmission of *M. tuberculosis* to health care workers resulted from workplace sources.

Individual Reports: Prisons and Jails

Of the outbreak reports that the committee found on organizations other than hospitals, most involve correctional facilities. The reports, however, often focus on inmates rather than correctional facility workers.

Prisons Three studies have reported on outbreaks in California prisons that involved the transmission of *M. tuberculosis* from inmates to correctional facility personnel. For one 1990–1991 outbreak, the skin test

---

[7]If Grady Memorial Hospital were a state, it would have ranked 28th in the number of tuberculosis cases for the period from 1991 to 1997 (Sotir et al., 1999). The state of Georgia ranked third for that period.

results for 2 of 11 previously skin test-negative physicians and nurses in a prison infirmary converted to positive during the period November 1990 through March 1991 after exposure to a prisoner with active multidrug-resistant tuberculosis (annual rate of infection, 6.4 percent) (Campbell et al., 1993). A report on two other outbreaks in 1995 and 1996 cited annual skin test conversion rates for previously negative employees of 2.8 percent for those exposed in one prison and 4.9 percent for those exposed in a second prison (Prendergast et al., 1999). No employees developed active tuberculosis.

A 1991 outbreak of tuberculosis among New York state prison inmates resulted in the transmission of *M. tuberculosis* to prison workers. The state then instituted a program of mandatory tuberculin skin testing for employees beginning in November 1991 (Steenland et al., 1997). For 1992, investigators concluded that approximately one-third of new tuberculosis infections among workers were due to occupational exposure, with higher rates for workers in prisons that reported cases of active disease among inmates. They suggested that 1992 was probably the peak year for transmission because the incidence of tuberculosis among prisoners dropped by about 40 percent during the next 3 years.

A report on a 1994 outbreak in a Texas prison found a clustering of cases of active tuberculosis including 15 cases in inmates and one case in a prison worker (an instructor in educational program) (Bergmire-Sweat et al., 1996). The report did not include skin test information for workers but found higher conversion rates for inmates in the wing on which the source case resided and for those having classes in the same classroom as the source case.

A recent outbreak in a South Carolina state prison is still being investigated, but investigators have indicated that a medical student exposed to infectious inmates developed active tuberculosis. A brief abstract describes the setting for this outbreak as a segregated dormitory for HIV-infected inmates (Spradling et al., 2000). Twenty-nine inmates in the population investigated developed active tuberculosis, and 26 of these inmates were housed in the same area of the segregated dormitory as the index case.

Prisons differ from hospitals in that they more often draw inmates from distant communities. For example, New York City residents convicted of violating state laws may be incarcerated in upstate prisons, whereas those convicted of violating federal laws may go to an out-of-state prison. Some prison systems actively seek to import prisoners from other states. For example, a private prison in Oklahoma, a state with a low prevalence of tuberculosis, has contracted to house prisoners from Hawaii, a high-prevalence state (Kakesako, 1998). Other inmates from Hawaii have gone to Minnesota and Tennessee prisons.

Although facilities that import prisoners may seek relatively low-risk offenders and screen them for tuberculosis and other medical problems, protocols and tests for the identification of individuals with infectious tuberculosis are not perfect and may also be imperfectly implemented. Recently, a Pennsylvania prison that contracts to house detainees of the U.S. Immigration and Naturalization Service (INS) received a detainee with infectious, multidrug-resistant tuberculosis following a "paperwork error" (Lang, 2000; Lebo and Scolforo, 2000). News stories have cited county officials as planning to improve the "sieve-like" system of transferring medical records. As noted in Chapter 1, INS was recently cited by OSHA for failing to protect workers from known hazardous conditions that put workers at risk of exposure to tuberculosis (OSHA Region 6, 2000).

Jails   A study of tuberculosis cases associated with a Nassau County (New York) jail found that 24 percent of the cases in the county were associated with the jail (Pelletier et al., 1993). Most of the cases involved prisoners, but one case involved a correctional officer. DNA analysis of *M. tuberculosis* isolates suggested that transmission of the disease was occurring within the jail. The jail did not screen detainees or workers for tuberculosis infection or active tuberculosis.

Jones and colleagues (1999) reported on an outbreak in the Memphis city jail that involved 38 inmates and five guards who were diagnosed with active tuberculosis between January 1995 and December 1998. Among the 24 inmates with positive cultures, DNA fingerprinting matched the isolates from 19 inmates to isolates found among 2 or more other inmates. For the two culture-positive guards, isolates from both individuals matched the dominant inmate strain. Among a randomly selected sample of 43 isolates from patients with tuberculosis identified in the community, 6 percent matched the dominant inmate strain and 4 of these came from individuals who had been incarcerated in the jail. Of 686 jailers evaluated in October 1997, 1.2 percent had a skin test conversion following a negative test the previous year.

In addition, the article of Jones and colleagues (1999) cited 14 published reports of outbreaks of tuberculosis in U.S. prisons since 1985 but identified only 2 published reports of outbreaks in U.S. jails, with one report dating back to 1977. It also noted that nearly 10 million individuals were admitted to local jails and that 6 percent of the nation's jails housed 50 percent of jail inmates.

Individual Reports: Long-Term-Care Settings

Nursing homes, chronic care units of hospitals for veterans, long-term psychiatric facilities, and other similar settings often serve elderly people and others at increased risk of tuberculosis. They also typically offer the opportunity for the sustained close contact that facilitates the transmission of tuberculosis.

Most reports on nursing homes have examined the transmission of *M. tuberculosis* in nursing home residents. Data from the mid-1980s suggest that the incidence of active tuberculosis may be almost twice as high among elderly nursing home residents as among elderly people living in the community (CDC, 1990b). In 1998, residents (all ages) of nursing homes and long-term-care facilities accounted for 3.5 percent of tuberculosis cases nationwide (CDC, 1999b).

In the early 1980s, two reports of tuberculosis outbreaks in nursing homes pointed to workplace transmission of tuberculosis infection and disease to workers (Stead, 1981; Munger et al., 1983). Another report on a skin testing program for workers on a chronic care ward in a Veterans Administration Medical Center found evidence of "occult" transmission of endemic tuberculosis (Brennen et al., 1988).

Since 1995, New York State has required acute-care hospitals and long-term-care facilities to report clusters of tuberculin skin test conversion and evidence of nosocomial tuberculosis transmission as well as cases of active tuberculosis (Rachel L. Stricof, Bureau of Tuberculosis Control, New York State Department of Health, personal communication, October 3, 2000). The number of reports and the seriousness of the events reported have declined over that period. Between 1995 and 1997, covered facilities reported 15 clusters of possible or confirmed tuberculin skin test conversion among health care workers. One of the 15 clusters involved a hospitalized patient who was considered no longer infectious and was transferred to a long-term-care facility that subsequently failed to maintain appropriate therapy for the person. The other clusters were associated with exposure to unsuspected or unconfirmed index cases. During this same period, eight pseudo-outbreaks were reported involving clusters of skin test conversions linked, for example, to atypical mycobacteria or deficiencies in the tuberculin skin test procedure. Since 1998, the state has undertaken numerous contact investigations but has not documented any further outbreaks involving patients or health care workers in recent years.

Recently, investigators at the Arkansas Department of Health reported on probable transmission of tuberculosis to two health care workers from a resident of a nursing home who died in a hospital with undiagnosed tuberculosis. Investigators later located a radiograph for the individual showing a cavitary lesion (Ijaz et al., 1999). The investigation started when the nursing home's surveillance program detected skin test conversions in four previously negative employees. The secondary cases of active tuberculosis included an employee in the nursing home where the source patient was a resident, a nurse in the hospital that treated the source patient, and a nursing home resident who moved from the nursing home that housed the source patient to a second jointly operated facility in the community. DNA fingerprinting found the same strain of *M. tuberculosis* in all three individuals. On-site investigation determined that the source resident was very mobile and had a persistent, spraying cough. Investigators also found that laboratory tests for possible tuberculosis were ordered but not performed during one of the resident's several hospital stays (Kevin Ijaz, Arkansas Department of Health, personal communication, August 23, 2000). In addition, investigators determined that an air intake for the air-conditioning system was located outside the resident's nursing home room.

The committee located one report of a skin test conversion in an employee of a residential substance abuse facility in Michigan following diagnosis of multidrug-resistant tuberculosis in a resident of the facility (Hoch and Wilcox, 1991). The facility had no health screening program for patients and a high attrition rate.

Individual Reports: Other Settings

Homeless Shelters The committee located only one published report on transmission of tuberculosis to workers in a homeless shelter. That report involved a 1987–1988 outbreak in a Syracuse, New York, shelter for men (Curtis et al., 2000). Investigators found that 70 percent of 257 clients and staff had positive tuberculin skin test results. Although skin test conversions were documented in 2 of 8 previously tuberculin skin test negative staff members, 52 other staff members who might have been exposed were not available for skin testing. Shelter workers are often previous shelter clients. They tend to be more transient and less available for follow-up than workers in many of the other settings reviewed in this chapter.

Hospice and Home Care Although the advent of effective treatment for people with HIV infection or AIDS has reduced their need for hospice care, hospice workers still care for many people at higher than average risk of tuberculosis. One outbreak of tuberculosis in a hospital-based hospice has been reported (Pierce et al., 1992). Eleven of 65 workers converted their skin tests after exposure to an AIDS patient with a delayed diagnosis of tuberculosis.

Ambulatory Care Setting The committee located one report of an outbreak in an ambulatory care setting. It occurred in 1988 among workers in a Florida clinic that reported skin test conversions for 17 of 30 (57 percent) workers with previously negative test results (Howell et al., 1989). Investigators identified four possible sources of transmission including 1 nurse with noncavitary pulmonary tuberculosis, 39 clinic patients with pulmonary tuberculosis (14 with at least one positive smear), sputum inductions for 13 culture-positive patients, and aerosolized pentamidine treatments for 2 culture-positive patients. The investigation identified ventilation problems in the facility that could have contributed to transmission.

Funeral Homes   Two cases of tuberculosis transmission from cadavers to embalmers have recently been documented (Lauzardo et al., 2000; Sterling et al., 2000a). Before death, one individual had been under treatment for AIDS and active tuberculosis. The employee who embalmed the body was diagnosed with active tuberculosis, and DNA fingerprinting showed that the strain matched that from the cadaver (Sterling et al., 2000a). Investigators suggested aerosolization from the airway during the embalming process as a possible means of transmission. In the other case of transmission related to embalming, DNA fingerprinting again linked the disease in the embalmer to a deceased person under treatment for AIDS and rifampin-resistant tuberculosis (Lauzardo et al., 2000).

COMMITTEE CONCLUSIONS

Context

Are health care, correctional, and selected other categories of workers at greater risk of infection, disease, or mortality due to tuberculosis than others in the community in which they reside? This question has no simple yes-or-no answer. Instead, conclusions must be qualified to reflect the

- changing epidemiology of tuberculosis,
- continuing geographic variation in tuberculosis case rates,
- evolving institutional and public responses to tuberculosis in the community and the workplace, and
- ongoing risk from people with undiagnosed infectious tuberculosis.

The *changing epidemiology of tuberculosis* encompasses both the decline in the number of tuberculosis cases and case rates since 1993 and the decline in the proportion of cases accounted for by multidrug-resistant disease, as described in Chapter 1. Overall, fewer cases of tuberculosis and less multidrug-resistant disease means less risk for nurses, doctors, correctional officers, and others who work for organizations that serve people who have tuberculosis or who are at increased risk of the disease.

Despite the general decline in rates of tuberculosis in recent years, marked *geographic variation* in tuberculosis case rates persists. Today, as in the past, a few states and cities account for a disproportionate share of cases of active tuberculosis. Nonetheless, even within areas with relatively high rates of tuberculosis, risks to health care and other workers are not equal. Some hospitals have policies to transfer rather than treat patients with suspected or confirmed tuberculosis. Many nursing homes, jails, and other facilities will not accept persons known to have active tuberculosis. Although these policies should reduce risk, workers may still be exposed to individuals with undetected disease. In contrast to these "transfer rather than treat" institutions are the so-called safety net hospitals whose workers care for a high proportion of people who are at increased risk of tuberculosis (e.g., those who are unemployed or homeless, recent immigrants from developing countries, and individuals with HIV infection or AIDS).

Workers' risk of tuberculosis is also affected by *employer and community efforts to prevent the spread of tuberculosis.* Investigations of workplace outbreaks of tuberculosis have typically identified lapses in infection control measures as probable contributors to transmission. As discussed in Chapter 6, much of the support for the effectiveness of tuberculosis control measures comes from outbreak investigations and subsequent studies of the implementation of administrative controls and other measures. In workplaces that have many workers in direct contact with infectious individuals, employers' policies and procedures affect the likelihood that employees will acquire tuberculosis infection or disease on the job.

Although Chapter 6 points to the importance of careful and alert application of protocols for identifying those likely to have infectious tuberculosis, application of such protocols does not guarantee that all cases will be promptly identified. *Unsuspected and undiagnosed tuberculosis is the primary threat to workers.*

The committee's conclusions about the workplace risk of tuberculosis must be understood against this backdrop. If the conclusions highlighted below are taken out of context, the occupational risk of tuberculosis may be misunderstood. Although the committee judged that the following conclusions were reasonably supported by the available literature, it notes that most of the studies that it consulted involved hospitals and were inconsistent in methods, reporting, and results.

Conclusions

Through at least the 1950s, health care workers were at higher risk from tuberculosis than others in the community. Before the development of effective treatments for the disease, several studies documented very high rates of infection for nurses and physicians. The available data do not allow conclusions about the historical risk to other categories of workers covered by the 1997 proposed OSHA rule.

Despite the availability of effective treatments, the last decade and a half has shown that *tuberculosis remains a threat to health care and other workers,* especially when workplaces neglect basic infection control measures and when multidrug-resistant disease is present. The primary risk today comes from patients, inmates, and others with unsuspected and undiagnosed infectious tuberculosis. Even with good tuberculosis control measures, some workers will still be exposed to people with unsuspected infectious disease, particularly in communities where the disease is common.

Available data suggest that where tuberculosis is uncommon or where basic infection control measures are in place, the occupational risk to health care work-

ers of tuberculosis infection now approaches the level in their community of residence. Tuberculosis risk in communities has been declining since 1993. Overall, rates of active tuberculosis among health care workers are similar overall to those reported for other employed workers. Comparable data are not available to compare mortality risk. Whatever the origins of their disease, health care workers and others with compromised immune systems are at high risk of death if they contract multidrug-resistant tuberculosis. The limited information available to the committee and the changing epidemiology of tuberculosis did not allow the committee to make quantitative estimates or comparisons.

The potential for exposure to tuberculosis in health care and other facilities varies within and across communities. In general, where the disease is more common, health care and others workers are at higher risk of coming into contact with people who have infectious tuberculosis. The U.S. population is, however, mobile, and visitors and new residents can bring tuberculosis with them into communities where the disease is rare. Should a hospital or other worker encounter such an unexpected person, she or he may be at higher risk than colleagues in high-prevalence inner cities, who are more likely to be familiar with and alert to the signs and symptoms of tuberculosis.

The occupational risk of exposure to tuberculosis varies with job category and work environment. Only some health care, correctional, and other workers are reasonably anticipated to have contact with people with tuberculosis, even in facilities that treat or admit such individuals. For example, many administrative and other personnel in hospitals have little contact with patients of any sort and little chance of exposure to contaminated air. For those with direct patient contact, the risk of tuberculosis infection and disease is also not uniform. Although data are not completely consistent, the risk tends to be higher for those who work on wards where patients with suspected or confirmed tuberculosis are admitted and for those whose jobs involve aerosol-generating procedures such as bronchoscopies. For these workers, in particular, *the effectiveness of workplace tuberculosis control measures matters.*

Workers at particular risk from occupationally acquired tuberculosis infection include those with HIV infection or AIDS or other conditions associated with suppression of normal functioning of the immune system. Data about cases of tuberculosis among health care and other workers are limited, but those with HIV infection or AIDS (or other conditions affecting the immune system) are disproportionately represented in reports of tuberculosis cases and deaths during hospital and prison outbreaks of multidrug-resistant disease. CDC guidelines recommend that health care workers with HIV infection be counseled about the risk of contact with patients who have tuberculosis and be offered assignments that minimize such contact (CDC, 1994b).

Many health care, correctional facility, and other workers are at increased risk of tuberculosis for reasons unrelated to their work. Most people spend more time in the community than at work. In general, low-income individuals, members of racial and ethnic minorities, immigrants from developing countries, and people living in low-income neighborhoods are at higher risk of community-acquired tuberculosis infection and active tuberculosis. This does not mean that the risk of workplace transmission of tuberculosis can be disregarded for workers with these demographic risk factors. It does mean, however, that workplace surveillance programs need to consider the likelihood of community exposure in assessing the results of tuberculin skin tests.

SUMMARY

Historically, health care workers were at higher risk from tuberculosis than others in the community. Since then, effective treatment has drastically cut tuberculosis case rates and consequently reduced health care workers' occupational risk of tuberculosis. Lower community case rates also mean that prison, jail, homeless shelter, and other workers are less likely to be exposed to tuberculosis than in the past.

Still, tuberculosis remains a threat, particularly when the disease is unsuspected and undiagnosed and when infection control measures are neglected. Other risk factors for health care, correctional, and other workers include work that involves direct contact with people who have infectious tuberculosis and work in communities with high prevalence of the disease.

6

Implementation and Effects
of CDC Guidelines

Neither voluntary guidelines nor government regulations implement themselves. Given factors such as competition within and among organizations for scarce resources and disagreements about problems and priorities, implementation cannot be assumed. The literature reviewed in Chapter 5 has already pointed to departures from recommended tuberculosis control measures as likely contributors to outbreaks of tuberculosis in health care facilities in the late 1980s and early 1990s.

This chapter reviews what is known about the implementation and effects of the 1994 Center for Disease Control and Prevention (CDC) guidelines to prevent worker exposure to tuberculosis in hospitals, correctional facilities, and other work settings. The review also covers information about the implementation of earlier tuberculosis control guidelines including those that were recommended by CDC in 1990. Although some specific recommendations have changed and technologies have been evolving, the basic elements have remained constant enough that studies that predate the 1994 guideines are still useful. In fact, most of the published reports located by the committee describe steps taken before publication of the 1994 guidelines.

In addition to the CDC's own efforts, recommendations and actions by other public and private agencies may also have influenced employer decisions about tuberculosis control measures in the 1990s. For example, in 1993 the Occupational Safety and Health Administration (OSHA) announced efforts to enforce the adoption of tuberculosis control measures under the agency's general-duty clause and its 1987 respiratory protection standard. The next year it issued a notice of proposed rulemaking on occupational tuberculosis. In addition, as noted in Chapter 4, some state regulatory agencies and some accrediting organizations included tuberculosis control measures in their regulations or standards for health care and correctional facilities.

The committee identified three general types of information on the implementation and effects of CDC guidelines: multi-institution surveys, multi-institution inspections, and reports on individual organizations. A few studies focus on the adherence of individuals (e.g., physicians and nurses) to recommended practices such as using personal respiratory protection devices. The literature review in Appendix D includes additional details, and Appendixes B and F also provide relevant information on two specific control measures: tuberculin skin testing and personal respiratory protections. The primary outcome measures reported are tuberculin skin test conversions and cases of active tuberculosis (including multidrug-resistant disease).

Again, nearly all the information that the committee located relates to hospitals. The committee found little on nursing homes, ambulatory care clinics, health units of correctional facilities, and other organizations covered by the 1994 CDC guidelines for health care facilities or by the 1996 CDC guidelines for correctional facilities.[1]

IMPLEMENTATION OF TUBERCULOSIS CONTROL GUIDELINES

Broadly, implementation refers to the practical activities and interventions undertaken to turn guidelines or policies into desired results. Implementation of the tuberculosis controls measures recommended by CDC calls for a complex set of actions at both the organizational and the individual levels.

The primary focus of the tuberculosis control measures is the organization as a whole rather than the individual. As described in Chapter 4, institutional responsibilities include the preparation and implementation of an overall tuberculosis control plan and record-keeping system; assessment of the tuberculosis risk in the facility; the development and application of written policies and protocols for the rapid identification, isolation, and treatment of individuals with infectious tuberculosis; the creation and maintenance of surveillance, education, and other programs for workers; the establishment and maintenance of appropriate engineering controls for negative-pressure isolation rooms and other areas; and the creation and monitoring of a respiratory protection program.

---

[1]The CDC recommendations for preventing tuberculosis in correctional facilities describe core activities of screening, containment, and assessment but are generally similar to the guidelines for health care facilities, taking into account differences in the purposes and operation of correctional facilities and health care facilities.

Policies are, of course, carried out by individuals. The personnel who provide clinical care, maintain engineering systems, and otherwise do the day-to-day work of the organization often have considerable discretion in following policies and recommended practices. In recent years, many health care and other organizations have attempted to design systems to minimize opportunities for unwanted variations in work practices. For example, some facilities have installed electronic monitoring systems that check whether doors to tuberculosis isolation rooms are closed, consistent with policy. Nonetheless, for many activities, universal standardization or monitoring of work practices would be viewed as impossible, offensive, counterproductive, or excessively expensive. Thus, individual adherence to organizational policies continues to be a concern.

Surveys of Organizational Implementation of Tuberculosis Control Measures

Mailed surveys are a relatively inexpensive way of collecting information about a large number of geographically dispersed institutions. When the surveyed institutions are familiar with both the surveying organization and the kinds of questions asked and when the topic is viewed as important, voluntary questionnaires can generate respectable response rates of 70 percent or more.

The potential limitations of survey data are, however, familiar. If all members of a population are not surveyed and the sample of the population is not properly selected, the subset chosen may be unrepresentative of the population. This limits generalizations from the surveyed population to the larger population. Whether surveys are directed to a universe or a representative sample, the lower the response rate, the greater the concern that responses will be unrepresentative. In addition, survey questions may be deliberately or unintentionally biased or otherwise formulated in ways likely to produce inaccurate and unrepresentative responses. Even if the questions are sound, those who respond may intentionally or unintentionally provide inaccurate or insufficient information. Bias is a particular concern if those surveyed know that important policy decisions may hinge on the survey results. Organizational surveys may also be misdirected to and returned by individuals who lack the knowledge to respond accurately.

Results from National Surveys of Hospitals

In 1992, while increases in tuberculosis cases and case rates were still being recorded, CDC surveyed hospitals about their tuberculosis control practices. Questionnaires went to all 632 federal, state, and local public hospitals in the United States and to a 20 percent random sample

(444 institutions) of hospitals with 100 beds or more that were listed in the American Hospital Association database (Manangan et al., 1998). The response rate was about 70 percent for each group (726 institutions total). (Note that Table 6-1, described in the next paragraph, covers only a subset of this survey's respondents.) Half of the respondents reported that their institutions had admitted six or more patients with tuberculosis. One-quarter said that their institutions had admitted patients with multidrug-resistant disease. Nearly all reported some kind of tuberculin skin testing program. Just over 70 percent reported having isolation rooms that met the 1990 CDC criteria for the isolation of patients with tuberculosis, but 60 percent of that group reported that their institutions did not routinely check the airflow in isolation rooms. Of those that did routinely check, few (13 percent) checked it at least monthly. One of five institutions allowed patients out of isolation for other than medical reasons. Although nearly 90 percent reported that their policy was to keep

TABLE 6-1. Comparison of Tuberculosis Control Measures for 103 Hospitals That Reported More than Six Admissions of Patients with Tuberculosis in 1992 CDC Survey and That Also Responded to 1996 CDC Survey

	1992 No. (%)	1996 No. (%)
Engineering Controls		
Isolation rooms meeting CDC criteria	59/92 (64)	99/103 (96)
Routine check of negative air pressure	42/85 (49)	96/99 (97)
Monthly check of negative air pressure[a]	5/35 (14)	76/90 (84)
Respiratory Protection[b]		
Nonfitted surgical mask	69/101 (68)	1/103 (1)
Soft mask, molded or fitted	34/101 (34)	NA
Particulate respirator	8/101 (8)	40/103 (39)
N95	NA	85/103 (83)
Tuberculin Skin Testing Program		
Testing by Worker Category		
Nurses	103/103 (100)	103/103 (100)
Respiratory therapists	102/103 (99)	103/103 (100)
House staff	65/81 (69)	65/73 (89)
Attending physicians	43/86 (50)	65/94 (69)
Students	55/95 (58)	74/97 (76)
Testing Elements		
After exposure incident	98/101 (97)	102/103 (99)
Two-step testing	NA	77/98 (79)
Maintain yearly reports	64/98 (65)	93/98 (95)

[a]When an isolation room is actually in use for a patient with suspected or confirmed tuberculosis, the 1994 CDC guidelines recommend that pressure be checked daily.
[b]Numbers add to more than one hundred because facilities may use more than one type of mask.
SOURCE: Manangan et al., 1998.

the doors of isolation rooms closed, a near majority reported that staff left doors open some or all of the time. Few (11 percent) reported negative-pressure isolation facilities for their emergency departments that met CDC recommendations.

In 1996, nearly 2 years after the 1994 CDC guidelines were released, CDC randomly selected and resurveyed half of the 272 hospitals that had reported six or more admissions of patients with tuberculosis in the 1992 survey (Manangan et al., 1998, 2000). Responses were received from 75 percent (103) of these facilities. Table 6-1 compares the 1992 and 1996 responses for these hospitals. The 1996 responses showed substantial improvement in all areas in which implementation of control measures had not already been near or at 100 percent.

CDC initiated a new survey of hospital tuberculosis control practices in 2000 (Pugliese, 2000). Final results were not yet available when the committee finished its work.

In 1993, the Society for Healthcare Epidemiology of America (SHEA) and the CDC surveyed members of SHEA to assess compliance with the 1990 CDC guidelines (Fridkin et al., 1995a,b). They obtained responses that were suitable for analysis for 210 hospitals, but not all respondents returned complete information. The researchers concluded that despite an increase in patients with multidrug-resistant tuberculosis, "TB infection control measures still did not meet the 1990 CDC guideline recommendations" (Fridkin et al., 1995b, p. 129).

Another analysis focused on tuberculosis control measures in emergency departments in a randomly selected sample of the hospitals responding to the 1992 CDC survey described above (Moran et al., 1995). Of the institutions responding (305, or 68 percent of 446 facilities contacted), more than half (53 percent) reported seeing tuberculosis patients at least monthly. More than 90 percent reported giving surgical masks to patients with suspected tuberculosis. Although 76 percent reported written patient isolation criteria for the emergency department, only 56 percent had such criteria for triage or waiting areas. (Some institutions may not have had separate triage areas.) Respondents reported tuberculosis isolation rooms in only 20 percent of emergency departments and 2 percent of triage and waiting areas. Air recirculation measures were reported for approximately 80 percent of emergency departments.

In 1992 and 1995 surveys of hospitals with 100 or more beds, Tokars and colleagues (1996) focused on the CDC recommendations for mycobacteriology laboratory methods and on rapid laboratory processing of smears and cultures. The 1992 survey of 1,076 institutions obtained a 70 percent response rate. In 1995, 20 percent of those responding to the earlier survey were surveyed again and 70 percent responded. Those responding to both surveys reported increased use of recommended testing procedures in 1995. They also reported drops in the median time for providing results from 2 days to 1 day for smear results, from 40 to 21 days for culture results, and from 45 to 35 days for drug sensitivity test results. Some of these improvements probably reflect the availability of better technologies.

Appendix D reports limited information from some dental schools. It suggests limited implementation of tuberculin skin testing and, probably, other protective measures.

Other Surveys of Health Care Facilities

As background for continuing efforts to develop tuberculosis control policies, researchers in Minnesota surveyed a voluntary sample of 18 hospitals to determine hospital practices and analyze tuberculin skin test results for the period from 1989 to 1991. Although the survey documented variable compliance with recommended practices of the time, the researchers concluded that practices were "reasonably consistent with the critical elements in the 1990 CDC guidelines" (Van Drunen et al., 1996).

The Maryland Hospital Association and the state of Maryland surveyed the state's hospitals in 1992, 1993, and 1997 to assess tuberculosis control practices (Fuss et al., 2000). The 1992 survey, which obtained responses from nearly three-quarters of the hospitals, found that about half reported having a routine (at least annual) tuberculin skin testing program for employees. About half also reported that they routinely checked isolation rooms for negative pressure. Subsequent site visits found deficiencies in isolation room performance. Less than a quarter of the hospitals reported that they supplied workers with respirators.

The 1997 Maryland survey also obtained responses from about three-quarters of the hospitals surveyed. This time 90 percent of the hospitals reported that they checked isolation rooms for negative pressure. All reported having a routine employee skin testing program and providing workers with respirators consistent with CDC recommendations. More than 90 percent had conducted a risk assessment consistent with CDC guidelines.

Manangan and colleagues reported on 1992 and 1996 survey results for New Jersey hospitals (1999). Again, the reports showed improved compliance with tuberculosis precautions. The committee also located a 1992 convenience survey of Texas hospitals that concluded that many hospitals had policies and practices that were inconsistent with the CDC guidelines in place at the time (Manangan et al., 1997).

Surveys of Correctional Facilities

In 1992–1993, 1994–1995, and 1996–1997, CDC and the National Institute of Justice (NIJ) sent surveys on tuberculosis control practices to the

Federal Bureau of Prisons, all 50 state systems, and a number of large local jail systems (37 for the first two surveys, 41 for the third survey) (NIJ, 1996, 1999). All of the federal and state systems responded to the surveys, as did approximately 80 percent of the local jail systems.

The first two surveys predated the official publication of CDC guidelines for correctional facilities (CDC, 1996b), although earlier agency and other guidelines covered high-risk populations and tuberculosis control measures applicable to facilities treating or housing people with tuberculosis (ATS, 1992; NCCHC, 1992; CDC, 1990b, 1994b). The survey questions for correctional facilities differed somewhat from those for hospitals, so comparisons are not always possible. For example, the first two surveys apparently did not include questions about screening of correctional facility staff. Responses to the third survey indicated that more than 90 percent of federal and state systems and almost all local jail systems reported screening of new employees. Roughly three-quarters reported periodic retesting. For each survey, reported use of negative-pressure rooms (in infirmaries or community hospitals, or both) for the isolation of inmates with suspected or confirmed infectious tuberculosis increased: from approximately 30 percent (1992–1993) to approximately 65 percent (1994–1995) to nearly all (98 percent) of the federal and state systems and 85 percent of the local jail systems (1996–1997). The reported use of directly observed therapy for all inmates with active tuberculosis also increased from 77 to 94 to 98 percent for federal and state systems and from 84 to 90 to 95 percent for local jail systems, for the three surveys, respectively.

The 1996–1997 survey included validation surveys of institutions within 13 systems. These surveys showed some differences between system-level and institution-level policies. For example, for systems with policies requiring four-drug initial treatment of active tuberculosis, only three-quarters of the individual institutions in those systems reported having the same policy.

In the 1996–1997 survey, nearly one-third of the federal and state systems failed to report whether or not they had cases of tuberculosis. Reporting on tuberculin skin testing programs was even more incomplete, with more than half of the state and federal prison systems and more than a third of the jail systems failing to report conversion data. The authors suggest that cases of tuberculosis in prisons may be undercounted because reporting is incomplete.

A separate survey of staff in Texas correctional facilities reported lack of knowledge of how tuberculosis is transmitted and how it can be prevented and treated (Woods et al., 1997). A survey of 225 health care workers in the Maryland Department of Corrections noted similar gaps in tuberculosis-related knowledge among frontline correctional health care workers (DeJoy et al., 1995). For example, 30 percent of the workers thought that a standard surgical mask would protect them from inhalation of aerosolized tuberculosis droplets, and 23 percent thought that correctional health care workers were not at risk for infection with multidrug-resistant tuberculosis. The researchers found that training on tuberculosis risk was inconsistent. Some prison facilities provided extensive training, whereas others provided almost no training. A third of all respondents said that they had received no workplace training at all on tuberculosis in the previous year. Eleven percent of the workers reported that they had not been offered tuberculin skin testing in the previous 12 months, which is in conflict with stated institutional policy. Almost a fifth of respondents reported that they had a positive skin test history, and roughly half of this group said that they had received some type of follow-up care.

A report on the Cook County Jail in Chicago underscores the logistical challenges of implementing tuberculosis control measures to protect jail inmates and staff in a large facility (McAuley, 2000). This jail admits more than 100,000 people a year and houses about 10,000 per day on average, more than the facility was designed to handle. All those detained have a medical evaluation that includes a tuberculin skin test (read within 48 to 72 hours) and a chest radiograph (read within 18 hours). Persons with suspected tuberculosis identified during or after the evaluation are sent to the jail's emergency room, which has negative-flow isolation rooms. Those who have a suspicious radiograph but are released before it is read are to be seen by a communicable disease investigator and brought to the tuberculosis clinic of the county health department. (An analysis of the experience with this system's screening strategy is reported later in this chapter.)

An article by Jones and colleagues (1999) about their experience at the Memphis city jail is also illuminating. From January 1995 through December 1998, the Memphis city jail admitted and discharged more than 173,000 individuals, an average of 159 a day. The median length of stay was 1 day, and four-fifths of those admitted had been incarcerated in the jail previously. Single cells held between 18 and 36 inmates, and mingling of inmates was extensive.

Other Surveys

In 1997, the American Federation of State, County, and Municipal Employees (AFSCME) developed separate but similar surveys to collect information about employer compliance with tuberculosis control recommendations affecting health care workers, law enforcement personnel, and social services workers (August, 1999).[2] They received responses for

---

[2]The survey went to approximately 100 district councils (which distributed them to local unions) and large unaffiliated local unions. Of the 170 responses, some came from employers, but most (145) came from workers. Reporting on skin test conversions and cases of tuberculosis was incomplete, but cases of disease were reported in all sectors.

170 workplaces including 94 health care facilities, 48 correctional and law enforcement facilities, and 28 social service agencies. The results reported for the 16 responding acute-care hospitals were, overall, the most consistent with the CDC guidelines. Just over half of the correctional and law enforcement facilities were reported to have a written tuberculosis control plan. Of the social service agencies (which were not covered by the 1994 CDC guidelines for health care facilities), only one respondent reported a written tuberculosis control plan or a worker training program. For all organizations, the lowest levels of practice consistent with the 1994 CDC guidelines were reported for respiratory protection programs. Half of the 16 hospitals, less than 10 percent of the 23 long-term facilities for the elderly, 20 percent of the 28 mental health facilities, and 20 percent of 48 correctional and law enforcement facilities reported such programs. The responses to the AFSCME survey come from a very small, nonrandom set of respondents and must be viewed with considerable caution. They do, however, help explain organized labor's continuing concern about the protections being offered workers, particularly those outside hospitals.

In 1997, researchers from Johns Hopkins University asked attendees at a national funeral director's convention to complete a risk assessment questionnaire and undergo tuberculin skin testing (Gershon, 1998). Approximately 800 funeral home employees completed the survey and consented to a tuberculin skin test. This group included 500 embalmers, who have the highest risk of exposure. Only 16 percent of the embalmers reported consistently wearing any kind of face mask during embalming procedures. About half reported some kind of training about tuberculosis during their career; less than 20 percent reported such training in the preceding 12 months. Nonetheless, the researchers concluded that most were reasonably knowledgeable about the disease. Overall, these data supported findings from a smaller pilot study of 123 Maryland embalmers that also showed limited adoption of measures for the prevention of transmission of M. tuberculosis (Gershon et al., 1995b).

Taken together, survey results suggest, at a minimum, two conclusions. First, institutional departures from recommended tuberculosis control policies and procedures were common, if not the norm, in the late 1980s and early 1990s. Second, institutions—at least hospitals and correctional facilities—were taking tuberculosis control measures more seriously and reporting substantially higher rates of implementation of recommended measures in later years. As discussed below, written policies may not be consistent with routine practices.

Facility Inspections or Visits

Although limited in some respects by the lack of a specific standard on occupational tuberculosis, OSHA can inspect health care and other facilities under its general duty (which provides that employers maintain a safe workplace) and its respiratory protection standard.[3] In addition, many state governments and private agencies periodically inspect health care and other facilities to determine compliance with regulations or voluntary standards. As described in Chapter 4, some of these regulations and standards include provisions related to tuberculosis control measures, although the committee found no overall summary of state regulatory requirements or accreditation requirements. Committee members were aware of institutions that had been cited or questioned by state agencies or accrediting organizations about tuberculosis control measures during visits by the state licensure agencies and the Joint Commission on the Accreditation of Healthcare Organizations.

In addition to such routine inspections, inspections may also be prompted by complaints by patients, families, health care workers, or others. The facilities involved in these kinds of complaint-generated inspections may not be representative. In addition, a few on-site inspections were specifically prompted by state concern about facility readiness to cope with the increasing rates of tuberculosis seen in the late 1980s and early 1990s.

Although inspectors often rely on responses to written questions and written records, they may have the opportunity to conduct more flexible, open-ended interviews with facility personnel and to view or test the physical plant, equipment, and work practices. Such inspections are labor-intensive and expensive, which limits their number and scope.

OSHA Inspections

Between May 1992 and October 1994, OSHA inspected 272 health care, correctional, and other facilities to assess compliance with the tuberculosis control measures that were described first in a May 1992 OSHA Region 2 directive and then in a nationwide enforcement policy (McDiarmid et al., 1996). Inspections in New York and New Jersey accounted for a substantial proportion of the total. Worker or union complaints prompted most inspections (71 percent). Hospitals accounted for almost half of the workplaces inspected. Basic citation data were available for nearly all the facilities, but detailed questionnaire data were available for only 149 facilities.

Inspectors found compliance with recommended tuberculosis control measures to be quite variable. It was best, overall, for administrative controls. For example, annual tuberculin skin testing was reported for better than three-quarters of hospitals, prisons, shelters, and nursing homes.

---

[3]As described in Chapter 4, OSHA revised its 1987 respiratory protection standard in 1998. Pending publication of the standard on occupational tuberculosis, the 1998 general standard did not cover tuberculosis, which instead was covered by special interim regulations.

Negative-pressure isolation rooms were reported for 33 of 56 hospitals (59 percent), 15 of 35 prisons (43 percent), and 4 of 9 nursing homes (44 percent) but no shelters. Respiratory protection was reported for nearly 60 percent of hospitals but less than 20 percent of prisons, shelters, and nursing homes. Overall, 42 percent of facilities received citations, most for noncompliance with respiratory protection requirements. (The inspections occurred before the National Institute for Occupational Safety and Health [NIOSH] had certified the N95 respirators, which were less expensive and generally more convenient and comfortable than the devices previously certified.) Again, because inspections were generally prompted by complaints, the results may reflect a negative bias.

State and Other Inspections

New York State officials examined tuberculosis isolation procedures in 22 New York City hospitals in 1992, 1993, and 1994 (Stricof et al., 1998). They reviewed medical and laboratory records to collect information about patient risk factors and history, signs and symptoms, length of time in the emergency department, turnaround time for laboratory reports, timing of isolation and treatment, and other information. They also directly observed and evaluated isolation rooms and isolation practices. From 1992 to 1994, they found that hospitals made substantial progress in correcting deficits in tuberculosis control measures. The percentage of isolation rooms with negative pressure increased from 51 to 80 percent. The number of patients with active tuberculosis sharing rooms dropped from 13 percent to zero, and the percentage of patients with suspected or diagnosed tuberculosis isolated upon admission increased from 75 to 84 percent. The number of facilities able to process smears 7 days a week increased from 40 to 95 percent. Despite improvements, the inspections also revealed continuing problems in some areas, including open doors and windows for isolation rooms and isolation rooms without negative pressure.

In addition to any state-specific requirements, states must survey and inspect nursing homes annually to assess compliance with Medicaid certification requirements set by the U.S. Health Care Financing Administration (HFCA). HCFA requires that nursing homes have an infection control program. Recent data (June 2000) showed that states had cited 10.8 percent of facilities for deficiencies in their infection control programs, 0.9 percent for deficiencies related to isolation of residents, 0.1 percent for deficiencies related to employees with (any) communicable disease, and 6.4 percent for hand-washing and infection control deficiencies (AHCA, 2000).

One on-site study (supported by NIOSH and the California Department of Health) compared written tuberculosis control policies with actual practices in three hospitals in high-incidence counties in California (Sutton et al., 1998, 2000). The investigators used questionnaires and reviews of written documents to assess policies. They then attended tuberculosis control meetings and training sessions, directly observed work practices for patient isolation, and measured the ventilation performances of isolation rooms. The first report indicated that of 67 rooms equipped with continuous airflow monitoring devices, devices in 8 rooms did not accurately reflect the direction of airflow. Of 62 workers observed using a respirator, 65 percent did not put it on properly. In the second report from the study, investigators found that only one hospital followed the CDC's recommendations for respiratory protection. Of the isolation rooms tested, 28 percent (7 of 25) were under positive pressure. In most of the rooms tested (26 of 27), air moved toward rather than away from workers. None of the three facilities regularly checked the performances of the isolation rooms.

In 1994, researchers associated with a midwestern hospital system combined a written survey with record reviews and on-site testing of isolation rooms in seven rural and six urban hospitals (Woeltje et al., 1997). All hospitals reported having tuberculosis control plans and performing annual tuberculin skin testing. Eleven of 13 hospitals had negative-pressure isolation rooms. The researchers found that the median percentage of rooms with effective negative pressure was 95 percent (with one institution reporting a median of only 44 percent). Three hospitals provided high-efficiency particulate air masks, and eight provided dust-mist or dust-mist-fume masks. This inspection occurred before NIOSH had certified the use of N95 respirators. Actual worker use of the masks was not observed.

Although reports of facility inspections cover relatively few institutions, the results may still provide some insights into the match between institutional policies and routine, day-to-day practices. In general, they suggest that departures from recommended tuberculosis control measures occur at both the institutional level (e.g., provision of appropriate respirators) and the individual level (e.g., appropriate use of respirators). Implementation is probably most complete for administrative controls including written plans and procedures. For engineering controls, implementation is likely better for the installation of isolation rooms than for their day-to-day operation in accordance with guidelines.

Implementation Lapses Mentioned in Outbreak and Other Case Reports

Rather than systematically describing the implementation of tuberculosis control measures, outbreak reports typically focus on factors that might have contributed to the outbreak, including the failure to implement specific controls. As discussed later in this chapter, most reports describe efforts to improve tuberculosis control practices and document the consequences.

Published case reports often involve organizations with particularly interesting situations or problems such as an outbreak of multidrug-resistant tuberculosis in a hospital or a case of disease in an atypical setting. Stable, nonoutbreak situations are less interesting to researchers, government agencies, and journals. Moreover, from the committee's personal experience and conversations with CDC staff, not all outbreaks are reported, and not all those reported are investigated. Of those investigated, not all result in published reports. Thus, published reports on outbreaks therefore cannot be treated as representative of all outbreaks, much less all employers.

Several articles have summarized information presented in case reports, and the committee's reading of the individual reports is consistent with these summaries. Menzies and colleagues (1995), for example, reviewed 13 incidents (all before 1993) of single or multiple cases of occupationally acquired tuberculosis infection or disease in hospitals. The reports on these incidents usually associated outbreaks with delayed diagnosis of hospitalized patients with infectious tuberculosis, inadequate therapy, or unrecognized drug resistance. The reports also frequently cited inadequate ventilation and isolation practices. In addition, the review authors noted other reports describing low levels of health care worker compliance with treatment for tuberculosis infection, which reduces the benefits of tuberculin skin testing programs.

Dooley and Tapper (1997) summarize reports on 21 inpatient facilities with episodes of tuberculosis transmission to patients or workers in inpatient facilities all before 1993. Most (17) involved patients with undiagnosed, untreated infectious tuberculosis, and most of the sustained outbreaks involved people with human immunodeficiency virus (HIV) infection and suppressed immune systems who were exposed to patients with undiagnosed infectious tuberculosis or unrecognized drug-resistant disease. Some reports cited isolation practices that departed from recommendations. Such departures included the ending the isolation before a response to treatment was documented, failure to close doors to isolation rooms, and failure to keep patients confined to isolation rooms. Many reports also cited inadequate engineering controls including use of recirculated air with no or few air changes and isolation rooms with positive or essentially neutral pressure. In at least two episodes, transmission occurred despite frequent air changes. Most reports did not describe respiratory protection policies or practices, although three described transmission to workers who had worn surgical masks during contact with a patient with tuberculosis.

A review by Garrett and colleagues (1999) includes 23 pre-1993 episodes of transmission of *M. tuberculosis* to patients or workers, most of which are covered by Tapper and Dooley. The review also covers five episodes between 1993 and 1996, two of which involved unrecognized active tuberculosis and two of which were associated with inadequate cleaning and disinfection of bronchoscopes (the latter involving patients only).

Nearly all of the reports summarized above involved inpatient facilities. A few reports have described apparent or documented transmission of tuberculosis in other settings including prisons, jails, funeral homes, and ambulatory care clinics. Most suggest the same general kinds of contributing factors described above. For example, a report on an ambulatory care clinic cites undiagnosed infectious tuberculosis and inadequate engineering controls including insufficient fresh air exchanges in the building and improper ventilation of rooms used for administration of aerosolized drugs (Howell et al., 1989).

Some reports point to unintentional error and inefficiency. For example, according to newspaper reports, a recent outbreak in a Pennsylvania prison involved the improper transfer by the U.S. Immigration and Naturalization Service (INS) of a prisoner with infectious, multidrug-resistant tuberculosis following a "paperwork error" (Hoover, 2000; Lang, 2000). The investigation of this outbreak is, however, incomplete and not yet described in any official report.

Overall, outbreak reports reinforce the picture of implementation presented by surveys and inspections of institutional practices. The reports from the late 1980s and early 1990s underscore the importance of administrative controls, especially respiratory isolation policies, by highlighting the role of undiagnosed infectious tuberculosis and the involvement of particularly susceptible patients as factors in transmission (e.g., those with HIV infection or AIDS). The reports also cite lapses in engineering controls (e.g., lack of isolation rooms and inadequate maintenance).

Worker Adherence to Tuberculosis Control Measures

Several studies suggest that health care workers—including physicians and other professionals—vary greatly in their level of adherence to recommended measures for preventing the transmission of tuberculosis. Chapter 2 has already discussed studies documenting the generally modest rate of compliance of health care workers—including physicians—with recommended treatment for latent tuberculosis infection (Fraser et al., 1994; Blumberg et al., 1996; Ramphal-Naley et al., 1996). Other studies have documented physicians' incomplete awareness of and adherence to guidelines for treatment of patients with tuberculosis (DeRiemer et al., 1999; Evans et al., 1999). The committee notes that neither the 1994 CDC guidelines nor the 1997 proposed OSHA rule stressed treatment for latent tuberculosis infection. The American Thoracic Society and CDC recently issued guidelines that emphasize the importance of such treatment when indicated (ATS/CDC, 2000b).

As described above in the three-hospital study by Sutton and colleagues, nearly two-thirds of workers observed using a respirator did not put it on properly. In another study at a single facility (the University of California at San Diego), researchers observed health care workers over a 14-week period (LoBue et al., 1999). They recorded 64 violations (during 541 observations) that included 36 failures to maintain isolation (e.g., leaving a door open) and 28 failures to use respirators properly. Medical students, residents, and fellows accounted for 17 percent of the study observations and 45 percent of the violations. (Eight of the 29 violations for this group were described as not clinically important; for example, isolation had been ordered discontinued, but a sign was still on the door.)

Asimos and colleagues (1999) reported results of a survey of emergency medicine residents conducted in 1998 in conjunction with the annual in-service examination of the American Board of Emergency Medicine. Nearly 90 percent of the residents responded to at least part of the survey. Half reported that they did not routinely wear a NIOSH-approved respirator during contact with patients at risk of having tuberculosis. Almost half reported that the reason for lack of compliance was a lack of easy availability of respirators, and about a third reported a lack of fit testing as the reason. Just under one-third reported they had not been offered fit testing, and 8 percent reported being offered but not going through fit testing.

The interplay between institutional and individual practices is also suggested by another observational study. During the investigation of 22 New York City hospitals described earlier, Stricof and colleagues found that the rate of use of approved respirators was higher when the respirators were placed outside isolation rooms rather than at nursing stations and when only approved respirators were available (i.e., surgical masks were not available) (Rachel Stricof, New York State Department of Health, personal communication, August 28, 2000).

A 1993 study of health care workers focused on knowledge rather than practice (Lai et al., 1996). Two hundred health care workers with patient contact were tested. Just under half reported some education on tuberculosis during the preceding 2 years. Nearly all (98 percent) knew that coughing or sneezing could spread tuberculosis, but more than a quarter (28 percent) thought that it could be transmitted by a handshake. The great majority (88 percent) knew that masks should be used in the rooms of patients with tuberculosis, but a third also thought that gowns were needed.

EFFECTS OF IMPLEMENTING TUBERCULOSIS
CONTROL MEASURES

Ideally, the 1994 CDC guidelines would have been based on rigorous, prospective, controlled studies demonstrating the effectiveness of each key recommended measure. In fact, there was in 1994 and there remains today little controlled research documenting the independent effects of these elements in preventing transmission of M. tuberculosis.[4] Instead, evidence of the effectiveness of tuberculosis control measures comes primarily from case reports, analyses of survey responses, and a few studies of specific precautions. For the most part, the case for the CDC recommendations and the proposed OSHA rule rests on these sources supplemented by logic, biologic plausibility, theoretical arguments, animal studies, laboratory simulations, and mathematical modeling.

Results Described in Case Reports Following Outbreaks

Methodologic Limitations

The committee identified several published reports on the experiences of hospitals with protective measures that were newly or more vigorously implemented after outbreaks of tuberculosis. Some of the limitations of case reports have already been described above and in Chapter 5. As already noted in the discussion of implementation, most studies identified by the committee describe steps taken before the release of the 1994 guidelines. It is often difficult to tell from published reports how well the specifics of control measures matched the recommendations in either the 1990 or the 1994 CDC guidelines.

Strategies for implementing the guidelines have often involved the nearly simultaneous implementation of multiple precautions. This makes judgments about the effectiveness of individual measures difficult. Although several reports present time series data, many institutions had such rudimentary tuberculin skin testing programs before the adoption of new measures that they could not report data on the preintervention period. In addition, reports vary in the way that they define time periods for study and sometimes report rates for unequal time periods. Some, for example, compare a preintervention period with an intervention period. Others compare an intervention period with a postintervention period, or they compare different periods during which different interventions were adopted.

With outbreaks of infectious disease, another concern is that subsequent decreases in disease rates might reflect not the result of implementation of control measures but rather the natural waning of infection after

---

[4]The kinds of rigorous scientific studies needed to document the effect on tuberculosis or health of hazard reduction strategies in the workplace often would be operationally infeasible, requiring very large numbers of test subjects followed for a very long period under relatively stable conditions. They would also likely raise ethical and political objections.

the pool of most susceptible individuals has been exhausted. Similarly, drops in infection in a workplace could result from the implementation of measures in the community that reduce the number of potential source cases. Some of the studies reviewed below note that new hiring partially refreshed the pool of tuberculin skin test negative workers, and some report that facilities continued to admit substantial numbers of patients with active tuberculosis.

Summaries of Reports

In their review of outbreak reports, Dooley and Tapper (1997) note that the responses to outbreaks have virtually always begun with administrative controls (as recommended and stressed by CDC) to improve prompt identification of people suspicious for active tuberculosis, to make respiratory isolation policies and practices more stringent, and to implement initial treatment regimens that cover the prevalent drug-resistant strains of tuberculosis. The next steps typically involve engineering controls (e.g., the installation, maintenance, and monitoring of negative-pressure isolation rooms). The timing of policies and the specific practices involving respiratory protections appears to be more variable, partly because recommendations about respirators changed several times in the first half of the 1990s.

Individual Reports

Below are summarized three of the more complete analyses of associations between facility implementation of tuberculosis control measures and worker risk of infection with *M. tuberculosis*. Three less complete studies are then briefly described.

Grady Memorial Hospital (Atlanta)   After an outbreak of drug-sensitive tuberculosis in 1991 and early 1992, Grady Memorial Hospital initiated a number of new tuberculosis control policies and practices during the period from March to July 1992 (Blumberg et al., 1995). The descriptions of the interventions and the subsequent monitoring of skin test conversions and other results are among the most thorough in the literature. The study's authors conclude that these practices halted the transmission of *M. tuberculosis*.

Beginning in March 1992, Grady Memorial Hospital implemented a new, more stringent policy of respiratory isolation of patients with known or suspected tuberculosis. Notably, respiratory isolation was required for all patients for whom smears for acid-fast bacilli (AFB) and culture were ordered and for all patients with HIV infection (or risk factors for HIV infection if serology results were unavailable) who had abnormal chest radiographs. In addition, isolation was to be stopped only after three negative AFB smears. At the same time, the hospital began to intensify its physician education efforts. As an interim measure, it also added window fans to 90 rooms to provide negative-pressure isolation. In June 1992, masks with submicron filters were adopted for personal respiratory protection. In July 1992, the hospital began requiring skin testing of non-employee health care workers including attending physicians, house staff, and medical students. A tuberculosis nurse epidemiologist joined the hospital that same month. (Since 1994, additional refinements including the use of N95 respirators have been adopted.) The study notes some problems, for example, an average failure rate of 16 percent for negative-pressure rooms during routine testing conducted every three months.

Table 6.2 summarizes the reported changes in patient admissions and exposure episodes at Grady Memorial Hospital. The number of tuberculosis patients admitted per month dropped slightly from a pre-intervention level of 23 per month to 20 per month for the period during and after the introduction of the new precautions. Nonetheless, exposure episodes and isolation failures dropped substantially, from a preintervention level of 4.4 (July 1991 through December 1991) to 0.6 per month during the last postintervention period studied (January 1994 through June 1994).

Nonetheless, skin test conversion rates for employees fell from a mean of 3.3 percent (July through December 1992) to 0.4 percent (January through June 1994) over the time interval studied. A later analysis reports that conversion rates also decreased for Emory University house staff whose rotation included Grady Memorial Hospital (Blumberg et al., 1998).

A subsequent analysis of skin test conversion rates for the period July 1994 through October 1998 suggests the continued effectiveness of Grady's

TABLE 6-2. Results of Interventions at Grady Memorial Hospital

Measure	Preintervention (7/91–2/92)	Intervention/ Postintervention (3/92–6/94)	P
No. of tuberculosis admissions	184	568	
No. of admissions/month AFB	23 (12.9)	20 (12.8)	
No. of exposure episodes/month	4.4	0.6	
No. of exposure days/month	35.4	3.3	< 0.001
No. of patients not appropriately isolated/total no. of patients isolated (%)	35/103 (34)	18/358 (5)	< 0.001
No. of HIV infected patient admissions associated with exposure episodes/total no. of episodes (%)	22/33 (67)	7/143 (5)	< 0.001

SOURCE: Blumberg et al. (1995) as summarized in Appendix D.

tuberculosis control measures (Blumberg, 1999). A multivariate analysis found no association between tuberculin skin test conversions and patient contact (frequent contact versus no contact). The analysis did, however, show an association between skin conversions and bacille Calmette-Guérin (BCG) vaccination, lower salary levels, and shorter time of employment. This suggests that community exposure was likely important for lower-salary workers, who probably come from parts of Atlanta with high rates of active tuberculosis.

Jackson Memorial Hospital (Miami)   From 1988 to 1990, Jackson Memorial Hospital in Miami experienced an outbreak of multidrug-resis-tant tuberculosis related to patient-to-patient transmission on an HIV ward (Beck-Sague et al., 1992; Fischl et al., 1992; Wenger et al., 1995). After reviewing their infection control policies and work practices, hospital managers implemented a series of more stringent tuberculosis control measures (Wenger et al., 1995). The first control measures, which were implemented in March 1990, included a four-drug initial treatment regi-men and more rigorous isolation policies on the ward (i.e., stricter isola-tion criteria for HIV infected patients, stricter criteria for discontinuing isolation; stricter enforcement of policies that infectious patients stay in their rooms unless medically necessary and wear surgical mask when out of their rooms, and restriction of sputum induction procedures to isola-tion rooms). In April 1990, the hospital repaired improperly functioning isolation rooms and improved the ventilation in other rooms. In June 1990, the hospital instituted a policy that aerosolized pentamidine would be administered only in isolation rooms. In the following months the hospital switched respiratory protections for health care workers from a surgical mask to a submicron mask (September 1990), established and staffed a separate unit for tuberculosis control (October 1990), added labo-ratory staff to improve turnaround times for specimen results (December 1990), required isolation for all patients with multidrug-resistant tubercu-losis (February 1991), and switched to dust-mist respirators (April 1992). NIOSH checked the ventilation in the isolation rooms, and hospital staff checked negative pressure daily. Implementation of other practices (e.g., keeping doors to isolation rooms closed, and wearing of respirators) was checked by observation.

The effects of these changes were monitored for three time periods: January through May 1990 (which overlaps the first interventions), June 1990 through February 1991 (which overlaps most of the remaining inter-ventions), and March 1991 through June 1992. The investigators found that all patients with multidrug-resistant tuberculosis who were admitted during the first monitoring period had been exposed to other such pa-tients while on the HIV ward. In contrast, none of the patients with multidrug-resistant disease admitted during the subsequent monitoring periods had infection traceable to their stay on the ward during those periods. When workers on the HIV ward were compared to workers on a control ward that did not admit HIV infected patients, the former group had significantly higher skin test conversions rates during the outbreak period from January 1988 through January 1990 (Beck-Sague et al., 1992). Rates for the two groups of health care workers did not differ significantly for the period from June 1990 through June 1992 (Wenger et al., 1995).

The study authors note that although the "density" of patients with multidrug-resistant disease declined after the initial monitoring period, "infectious patients were still present and the potential for transmission still existed" (p. 239). Indeed, two of the three skin test conversions in the follow-up period occurred in workers who were exposed to a patient who had previously been diagnosed with tuberculosis but who was thought to be no longer infectious. This led to a requirement that all patients with multidrug-resistant tuberculosis be isolated upon admission. Following the implementation of this policy, no further tuberculin skin test conversions were reported among health care workers. The study authors concluded that most of the effect of the controls came before complete implementation of the engineering controls and respiratory protections and, thus, were likely due to administrative controls.

Cabrini Medical Center (New York City) Another report following an outbreak of multidrug-resistant tuberculosis tracked the sequential adoption of tuberculosis control measures from June through October 1991 (Maloney et al., 1995). The control measures included stricter isolation criteria and use of molded surgical masks for employees (June), improved laboratory services (July), increase from no isolation rooms (0 of 10) with negative pressure to a majority of rooms (16 of 27) with negative pressure (September), and use of an isolation chamber for sputum induction and administration of inhaled pentamidine (October).

The initial assessment of worker tuberculin skin test conversions found similar conversions rates during the preintervention period (January 1990 to June 1991) and the intervention period (July 1991 through August 1992). When the analysts categorized workers by job category and ward location, however, they found higher conversion rates during the 18-month preintervention period for workers on wards serving tuberculosis patients than for workers on other wards (16.7 versus 2.8 percent). In contrast, during the 13-month intervention period, rates for the comparison groups differed little (5.1 versus 4.0 percent). When analysts categorized workers by whether or not they had direct patient contact, the difference in rates was smaller for the preintervention period (6.4 percent for those with patient contact and 1.0 percent for those without patient contact) and the change during the intervention period was less (4.7 percent compared with 2.3 percent). Analysts examined worker age, race, and BCG vaccination status and concluded that these factors could not account for the differences in skin test conversion rates. They also found no clustering of conversions by the worker's zip code of residence. The analysts concluded that "the combination of source and environmental controls together with the use of molded surgical masks were all effective in reducing tuberculin skin test conversions among health care workers" (p. 94). The individual effects of different measures could not be isolated.

Other New York City Studies   Three additional studies in different New York City hospitals also suggest the effectiveness of tuberculosis control measures. The first report (from Roosevelt Hospital) had insufficient data to analyze skin test conversions for workers (Stroud et al., 1995). For patients, it concluded that the implementation of stricter isolation policies was associated with reduced delays in initiating isolation and reduced rates of patient-to-patient transmission of tuberculosis.

In a second study at St. Clare's Hospital, analysts reported decreases in skin test conversions for medical house staff concurrent with the adoption of more stringent isolation policies, the initial installation of negative-pressure isolation rooms, and adoption of a new kind of respirator. The conversion rates fell from 20.7 percent for the 6-month preintervention period to 7 percent during next 6 months (Fella et al., 1995). Subsequent adoption of particulate and then dust-mist-fume respirators was not associated with any further consistent pattern of decreases in conversion rates. The report did not include information on employee demographics. The study's authors commented that they had a steady inflow of new workers with negative tuberculin skin tests, so "we do not think that our decrease in [tuberculin skin test] conversions is simply the result of an exhaustion of susceptible persons" (Fella et al., 1995, p. 355). However, given inadequacies in the previous skin testing program it was possible that there was "a backlog of 2 years of conversions" in the 20.7 percent rate reported for the first period studied (Fella et al., 1995, p. 355).

A third study at Columbia-Presbyterian Medical Center of the sequential adoption of stricter tuberculosis control measures examined skin test conversions for medical house staff from June 1992 to June 1994 (Bangsberg et al., 1997). The largest drop (from 5.1 to 0 conversions per 100 person-years) occurred after the adoption of a more rigorous isolation policy (administrative controls) and the construction of isolation rooms in the emergency department (engineering controls). This drop occurred before the adoption of new respiratory protections. The number of tuberculosis patients seen remained steady. The authors conclude that stricter isolation policies contribute the most to decreases in skin test conversion rates. They did not report information on employee demographics.

Summary of Individual Reports Notwithstanding their limitations, taken together, the studies reviewed above suggest that implementation of tuberculosis control measures can help end outbreaks and prevent new transmission of *M. tuberculosis*. They support the logic of CDC's emphasis on the primacy of administrative controls, in particular, rigorous respiratory isolation policies to reduce exposure opportunities by promptly identifying, evaluating, and isolating people with signs and symptoms suspicious for tuberculosis. The studies suggest some positive effects from engineering controls, which come second in CDC's hierarchy of controls, but their contributions are hard to disentangle from the effects of previously or simultaneously adopted administrative controls. Personal respirators did not appear to play a significant role in ending outbreaks of tuberculosis.

In recent years, hospitals may also have benefited from changes in the treatment patterns including both a shift from inpatient to outpatient treatment for people with infectious tuberculosis and the availability of more effective treatments for AIDS that have reduced the need for inpatient care. Continued reports of outbreaks in correctional facilities in South Carolina and Pennsylvania (see Chapter 5) suggest the need for better information on surveillance programs and other tuberculosis control measures in these settings.

Other Studies and Reports

In addition to the reports reviewed above, the committee found some additional relevant studies that involved mostly low-risk or stable settings.[5] One study reviewed tuberculosis control measures in 13 midwestern hospitals, all but one of which were categorized as low or very low risk for transmission of tuberculosis. The researchers did not find an association between the kinds of tuberculosis control measures adopted and worker skin test conversion rates (Woeltje et al., 1997). The study did not examine isolation policies, and the authors noted that compliance with written policies for other measures was imperfect.

In one of the few studies examining a single control measure, Behrman and Shofer (1998) report on an emergency department that adopted improved engineering controls while leaving isolation and respiratory pro-

---

[5]Appendix D reviews several surveys that asked questions about the implementation of tuberculosis control measures and about results of worker skin testing programs. Analyses of the association between control measures and conversion rates produced inconsistent results. Given the variations in response rates, the limited detail possible in survey responses, and similar concerns, the committee did not find that these analyses contributed to its understanding of the effects of the CDC guidelines.

tection protocols unchanged.[6] The controls included installation of four isolation rooms, improved general-area ventilation, and installation of Plexiglas shields for registration personnel. The researchers compared skin test conversion rates for emergency department personnel and other hospital personnel. (The two groups did not differ significantly in age, ethnicity, foreign birth, county of residence, BCG vaccination status, or initial tuberculin skin test status.) The department implemented tuberculosis control measures at the end of the first year for which conversion rates were compared. In that year, emergency department personnel had significantly higher conversion rates than other hospital personnel (12 versus 2 percent). In the year after the measures were adopted, the rates did not differ significantly (0.0 percent for emergency department personnel compared with 1.2 percent for other workers).

In one of the few studies in a correctional facility, Puisis and colleagues (1996) reported on the introduction of radiographic screening in the Cook County Jail as part of the intake medical evaluation process. The new technology reduced the time from jail entry to isolation to 2.3 days from 17.5 days. During the period from March 1992 through December 1997, jail health care staff screened more than 445,000 inmates and found 206 cases of active tuberculosis (46.2 per 100,000 population) from the radiographic screening alone (McAuley, 2000). Staff concluded that screening had been cost-effective but noted that decreasing tuberculosis case rates could change the picture in the future.

Finally, a few studies have attempted to model the contributions of engineering controls and respiratory protections to preventing transmission of tuberculosis.[7] Summarizing the results of one such effort, Fennelly and Nardell (1998) suggest that the "risk of occupational tuberculosis probably can be lowered considerably by using relatively simple respirators combined with modest room ventilation rates for the infectious aero-

---

[6]Menzies and colleagues, in an article published after the committee concluded its analyses, reported a cross-sectional study of 17 Canadian hospitals. It showed skin test conversions "strongly associated with inadequate ventilation in general patient rooms [and bronchoscopy rooms] and with type and duration of work, but not with ventilation of isolation rooms" (Menzies et al., 2000, p. 779). The authors suggest that this association reflects the "exposure in nonisolation rooms of undiagnosed patients . . . [who] are known to pose the greatest risk to hospital workers" (p. 788). In the higher risk hospitals, the room changes per hour in the negative-pressure isolation rooms averaged between 6.1 and 9.4. The 1994 CDC guidelines recommend a minimum of 6 air changes per hour for negative-pressure isolation rooms and 12 air changes per hour where feasible (CDC, 1994b).

[7]Modeling studies are important for the assessment of risk in a number of situations, for example, when levels of a hazard are low, slow to produce observable effects, or difficult to measure directly. They may likewise be useful when the effect of an intervention is expected to be small. In such situations, clinical studies may be impractical or ethically dubious, and epidemiologic studies may be of limited use because they can not detect effects of intervention without very large numbers of subjects or very long periods of time, or both.

sols likely to be present in isolation rooms of newly diagnosed patients" (p. 754). For workers involved in cough-inducing procedures for infectious patients, more sophisticated respirators may be needed to protect workers adequately. The benefit to workers of using respirators is probably minimal if patients are being properly treated in properly ventilated isolation rooms.

Another modeling exercise reported by Barnhart and colleagues (1997) came to generally similar conclusions but placed greater emphasis on cumulative risk over a worker's lifetime. The authors concluded that higher-level respiratory protection (more than a disposable mask respirator) was reasonable for workers in higher-risk situations (e.g., those performing bronchoscopies or those treating highly infectious patients or patients with multidrug-resistant disease).

A Chicago study suggests the ineffectiveness of personal respirators when adequate administrative and engineering controls are lacking. Kenyon and colleagues (1997) reported an outbreak of multidrug-resistant tuberculosis in a facility that provided and fit tested workers with high-efficiency particulate respirators but that had no isolation rooms that met CDC criteria. Three of the 11 previously skin test-negative workers whose tuberculin skin test result converted to positivity (including a ward secretary with no patient care responsibilities) had no contact with the source case patients. The authors conclude that a respiratory protection program alone cannot protect all workers. In the absence of appropriate isolation rooms, air that escapes from rooms housing infectious patients can infect those outside the room. Delays in recognizing and treating infectious patients also contributed to the outbreak. (Appendix F presents additional background on personal respiratory protection as a tuberculosis control measure.)

COMMITTEE CONCLUSIONS

When the resurgence of tuberculosis began in the mid-1980s in the United States, communities and workplaces were generally not prepared. After years of effective treatment and declining tuberculosis case rates, tuberculosis control measures—including those recommended by CDC in 1983—were not priorities for either public or occupational health programs. The epidemic of HIV infection and AIDS and public health and medical responses to the epidemic were still emerging issues, and the interaction of that epidemic with tuberculosis was not well documented or understood. Similarly, the threat of multidrug-resistant disease was not yet clearly appreciated.

Much has happened in the past 15 years. Certainly, the epidemiology of tuberculosis has changed, with case rates again in decline since 1993. Virtually all states have shown decline, although relatively high rates of tuberculosis persist in a number of states and communities. The special vulnerability of people with suppressed immune systems is now recognized, and the threat of multidrug-resistant disease and the conditions that give rise to it (primarily, incomplete and inadequate treatment of tuberculosis) are clearly understood. The tuberculosis control components of community health programs are better funded and better focused on measures that prevent spread of the disease including directly observed therapy for patients with active tuberculosis.

For most hospitals, prisons, and other facilities, these external changes have decreased the likelihood that employees will see someone with diagnosed or undiagnosed active tuberculosis. These changes have also raised the visibility and understanding of the disease.

Nonetheless, with more than 17,000 cases reported nationally in 1999, tuberculosis remains a threat. Inattention to community and workplace measures to control and prevent transmission of *M. tuberculosis* could lead to another, potentially more serious resurgence of tuberculosis. Thus, it is important to assess how workplace tuberculosis control measures are being implemented and how well they are working.

The changing environment for workplaces makes it difficult, however, to assess the effects of workplace tuberculosis control programs. This difficulty is compounded by the practical problems of conducting rigorous, well-controlled research on these programs, which have often implemented multiple measures simultaneously. Nonetheless, after reviewing the literature (including theoretical arguments and mathematical models), considering discussions during the committee's public meetings, and drawing on its members' experiences and judgments, the committee reached several conclusions about, first, the implementation and, second, the probable effects of workplace tuberculosis control measures. Whether regulations may be needed to sustain or increase rates of compliance with tuberculosis control measures is considered in Chapter 7.

Implementation of Tuberculosis Control Measures

The information base for the following conclusions applies mainly to hospitals and to a lesser extent to prisons. The committee expects that the consistent, correct implementation of control measures may be more difficult in other institutions such as jails and homeless shelters, which generally lack the resources, oversight, and expertise available to hospitals. These workplaces may also differ in the degree to which managers and workers understand and accept tuberculosis as a risk and tuberculosis control measures as necessary.

Most reports reviewed by the committee predate the 1994 guidelines, but the basic measures recommended have remained reasonably stable.

The conclusions below relate only to the implementation of tuberculosis control measures; the following section considers their effects.

Institutional departures from recommended tuberculosis control policies and procedures were common, if not the norm, in the late 1980s and the early 1990s. In large measure, the neglect that characterized community tuberculosis control programs (IOM, 2000) appears to have been duplicated in hospitals, correctional facilities, and, probably, but with less documentation, other facilities that serve people at increased risk of the disease. Even after public health authorities and newspapers were describing the resurgence of tuberculosis in the latter half of the 1980s, surveys in the early 1990s suggested that hospitals and prisons were neglecting recommended surveillance, isolation, and other measures that had been reinforced in 1990 CDC guidelines. Reports of tuberculosis outbreaks in hospitals also document lapses in infection control measures.

Hospitals and correctional facilities reported increased implementation of tuberculosis control measures by the mid-1990s. By 1996, for hospitals and correctional facilities, responses to national surveys and some other studies were showing much more complete and consistent reported compliance with recommended tuberculosis control measures. The hospitals experiencing outbreaks in the early 1990s clearly had a stimulus to implement control measures earlier. For other institutions, increased implementation likely reflects the impacts of further and more complete reports on workplace outbreaks of tuberculosis, the CDC's increased effort to educate health care managers and clinicians about tuberculosis and tuberculosis control measures, the pressure for action exerted by unions on both employers and public agencies, and the initiation by OSHA of enforcement procedures and rulemaking processes for occupational tuberculosis. Data do not allow the committee to draw conclusions about trends for other settings.

Implementation appears to be most complete for administrative controls including respiratory isolation policies. For engineering controls, the installation of negative-pressure isolation rooms has increased, but ventilation performance and performance monitoring may still fall short of recommendations. Information about organizational implementation of the various elements of personal respiratory protection programs is limited. Most studies suggest that most employers have been providing some kind of protection (surgical masks or respirators) and that they have changed the devices provided as new options, such as N95 respirators, have been certified.

Written policies have not necessarily been translated into routine practice. High levels of compliance with control measures, as reported in surveys, may not be matched by high compliance on a day-to-day basis. Although on-site reviews that match hospital policies to actual practices are limited, they suggest the need for some caution in accepting survey responses as conclusive. Departures from guidelines occur at both the institutional level (e.g., provision of respirators and installation of negative-pressure isolation rooms) and the individual level (e.g., use of respirators and closing doors of isolation rooms). Whether less than total compliance makes a practical difference in preventing workplace transmission of tuberculosis is a separate question.

Effects of Tuberculosis Control Guidelines

The caveats cited for implementation also apply to the following conclusions about the effects of tuberculosis control measures. In addition, the committee could not readily disentangle the effects of the CDC guidelines from environmental influences including the effects of community public health measures, regulatory actions by OSHA and others, and the changing epidemiology of the disease. Furthermore, because control measures were often introduced simultaneously or close in time, the relative contribution of individual measures is difficult to distinguish. Finally, the committee could reach no conclusions about what level of compliance with different measures might be sufficient to prevent transmission of *M. tuberculosis* under different workplace conditions.

Again, the conclusions presented below apply primarily to hospitals. The picture for other workplaces is less clear.

Overall, the measures recommended by CDC for prevention of the transmission of tuberculosis in health care facilities have contributed to the ending of outbreaks of tuberculosis and the prevention of new outbreaks. This conclusion rests primarily on several outbreak reports and on information from institutions that did not report outbreaks but reduced skin test conversion rates after implementing control measures. Although each report has its limitations, taken together they show consistent results.

The hierarchy of control measures recommended by CDC is supported by studies of tuberculosis outbreaks in hospitals as well as by logic and biologic plausibility. Outbreak studies support CDC's stress on administrative controls, in particular, application of protocols to reduce opportunities for worker or patient exposure to *M. tuberculosis* through prompt identification and isolation of people with signs and symptoms suspicious for infectious tuberculosis. Outbreak studies and modeling exercises suggest that engineering controls also make a contribution in limiting the transmission of tuberculosis. Although outbreak studies suggest that most of the benefit of control measures comes from administrative and engineering controls, modeling exercises support the tailoring of personal respiratory protections to the level of risk faced by workers—that is, more stringent protection for those in high-risk situations and less stringent measures for others.

The Limits of Control Measures

Tuberculosis control measures cannot be expected to prevent all worker exposure to tuberculosis, especially in areas with moderate to high rates of tuberculosis. Although control measures have helped end workplace outbreaks of the disease and prevent transmission of M. tuberculosis, they cannot be expected to prevent all exposures. Not all individuals with infectious tuberculosis have evident symptoms or signs of the disease, so workers may be exposed to them for some time before tuberculosis is suspected and a diagnosis is made. In addition, opportunities will exist for exposure in emergency departments and elsewhere before infectious individuals are recognized and isolation protocols can be applied and completed. Conscientious implementation of guidelines does not guarantee that transmission will never occur, but it appears to reduce risk significantly, especially in high-prevalence areas.

In communities with little or no tuberculosis, the effectiveness of control measures is necessarily limited. If success in community control of tuberculosis continues, more communities can be expected to join this low-prevalence group. Nonetheless, given the mobility of the U.S. population including immigrants from high-prevalence countries, it can be expected that people with infectious tuberculosis will occasionally appear in low-prevalence communities and their health care facilities. For example, in 1997, just 2 percent of the U.S. population lived in counties that had had no reported cases of tuberculosis in 5 years (Geiter, 1999).[8]

As noted in Chapter 5, workers in low-prevalence areas who encounter someone with infectious tuberculosis may be at higher risk of exposure than their colleagues in high-prevalence areas. They are less likely to be familiar with and alert to the disease's signs and symptoms and may be less likely to have protective engineering controls in place in the emergency departments and other areas where such individuals are first encountered.

SUMMARY

In the late 1980s and early 1990s, institutional departures from recommended tuberculosis control policies and procedures were widespread.

---

[8]By using CDC data and a definition of tuberculosis elimination as no cases in 5 years, 587 of 3,142 (19 percent) counties in the United States could be considered tuberculosis free as of 1997 (Geiter, 1999). Of the counties with no tuberculosis from 1993 to 1995, 75 percent had no cases in the next 2 years and an additional 19 percent only had one case in either 1996 or 1997. Another definition of tuberculosis elimination is a case rate of less than 1 per 1 million population. Starting from a case rate of 74 per 1 million population in 1997, it would take 50 years to reach the elimination target if case rates were declining at an average annual rate of 5 percent and 41 years to reach the elimination target if case rates were declining at an average annual rate of decline of 10 percent. The average yearly rate of decline in recent years has been about 7 percent.

By the mid-1990s, hospitals, correctional facilities, and possibly other facilities began to report higher levels of adherence to CDC recommendations. On-site inspections and other data suggest the need for caution in assuming that written tuberculosis control policies represent routine institutional or worker practice.

Implementation of tuberculosis control measures appears to have contributed to ending outbreaks of tuberculosis and preventing new ones. Outbreak studies as well as logic, biologic plausibility, and modeling exercises support CDC's hierarchy of tuberculosis control measures. That hierarchy stresses administrative controls (in particular, rigorous application of protocols to promptly identify and isolate people with signs and symptoms suspicious for infectious tuberculosis), followed by engineering controls and, finally, by personal respiratory protections. Especially in high-prevalence areas, occasional worker exposure to patients with infectious tuberculosis can still be expected, despite the implementation of generally effective protocols for respiratory isolation.

7

Regulation and the Future of Tuberculosis in the Workplace

Of the three questions considered by the Institute of Medicine, the most difficult was: what will be the likely effects on tuberculosis infection, disease, or mortality of an anticipated Occupational Safety and Health Administration (OSHA) standard to protect workers from occupational exposure to tuberculosis? The committee quickly realized—on the basis of conversations with OSHA staff and others—that the final standard on occupational tuberculosis would likely differ from the proposed rule in some important respects. The committee could not, however, be certain of the specific ways in which the proposed rule and the final standard would differ or when the standard would be published.

Therefore, rather than concentrate narrowly on individual features of the proposed rule, the committee decided to consider more generally the potential for a final standard to affect the transmission of tuberculosis. Possible effects include both benefits (e.g., cases of active tuberculosis prevented) and harms (e.g., unnecessary treatment following a false-positive tuberculin skin test result). The committee's charge and the time and resources given to it did not provide for an assessment of the costs or cost-effectiveness of implementing an OSHA standard or for an evaluation of policy options and recommendations.

During its 6 months of study and deliberation, the committee considered both positive and negative assessments of the need for OSHA regulations on occupational tuberculosis. On one side is the view that regulation is necessary to (1) achieve more complete, consistent, and long-term compliance with recommended tuberculosis control measures, especially in nonhospital settings, (2) prevent the kind of complacency about tuberculosis that characterized public health and workplace programs in the 1980s, and (3) extend additional financial and other protections to workers not provided for by voluntary tuberculosis control guidelines. On the other side is the view that (1) the rate of compliance with the tuberculosis control measures recommended by the Centers for Disease Control and Prevention (CDC) is already high; (2) even with the less than full compliance, the measures implemented have been effective; and (3) an OSHA standard would be inflexible, unnecessarily burdensome, and not easily changed to reflect revisions that might result from CDC's recently initiated review of its 1994 guidelines for health care facilities.

The next section of this chapter examines the context in which an OSHA standard would be implemented and the conditions that would need to be met for the standard to have positive effects on tuberculosis infection, disease, or mortality. The section also reviews OSHA's projections of the number of workplace cases of tuberculosis infection, disease, and mortality that would be prevented if the 1997 proposed rule were implemented. The final section of the chapter considers the relationship between workplace and community tuberculosis control programs. As in previous chapters, most of the available information concerns hospitals.

POTENTIAL EFFECTS OF AN OSHA STANDARD ON OCCUPATIONAL TUBERCULOSIS

Changing Environment

Any assessment of the potential effects of an OSHA standard must recognize the changes in communities and workplaces since OSHA announced its rule-making process in 1994. Even though only 3 years have passed since the proposed rule was issued in 1997, much of the analysis for the rule was developed earlier and relied on 1994 or older data. The epidemiology of tuberculosis has changed substantially in recent years. In addition, health care and correctional facilities appear to have more fully adopted the kinds of tuberculosis control measures described by CDC and OSHA.

As described earlier in this report, declining tuberculosis case rates have now been confirmed for the United States for 7 straight years. After increasing by 13 percent between 1985 and 1992, tuberculosis cases rates declined by 35 percent between 1993 and 1999. The rates of multidrug-resistant tuberculosis have also decreased significantly in recent years, from 3.5 percent in 1991 to 1.2 percent in 1999. (Resistance to isoniazid dropped from 8.4 in 1993 to 7.2 in 1999.) These improvements can be attributed at least in part to better funding of community tuberculosis control programs, increased attention to AIDS patients and other groups at increased risk, wider adoption of directly observed therapy, declining rates of human immunodeficiency virus (HIV) infection or AIDS, and improved implementation of tuberculosis control measures in hospitals, prisons, and, perhaps, other congregate settings.

Despite progress in efforts to control and prevent tuberculosis in the community, a few big cities still count hundreds of cases each year and occasional workplace outbreaks of the disease continue to be documented. In 1997, only two percent of the U.S. population lived in counties that might be described as "tuberculosis free," meaning that they had had no cases of tuberculosis in 5 years (Geiter, 1999; see also note in Chapter 6). Continued community and workplace efforts to prevent and control tuberculosis should help enlarge this percentage. Conversely, neglect of tuberculosis control measures could help create the conditions for a new, potentially more dangerous resurgence of the disease.

Conditions for an Effective OSHA Standard

Given the limited information and time available to the committee as well as the uncertainty about the actual content of a final standard, the committee concluded that it could not reasonably develop any quantitative estimate of the likely health effects of an OSHA standard. Instead, it identified three assumptions or conditions that would have to be met for an OSHA standard to have positive effects on tuberculosis infection, disease, and mortality.

Condition 1. Implementation of workplace tuberculosis control measures as recommended by CDC and proposed by OSHA must contribute meaningfully to prevention of the transmission of *Mycobacterium tuberculosis* in hospitals and other covered workplaces.

Condition 2. An OSHA standard must sustain or increase the level of adherence to workplace tuberculosis control measures, especially in high-risk institutions and communities.

Condition 3. An OSHA standard must allow reasonable flexibility to adapt tuberculosis control measures to fit differences in the level of risk facing workers.

Condition 1. Does implementation of tuberculosis control measures as recommended by CDC and proposed by OSHA help prevent transmission of M. tuberculosis in hospitals and other covered workplaces?

Overall, the committee finds that recommended tuberculosis control measures are effective. In Chapter 6, the committee concluded that more attentive implementation of these measures contributed to the ending of outbreaks of tuberculosis in hospitals and to the prevention of new outbreaks.

The most important measures appear to be administrative controls, in particular, policies and procedures aimed at promptly identifying, isolating, and treating people with infectious tuberculosis.

In addition to the CDC guidelines, hospitals may have been influenced by OSHA's efforts to enforce the adoption of tuberculosis control measures under the agency's general-duty clause and its respiratory protection standard. Likewise, after 1997, the expectation that a permanent OSHA standard would be issued may have played a role. Some state regulatory agencies and private accrediting organizations were also enforcing infection control requirements during the 1990s.

Because most of the information located by the committee dealt with hospitals, the committee could not reach conclusions about the effectiveness of tuberculosis control measures in these workplaces. To various degrees, these workplaces differ from hospitals and each other in physical environments, resources available, populations served, and range of tasks undertaken by different categories of workers. These workplaces may also differ in the level of management and worker understanding and acceptance of the threat of tuberculosis and the need for control measures. In principle, however, basic control measures such as screening to promptly identify and isolate those with symptoms and signs of tuberculosis should help prevent transmission of M. tuberculosis in prisons and other congregate settings serving populations at increased risk of tuberculosis.

Tuberculosis control measures cannot be expected to prevent all worker exposure to the disease. In areas with moderate to high levels of tuberculosis, occasional worker exposure to patients with infectious tuberculosis can be expected. For example, opportunities for exposure will exist in emergency departments and other "intake" areas before infectious individuals are recognized and isolation protocols can be applied and completed. Furthermore, not all individuals with infectious tuberculosis have easily recognized symptoms or signs of the disease, so workers may be exposed to them for some time before tuberculosis is suspected and diagnosed. Conscientious implementation of tuberculosis control measures does not guarantee that transmission will never occur, but it appears to reduce risk significantly, especially in high-prevalence areas.

Condition 2. Will an OSHA standard help sustain or increase the level of adherence to effective workplace tuberculosis control measures?

As the past decade's outbreaks of tuberculosis recede in memory and cost control continues as a priority for community and occupational health programs, the potential once again exists for communities and workplaces to neglect the control measures that helped end workplace outbreaks and reverse increases in tuberculosis case rates. The information reviewed in Chapters 5 and 6 suggests that the 1982 and 1990 CDC guidelines were not widely implemented and that lapses in infection control likely contributed to the workplace outbreaks of tuberculosis reported in the late 1980s and early 1990s. The 1994 CDC guidelines appear to be more widely accepted and adopted, albeit with some gaps between formal policies and day-to-day practices. Except to the extent that they have been incorporated as requirements by other public or private agencies, the steps recommended by CDC are voluntary.

On the basis of logic and experience, the *committee expects that an OSHA standard would sustain or increase the rate of compliance with mandated tuberculosis control measures*. First, a national standard is likely to motivate more organizational adherence to tuberculosis control measures than can be achieved by voluntary guidelines, variable state laws, or the threat of bad publicity or litigation in the event of a tuberculosis outbreak. The committee believes that most organizations want to do right as defined by laws, guidelines, ethical principles, and lessons of science or experience. It also believes that compliance with recommended practices can usually be increased by the threat of citation and financial penalties that lies behind regulations.

Second, as argued by OSHA, the committee agrees that a standard will be clearer, more hazard specific, and easier to enforce than either the general-duty clause in OSHA's statute or OSHA's existing standards on respiratory protection. Unlike OSHA's general-duty clause, a standard allows the agency to identify and require actions to abate workplace risks in advance. Unlike OSHA's general standard on respiratory protections, a tuberculosis standard would, in certain respects, be specific to this biologic hazard (e.g., by describing types of hazardous situations—such as entering an isolation room—and identifying respirators or respirator characteristics appropriate to these situations).

Third, by providing a firmer basis for OSHA enforcement actions, a standard should also put workers on stronger ground in identifying and challenging an employer's inadequate implementation of the tuberculosis control measures specified by the standard. Such a challenge need not involve an actual complaint to OSHA. Notifying an employer of deficiencies may be sufficient to prompt corrective action.

One caveat needs to be mentioned, however. State and local government hospitals and other facilities would not be covered by an OSHA standard unless a state had an approved OSHA plan for enforcing the standard in these facilities. The facilities might, however, be subject to other infection control requirements, for example, those set forth in state licensure laws. Also, if a facility such as a state or local correctional used a private contractor to run the facility's medical department, that private contractor would be covered by the standard for its activities and employees.

Condition 3. Will an OSHA standard allow reasonable adaptation of control measures to fit different organizational situations or changing environmental circumstances?

In general, regulations tend to reduce organizational flexibility. Revisions in regulations may also lag behind important changes in the environment or in the problem that gave rise to the regulation in the first place. Although much of the controversy about the flexibility of an OSHA tuberculosis standard focuses on costs or cost-effectiveness, some criticisms—mainly those relating to tuberculin skin testing requirements—involve the potential for inflexible requirements to harm workers' health. (As discussed earlier and below, CDC is reexamining its recommendations on tuberculosis control in health care facilities, including its statements about baseline and periodic tuberculin skin testing.)

The voluntary character of the CDC guidelines ultimately gives employers at any risk level the discretion to tailor their responses to the particular risks faced by their workers. Although some provisions of the 1994 guidelines are described as requirements, CDC has no enforcement power. Also, many statements are not phrased as "shoulds" (much less "musts") but, rather, are presented as suggestions for organizations to consider.

The following discussion compares the flexibility offered by the 1994 CDC guidelines and the 1997 proposed OSHA rule in three areas. The first and most important area involves the provisions of each for assessing the workplace risk of tuberculosis transmission, categorizing workplaces by the level of risk facing workers, and matching tuberculosis control measures to the level of risk. The other two areas involve tuberculin skin testing programs and respiratory protection programs.

Matching Requirements to Risk Level: Facility Risk Assessment

Chapters 1 and 5 make clear that the incidence of tuberculosis varies substantially among communities and that the risk of acquiring infection with *M. tuberculosis* has varied among hospitals and other workplaces. As described in Chapter 4, the 1997 proposed OSHA rule provides some very limited risk-related flexibility by distinguishing two categories of organizations, one of which would face fewer regulatory requirements. To qualify for the "lower risk" category (a label not used in the proposed rule), an organization would have to (1) neither admit nor provide medical services to individuals with suspected or confirmed tuberculosis, (2) have had no confirmed cases of infectious tuberculosis during the previous 12 months, *and* (3) be located in counties that have had no confirmed cases of infectious tuberculosis during 1 of the previous 2 years and fewer than six cases during the other year. Any facility that did not meet all of these criteria would have to meet all of the proposed rule's requirements applicable to its type of work environment.

In contrast, the 1994 CDC guidelines provide for a more complex risk assessment process for health care facilities. That process incorporates more information and differentiates facility risk level and related control measures more finely.[1] The guidelines specify that a health care facility or an area within a facility may be assigned to one of five risk categories: minimal, very low, low, intermediate, and high. For the facilities in the two lowest risk categories, the guidelines recommend considerably fewer control measures.[2]

Even if a facility had admitted no tuberculosis patients, had no tuberculosis cases in its community, and had a policy of referring those with diagnosed or suspected tuberculosis, that facility could not qualify for OSHA's "low risk" category if the surrounding county had reported one case of tuberculosis in each of the preceding 2 years. As discussed in Chapter 4, a facility's service area may not match county boundaries and may have a much different incidence of tuberculosis.

Reasonable flexibility in adoption of tuberculosis control measures does not imply lack of attention to the risk of tuberculosis in low risk facilities. Both the CDC guidelines and the proposed OSHA rule specify that all facilities—even those that have not recently encountered someone with active tuberculosis—should have protocols and trained individuals in place to identify the unexpected infectious individual and then transfer or otherwise manage the person in ways that minimize risks to workers and others. The issue is the degree to which control measures can be matched to tuberculosis risk in the community and in the facility, taking into account the facility's experience in preventing transmission of tuberculosis. The risk assessment criteria described in the CDC guidelines allow for a more sensitive match between control measures and tuberculosis risk than do the criteria in the proposed OSHA rule.

Overall, *the committee concludes that if an OSHA standard follows the 1997 proposed rule it may not offer sufficient flexibility for organizations to adopt control measures appropriate for the level of risk facing workers.* To the extent that an OSHA standard inflexibly extends requirements to institu-

---

[1]As described in Chapter 4, the CDC risk assessment process includes a review of the community tuberculosis profile, the numbers of patients with tuberculosis examined or treated in different areas of the facility, the tuberculin skin test conversion rates for workers in different areas of the facility or in different job categories, and evidence of person-to-person transmission of *M. tuberculosis* resulting in active disease. The process also includes review of medical records to identify possible delays or deficiencies in identifying or treating individuals with infectious tuberculosis. In some cases, it calls for observation of infection control practices.

[2]For the three higher-risk categories, the CDC recommendations differ primarily in whether they call for certain steps to be taken yearly or more frequently.

tions that are at negligible risk of occupational transmission of *M. tuberculosis*, the standard is unlikely to benefit workers at the same time that it would impose significant costs and administrative burdens on covered organizations and absorb institutional resources that could be applied to other, potentially more beneficial uses.

Requirements for Baseline and Serial Tuberculin Skin Testing

In addition to the broad concerns about whether an OSHA standard would allow sufficient flexibility for organizations to match tuberculosis control measures to the risk facing workers, a narrower question is whether a standard would allow organizations reasonable flexibility to adjust tuberculin skin testing programs to reflect the changing epidemiology of tuberculosis and, possibly, changing CDC recommendations. As described in Chapter 2 and Appendix B, when the prior probability of tuberculosis infection is low because of low prevalence, Bayes' Theorem shows that the probability of false positive test results increases. When prevalence decreases to very low levels, the majority of those with positive tests will not in fact be infected. This, in turn, increases the potential for workers to be treated unnecessarily for latent tuberculosis infection. The most serious possible harm of unnecessary treatment involve a very small risk of liver damage, although this risk is lower than previously thought (Nolan et al., 1999, as discussed in Chapter 2). Less serious potential harms include rashes, gastrointestinal upsets, fever, and joint pain. In addition, some people may suffer needless anxiety or fear related to a false-positive test result or subsequent treatment. Furthermore, the less an individual's social contacts understand about the meaning of a positive test result, the greater the potential for a person's social relationships to be compromised by such a result. Excessive workplace testing and treatment efforts would also waste resources that could be constructively used to support other aspects of a workplace tuberculosis control program.

That the tuberculin skin test has some limitations, especially in low-prevalence environments, does not mean that it is a poor test. It has been a valuable element in tuberculosis control programs, including in outbreak situations and as part of surveillance programs in health care and other facilities in high prevalence areas. Nonetheless, as recommended by the IOM report *Ending Neglect: The Elimination of Tuberculosis in the United States* (IOM, 2000), better diagnostic tests for both infection and active disease are needed.

Recognizing that the circumstances that prompted the 1994 guidelines have changed, the CDC's Advisory Council for the Elimination of Tuberculosis recently recommended that CDC review and, if appropriate, revise the guidelines, including the recommendations for tuberculin skin testing. Such a review is now under way, and the committee understands that new recommendations may be published sometime in 2002. OSHA could adapt its requirements for tuberculin skin testing to changes in CDC recommendations, for example, by declaring departures from the testing requirements in the standard to be *de minimus* violations (i.e., unimportant and not subject to citation or penalty). More straightforward, the standard could be revised to state that OSHA requirements for skin testing would follow CDC recommendations.

Requirements for Respiratory Protection Program

Much of the concern about the 1997 proposed OSHA rule has focused on the requirements for personal respiratory protection. When the CDC guidelines were published in 1994, they, too, were criticized for their recommendations for respiratory protection. Some of the criticism involved the cost and complexity of the limited choice of personal respirators that met the criteria set forth by the CDC in 1994. Much of that criticism abated soon thereafter when the National Institute for Occupational Safety and Health approved the relatively inexpensive and simple N95 respirators.

Earlier sections of this report describe personal respiratory protections as the third element in CDC's hierarchy of tuberculosis control measures. As discussed in Chapter 6, outbreak studies support this hierarchy and suggest that most of the benefit of control measures comes from administrative and engineering controls. Modeling exercises support the tailoring of personal respiratory protections to the level of risk faced by workers—that is, more stringent protection for those in high-risk situations and less stringent measures for others.

The following discussion considers first the workers targeted for respirator use by the 1994 CDC guidelines and the 1997 proposed OSHA rule. It then examines the requirements for fit testing of personal respirators.

Requirements for Respirator Use   Although the respiratory protection requirements of the 1997 proposed OSHA rule have been criticized for inflexibility, the proposed rule and the 1994 CDC guidelines mostly target the same types of workers for use of personal respirators. The wording differs, but both essentially call for workers to be provided personal respirators if they (1) enter isolation rooms housing people with known or suspected infectious tuberculosis, (2) are present when certain high-hazard procedures such as bronchoscopies are performed on individuals with known or suspected tuberculosis,[3] (3) transport such indi-

---

[3] The CDC guidelines (but not the proposed OSHA rule) also mention that workers performing such procedures might sometimes need more protective respirators (e.g., powered air-purifying respirators).

viduals, whether masked or not, in enclosed vehicles, or (4) otherwise work in areas where they may be exposed to contaminated air.[4]

The 1994 CDC guidelines are ambiguous for one low-risk situation involving facilities that are located in communities with tuberculosis, that have a policy of referring tuberculosis patients, and that have not admitted a tuberculosis patient within the preceding year. Workers in such facilities may be exposed to infectious tuberculosis while evaluating a patient in an emergency department or other area. The guidelines advise that these workers "may" need to be included in a respiratory protection program. The 1997 proposed OSHA rule appears to require explicitly that employers provide respirators to such workers if a patient is being evaluated because tuberculosis is suspected.

Although the proposed OSHA rule seems to require the use of personal respirators for workers in a few situations that are not clearly covered by the CDC guidelines, the committee could not determine how many additional employers or employees might be affected. In general, both the proposed rule and the guidelines focus their respirator use provisions on the worker's reasonably anticipated risk of exposure rather than the facility's risk category.

Requirements for Fit Testing   As described in Chapter 4, both the 1994 CDC guidelines and the 1997 proposed OSHA rule provide for initial training and fit testing for workers who use personal respirators. Consistent with the then-applicable 1987 OSHA respiratory protection standard, the 1994 guidelines do not mention annual fit testing. Consistent with the 1998 respiratory protection standard (see Chapter 4), the 1997 proposed OSHA rule provides for an overall respiratory protection program that includes both initital and annual fit testing.

In general, it seems rather a common-sense proposition that any workers who are provided with new safety equipment (such as a personal respiratory device) should also be provided some initial training in the equipment's proper use and maintenance and some continuing education to remind them about when and how it is to be used. Likewise, if the equipment differs by size, shape, or other characteristics to accommodate individual physical differences, then some kind of initial fit evaluation also seems generally plausible.

Administratively, a program for fit of testing personal respirators requires trained personnel to conduct a complicated series of tests. New

---

[4]The CDC guidelines do not specifically mention workers repairing air systems likely to contain airborne *M. tuberculosis*. Such workers would, however, seem to be covered under the guideline's more general language specifying the use of personal respirators by workers in "other settings where administrative and engineering controls are not likely to protect them from inhaling infection airborne droplet nuclei" (CDC, 1994b, p. 97).

equipment reduces the time required to administer the test, but the equipment is expensive and not yet in general use. Scheduling for an annual fit test must allow time for the test as well as time for workers to get to and from the test site (which may be on another floor or in another building). If a worker misses the test, he or she must be rescheduled. If the test itself cannot be provided when scheduled, new times must be scheduled for multiple workers. A requirement for annual retesting multiplies the number of people who must be scheduled and tested each year. The more workers who are covered by an employer's respiratory protection program, the more complex will be the employer's administrative burden and the greater the expense. For large medical centers that treat substantial numbers of tuberculosis patients, annual fit testing can be a major undertaking that involves thousands of workers.

Employers now have two fit testing options. In a *qualitative fit test*, the respirator user reports whether he or she can detect an external aerosol. For example, if the test substance is a saccharin aerosol, users can detect a sweet taste if the respirator does not fit properly (e.g., because of leakage at the face seal surface). In a *quantitative fit test*, the concentration of a marker material inside and outside the mask is determined by relatively complex equipment that produces more accurate results.

In a recently reported laboratory test, McKay and Davies (2000) compared two substances, Bitrex and saccharin, which are commonly used in qualitative fit testing. The researchers found that all 26 test subjects accurately detected leaks in respirators when exposed to Bitrex but that one-third did not identify leaks when saccharin was used. A second study by the same researchers (reported so far only in an abstract), now appears to cast doubt on the use of Bitrex as a fit-testing agent in certain situations (McKay, 2000).

Coffey and colleagues (1999) quantitatively tested the performance of N95 respirators in a simulated workplace setting. They made direct measurements of ambient particles both outside and inside the masks of 25 subjects who wore different types of commercially available respirators. The investigators report considerable model-to-model variability in the degree of protection against filter penetration by the test particles. Additionally, when testers applied the 1 percent pass-fail criterion required by OSHA, a substantial majority of test subjects failed the fit test for 17 of the 21 devices tested, that is, most subjects could not be successfully fitted. (The 1 percent pass-fail criterion is thought to be needed to achieve no more than 10 percent respirator face-seal leakage during normal use in the work place.) A determination that qualitative fit testing is ineffective and that quantitative fit testing is required could add substantial costs to a respiratory protection program, especially one that included annual testing for large numbers of workers. The findings by Coffey and colleagues raise a further serious concern that with quantitative fit testing, most workers might not pass a fit test with the currently available models of the widely used N95 respirator. This suggests that more attention should perhaps be paid to mask performance at the manufacturing and premarketing stage.

A determination that qualitative fit testing is ineffective and that quantitative fit testing is required could add substantial costs to a respiratory protection program, especially one that included annual testing for large numbers of workers. The findings by Coffey and colleagues raise a further serious concern that with quantitative fit testing, most workers might not pass a fit test with the widely used N95 respirator.

The committee found no epidemiologic studies that have evaluated whether qualitative or quantitative fit testing (either initial or annual) for N95 or other respirators used for tuberculosis control improves respirator fit in normal practice as workers treat, transport, guard, or otherwise have contact with people who have known or suspected tuberculosis. Given the relatively small numbers of workers with skin test conversions, it is unlikely that field studies would be sensitive enough to demonstrate whether initial or annual fit testing reduced worker's occupational risk of acquiring tuberculosis infection or active tuberculosis. The committee located no modeling studies that focused specifically on the potential health effects of fit testing.

One small, single-site study has suggested that education about proper fit may be as effective as physical fit testing (Hannum et al., 1996). In that study, a hospital recruited workers to participate in one of three respirator training programs. Researchers then tested the workers on their ability to correctly adjust their respirator's fit and seal. They concluded that training was important but that it did not matter much whether the training included direct fit testing or a classroom demonstration of how workers should fit check their respirator before each use. The devices used in the study were high-efficiency particulate air (HEPA) respirators, which differ from the now widely used N95 respirators. Thus, this study is not directly relevant to N95 respirators.

Flexibility of Respiratory Protection Requirements   Perhaps paradoxically the committee's most daunting challenge was to assess whether the 1997 proposed OSHA rule allowed employers reasonable flexibility to match respiratory protections to the level of risk. Although the group agreed that respiratory protection is the least important of the hierarchy of tuberculosis controls, it also agreed that respirators and respiratory protection programs have a role to play when an occupational risk of tuberculosis exists.

As described in Chapter 6, modeling studies suggest that the benefits of respiratory protection are directly proportional to the presence of risk. In facilities that admit only the occasional individual with tuberculosis or that have a policy of transferring such individuals, workers are likely to see no or very marginal additional protection from an extensive respiratory protection program. In a high-risk setting with many tuberculosis admissions, questionable administrative and engineering controls question, and, especially, cases of multidrug-resistant disease, a rigorous respiratory protection program may be beneficial.

The 1997 proposed OSHA rule allows little flexibility for organizations to adopt respiratory protection programs that reflect the variability in the level of risk facing workers. For low-risk institutions, a proportionately modest program might include the availability of N95 respirators and the training of key individuals in their appropriate use. In high-risk facilities, a program might include a spectrum of respiratory protection devices including N95 respirators for most situations and a more protective respirator for selected high-hazard procedures such as bronchoscopy and autopsy. The education and fit-testing elements of a respiratory protection program would then be tailored to the risk facing different employees.

In both high- and low-risk institutions, the highest priority would still be administrative controls that promote prompt identification and isolation of those with signs and symptoms suspicious for tuberculosis. For institutions that may admit those with tuberculosis, engineering controls are also important.

Given the variability of masks from different manufacturers that was noted earlier, it may be appropriate for policymakers to focus more attention on manufacturers so that generally poor-fitting respirator models are not marketed. In addition, further research and analysis may be useful to examine fit-testing criteria and methods in laboratory versus operational settings and to determine levels of respiratory protection that will reasonably reduce risk in environments posing different degrees of risk to workers.

Summary: Conditions for an Effective OSHA Standard

Overall, the committee concludes that an OSHA tuberculosis standard can have a positive effect if it meets three basic conditions: (1) it is consistent with tuberculosis control measures that appear to be effective, (2) it sustains or increases the level of compliance with those measures, and (3) it allows employers appropriate flexibility to adopt control measures that are matched to the level of risk facing their workers. The committee expects that a standard will meet the first two conditions by sustaining or increasing the rate of use of tuberculosis control measures that appear to be effective. The committee is, however, concerned that if an OSHA standard follows the 1997 proposed rule, it will not meet the third condition of allowing organizations reasonable flexibility to adopt measures appropriate to the level of risk facing their workers.

OSHA's Projections of Averted Infections, Disease, and Mortality from Implementing a Standard on Occupational Tuberculosis

As discussed in Chapter 3, courts have directed OSHA to undertake quantitative risk assessments to justify its standards. Such risk assessments are often difficult because relevant data about the full extent of a workplace hazard and the consequences of control measures are very limited. These difficulties are present in full measure for the assessment of the 1997 proposed rule on occupational tuberculosis.

In the 1997 proposed rule, OSHA presented a quantitative risk assessment that estimated the number of infections, cases of disease, and deaths due to tuberculosis that would be averted by adoption of the rule. OSHA staff had four experts review an earlier version of the risk assessment, and they made some revisions on the basis of the reviewers' comments. In preparation for the issuing of a final standard on occupational tuberculosis, OSHA staff have again revised and updated their estimates. This new analysis was not, however, available to the committee pending publication of the final standard. Therefore, the following comments necessarily apply to the earlier analysis included in the 1997 proposed rule.

Although OSHA published the proposed rule in 1997, much of the data on which it relied were several years older (e.g., a 1994 Washington State survey, 1991 data from Jackson Memorial Hospital in Miami, and a 1984–1985 North Carolina study). As summarized in this chapter, tuberculosis cases, case rates, and deaths have been declining since 1993, and recent studies also suggest low levels of occupational transmission of *M. tuberculosis*. The changing epidemiology of tuberculosis reflects both community and workplace tuberculosis control measures. Given this change, it is not surprising that the assessment presented with the 1997 proposed rule is outdated and that OSHA has revised it. (Again, the revised analysis was not available to the committee.)

Infection with *M. tuberculosis*

In 1997, OSHA defined infection with *M. tuberculosis* as the "material impairment of health." It did so on the basis of both the potential for latent infection to progress to active disease (which is discussed further below) and the risk for adverse health effects from treatment of the infection. As described earlier, although treatment is not risk free and individuals offered treatment should be informed of both benefits and risks, recent data suggest that the risk of liver damage from carefully monitored treatment of latent infection using isoniazid is quite low and is less than that described in the proposed rule.

Estimation of levels of tuberculosis infection and potential reductions in such infections as a result of an OSHA standard is particularly difficult in the absence of any recent systematic data on infection levels on a national or state-by-state basis. The last national survey of infection was undertaken in the early 1970s. As discussed in Chapters 5 and 6 and Appendixes C and D, all studies used to estimate the occupational risk of infection and the effects of tuberculosis control measures have their limitations.

The committee recognizes OSHA's efforts to take some criticisms of its estimating strategy into account. For example, after reviewers criticized the use of 1982 and 1984 Washington State data, in part, because the data were more than 10 years old, OSHA staff substituted data from a 1994 survey. Similarly, after data from a 1984–1985 North Carolina survey were criticized as likely being confounded by cross-reactions to atypical mycobacteria in the central and eastern parts of the state, the analysts used only data from hospitals in western North Carolina. The analysts also adjusted the 1984 data to reflect subsequent decreases in active tuberculosis in the state.

Nonetheless, the committee concludes that OSHA's original estimate that the proposed regulations would reduce yearly work-related tuberculosis infections by 90 percent from 1994 levels (thereby averting 21,400 to 25,800 infections) is overstated.[5] As discussed above, tuberculosis cases and case rates have declined substantially since 1993. Further, the committee is concerned that OSHA's analysis did not adequately recognize the contributions to worker infections of (1) unsuspected and undiagnosed cases of active tuberculosis in the workplace or (2) exposure in the community. One concern involves the choice of the definition for internal control and exposed groups for Washington State data (definition 1 as discussed in 62 FR 201 at Table V-3). Another concern is the use of North Carolina data flawed by very low hospital response rates and inconsistent skin testing procedures.

The committee also has some concerns about OSHA's use of 1991 data from Jackson Memorial hospital, which experienced a 1989 to 1990 outbreak of tuberculosis among patients on an HIV ward. Although the data used were for the year after the conclusion of the outbreak, skin test conver-

---

[5]The agency's state-by-state estimates of the "annual excess risk of tuberculosis infection due to occupational exposure" were defined as "a multiplicative function of the background rate of infection" (62 FR 201 at 54192). The agency then derived its estimates of the background rate of infection on the basis of a mathematical model that assumes that the rate of infection in an area can be "expressed as a numerical function of active tuberculosis cases reported in the same area" (62 FR 201 at 54197). Given the limited time and resources available to it, the committee did not evaluate this mathematical model. In the 1997 proposed rule, OSHA estimates the occupational risk of tuberculosis infection over a 45-year working lifetime to range from 4 to 723 per 1,000 population for hospital workers (with the lowest estimates based on the Washington State data and the highest based on the Jackson Memorial Hospital data).

sions among hospital workers exposed on the HIV ward in late 1990 were recorded in early 1991 (Wenger et al. 1995). Also, tuberculosis control measures (e.g., stricter isolation protocols) were still being implemented on the HIV ward in 1991. The committee questions the appropriateness of using outbreak-affected data as a basis for the high-end estimates of the effects of the proposed regulations on occupationally acquired infections.

Active Tuberculosis

Based on its estimating procedures and assumptions, OSHA concluded that implementation of the proposed rule would prevent each year between 1,477 and 1,744 cases of active tuberculosis among workers covered by the rule (p. 54219, Table VII-3). CDC data raise some questions about the plausibility of these estimates. In its surveillance report for 1999, CDC lists a total of 551 cases of tuberculosis among health care workers and 16 cases among correctional facility workers (CDC, 2000b).[6] This figure is less than two-thirds the number of cases that OSHA predicted would be prevented yearly by the implementation of its proposed rule. Moreover, of the reported cases of active disease reported, some proportion will have been the result of community rather than workplace exposure.

Although the figure is widely cited and used (including by the CDC), the committee also questions OSHA's estimate that 10 percent of workers infected with *M. tuberculosis* would progress to active disease over their lifetimes. Two reviewers of the initial OSHA risk assessment (George Comstock and Bahjat Qaqish) questioned whether this estimate was too high, although a third reviewer (Neil Graham) noted that it was widely accepted (see 62 FR 201 at 54198). In this report's background paper on the occupational risk of tuberculosis (Appendix C), the author (Thomas M. Daniel) likewise questions the 10 percent figure based on data analyses indicating that the rate of progression is probably half that figure or less, especially in populations more likely than average to be treated for latent infection. Most health care workers constitute such a population, although home health workers, workers in homeless shelters, and certain other groups covered by the proposed rule may have less access to health insurance and health care. The committee recognizes that the rate of compliance with treatment for both latent infection and active disease is often

---

[6]Health care and correctional workers account for about 95 percent of those covered by the proposed rule. The CDC data are based on reported occupation within the past 24 months (CDC, 2000b). Most of the progression from infection to active tuberculosis occurs within the first two years following infection. CDC first began collecting occupational data in 1993, but the initial reports are considered less reliable than subsequent ones. In recent years, approximately 500 to 600 cases of tuberculosis among health care workers have been reported yearly.

low, but well-structured programs involving education and directly observed therapy can improve rates of completion of treatment for both conditions (Camins et al., 1996). Recent guidelines from the CDC and the American Thoracic Society strongly recommend treatment for latent infection (ACT/CDC, 2000b).

In sum, the committee believes that the 1997 estimates of cases of active tuberculosis that a rule will avert are overstated on three grounds. First, the estimate is inconsistent with reported data on tuberculosis cases by occupation. Second, the rate of progression from infection to active disease is likely lower than traditionally cited. Third, the estimate of infection levels to which the progression rate is applied is too high. One committee member disagreed with this general assessment. That member argued that the validity and reliability of CDC's own data on tuberculosis case rates by occupation are questionable and that the 10 percent progression figure is reasonable since it continues to be cited by CDC.

Tuberculosis Mortality

In the 1997 proposed rule, OSHA estimated that the proposed rule would prevent between 115 and 136 tuberculosis-related deaths among covered workers each year. (It also estimated that the rule would also avert 23 to 54 additional deaths among family and other contacts of workers.) The committee concludes that the mortality estimates are overstated. First, as discussed above, the committee believes that the estimates of number of tuberculosis cases that would be averted by a standard are too high. Second, the estimated mortality rate used in the assessment does not take into account demographic factors or the effects of treatment.

In the 1997 proposed rule, OSHA estimated that 7.8 percent of all active tuberculosis cases among workers would end in death. It based the estimate on the 3-year average of mortality data reported by CDC for 1989 to 1991 (62 FR 201 at 54207). (More recent CDC surveillance reports apparently include revised numbers for tuberculosis cases and deaths for these years. Based on these numbers, the average case death rate for 1989–1991 is 7.3 percent.) Case mortality rates reported by CDC for recent years are lower: 6.0 percent in 1998, 5.9 percent in 1997, and 5.6 percent in 1996 (CDC, 2000b). (Population mortality rates dropped from 0.8 per 100,000 population in 1989 to 0.6 in 1994 to 0.4 in 1998.) Thus, use of revised and recent tuberculosis case mortality data would reduce the OSHA estimates.

More important, estimates of deaths among health care and other workers should take into account the effects of treatment. The majority of deaths due to tuberculosis occur in individuals in whom the disease is first recognized after death, meaning that their disease was not being treated (Rieder et al., 1991). In addition, the majority of cases of tuberculosis occur among unemployed individuals (CDC, 2000b). Such individuals are likely to have poor access to health care and, thus, to experience serious delays in diagnosis and treatment or to go untreated altogether. Even if all cases of tuberculosis among health care workers were due to occupational acquisition, which is clearly not the case, OSHA's estimates translate into an unrealistic 20 to 25 percent rate of tuberculosis-related mortality based on the number of cases of disease reported by CDC for health care and correctional workers in recent years.

For people with drug-sensitive disease who are diagnosed early and treated fully, the risk of death is very low (Cohn et al., 1990; Combs et al., 1990; Appendix C). Those who have both suppressed immune systems and multidrug-resistant disease, however, run a very high risk of death (Garrett et al., 1999, Appendix C). Fortunately, levels of multidrug-resistant disease are low in the United States and have been declining in recent years.

Unlike unemployed individuals, many workers covered by the proposed OSHA rule tend to have good access to health care and to spend their working day among health care professionals. In general, they should be more likely to be diagnosed relatively early and to be offered prompt, appropriate treatment. The financial protections for workers provided for in the 1997 proposed rule also should encourage workers to seek evaluation and treatment if they suspect they have contracted tuberculosis.

THE WORKPLACE AND THE COMMUNITY

Unlike typical occupational health problems such as those involving hazardous chemicals or dust exposures, the occupational risk of tuberculosis has a close connection to the risk of tuberculosis in the surrounding community. A theme throughout this report has been the interconnection between community risk and workplace risk and the challenge of fitting workplace tuberculosis control measures to these risks and to changes in risks over time.

The committee draws a parallel between the circumstances facing occupational health programs and the circumstances described in the recent report *Ending Neglect: The Elimination of Tuberculosis in the United States* (IOM, 2000). That report attributed the resurgence in tuberculosis in the 1980s to complacency resulting from the striking reduction in disease resulting from effective treatments introduced after World War II. Complacency led to disinterest in the goal of tuberculosis elimination and to the dismantling of tuberculosis control programs. Basic public health measures were neglected, including surveillance activities, contact tracing, outbreak investigations, and case management services to ensure completed treatment of latent infection and active disease. This helped set the stage for the resurgence of tuberculosis in the 1980s when new circumstances emerged—including the HIV and AIDS epidemic, the increase in the rate of multidrug-resistant disease (largely due to incomplete treatment), and expanded immigration from areas with high rates of tuberculosis.

For health care facilities, prisons, and other organizations that serve people at high risk of tuberculosis, a similar pattern of workplace neglect in the late 1980s and early 1990s contributed to workplace outbreaks of tuberculosis. Surveys, investigations of outbreaks, and facility inspections all point to institutionalized lapses in tuberculosis control including inattention to signs and symptoms of infectious tuberculosis, delays in initiating appropriate evaluations and treatments, and improper ventilation of isolation rooms and areas. Outbreaks were, however, concentrated in a relatively small number of states that account for a large proportion of people with HIV infection, immigrants from high-prevalence countries, and cases of multidrug-resistant disease.

Just as community neglect interacted with workplace neglect to set the stage for workplace outbreaks of tuberculosis, it now appears that community control measures have interacted with workplace control measures to help end outbreaks and reduce the potential for new ones. For example, public health efforts to ensure completed treatment of active tuberculosis can be credited with reducing the number and proportion of people appearing in hospitals and other workplaces with highly lethal, multidrug-resistant disease. This has reduced the risk to workers in these settings. At the same time, the implementation in hospitals of better tuberculosis control measures as recommended by CDC has almost certainly reduced the rates of transmission of drug-sensitive and multidrug-resistant tuberculosis not only within hospitals but also in the broader community into which patients are discharged.

The challenge now is to understand and adapt to the decreasing incidence of tuberculosis without re-creating the conditions that will make institutions and workers vulnerable to new and possibly more deadly outbreaks of the disease. Maintaining expertise and vigilance will not be easy assuming that tuberculosis case rates continue to decrease.

Ending Neglect set out a strategy for maintaining long-term vigilance and moving toward the elimination of tuberculosis in the United States. (The report's recommendations are listed in Appendix G.) This strategy stresses (1) better methods for identifying people with recently acquired tuberculosis infection, (2) stronger efforts to effectively treat those who could benefit from treatment of infection, (3) research to develop effective vaccines, (4) more active product development initiatives focused on diagnostic and treatment technologies, and (5) research to tackle the problem of patient and provider failure to follow treatment recommendations.

Many of the recommendations from the earlier report would, if implemented, benefit workplace- as well as community-based tuberculosis control programs. One recommendation calls for research to develop better diagnostic tests and treatments for latent tuberculosis infection and active tuberculosis, a need identified in Chapter 2.[7] Another recommendation is for research on nonadherence to treatment regimens that could be used to develop more effective strategies to promote acceptance and completion of treatment.[8] A third recommendation proposes new approaches to identifying and treating latent tuberculosis infection among high-risk immigrants, who are well represented in the health care workforce.[9] The report stresses that after treatment of active disease, "the second priority is targeted tuberculin skin testing and treatment of latent infection" (IOM, 2000, p. 8). In addition to immigrants from high-prevalence countries, the high-risk groups targeted include prison inmates, people with HIV infection, and homeless individuals. The report also calls for the United States to increase its support for global tuberculosis control. With more than 40 percent of tuberculosis cases in the United States and among health care workers involving people born in other countries, policymakers and public health authorities cannot ignore the international problem of tuberculosis.

In sum, just as tuberculosis risk in the workplace is linked to tuberculosis risk in the community, the risk in American communities is affected by the risk of tuberculosis elsewhere in the world and by migration within and across the nation's borders. Effective tuberculosis control measures in the workplace are one element of a much larger strategy to prevent and eventually eliminate the disease.

---

[7]*Recommendation 5.2.* To advance the development of diagnostic tests and new drugs for both latent infection and active disease, action plans should be developed and implemented. CDC should then exploit its expertise in population-based research to evaluate and define the role of promising products (IOM, 2000).

[8]*Recommendation 5.3.* To promote better understanding of patient and provider nonadherence with tuberculosis treatment recommendations and guidelines, a plan for a behavioral and social science research agenda should be developed and implemented (IOM, 2000).

[9]*Recommendation 4.1* calls for preimmigration tuberculin skin testing of visa applicants from countries with high rates of tuberculosis. Once they have arrived in the United States, those with positive skin tests would, when indicated, be required to complete an approved course of treatment for latent tuberculosis infection before being issued a permanent residency card ("green card"). (Screening and treatment for active tuberculosis are already required.) The report also recommends that the federal government support the cost of such treatment rather than putting the burden on local communities.

References

ACCP (American College of Chest Physicians)/ATS (American Thoracic Society). ACCP Consensus Statement: Institutional control measures for tuberculosis in the era of multiple drug resistance. *Chest* 108:1690–1710, 1995.

Addington WW. Patient compliance: The most serious remaining problem in the control of tuberculosis in the United States. *Chest* 76(6 Suppl):741–743, 1979.

Aguado JM, Ramos JT, and Lumbreras C. Transmission of tuberculosis during a long airplane flight. *New England Journal of Medicine* 335(9):675, 1996.

AHA (American Hospital Association). Technical comments [on] OSHA proposed standard for occupational exposure to tuberculosis. Attachment to letter to Jeffress CN from Pollack R, Washington, D.C., October 5, 1998.

AHCA (American Health Care Association). Written statement submitted to Institute of Medicine Committee on Regulating Occupational Exposure, Washington, D.C., August 31, 2000.

Aitken ML, Anderson KM, and Albert RK. Is the tuberculosis screening program of hospital employees still required? *American Review of Respiratory Diseases* 136:805–807, 1987.

APIC (Association of Professionals in Infection Control and Epidemiology). Comments on the proposed OSHA TB rule. Letter to Docket Officer from Frances Slater, Washington, D.C., February 13, 1998.

Asimos AW, Kaufman JS, Lee CH, Williams CM, Carter WA, and Chiang WK. Tuberculosis exposure risk in emergency medicine residents. *Academic Emergency Medicine* 6(10):1044–1049, 1999.

ATS (American Thoracic Society). Control of tuberculosis in the United States. *American Review of Respiratory Diseases* 145:1623–1633, 1992 (http://www.thoracic.org/-statementframe.html, accessed).

ATS. Respiratory protection statement. *American Journal of Respiratory and Critical Care Medicine* 154:1153–1165, 1996.

ATS/CDC (Centers for Disease Control and Prevention). Diagnostic standards and classification of tuberculosis in adults and children. *American Journal of Respiratory and Critical Care Medicine* 161:1376–1395, 2000a. (Earlier statement, Diagnostic standards and classification of tuberculosis. *American Review of Respiratory Diseases* 142:725–735, 1990.)

ATS/CDC. Targeted tuberculin testing and treatment of latent tuberculosis infection. *American Journal of Respiratory and Critical Care Medicine* 161:S221–S247, 2000b.

August J. Employer compliance with recommendations to control tuberculosis in the workplace: The need for an OSHA TB standard. *Journal of Healthcare Safety, Compliance & Infection Control* 3(10):471–479, 1999.

Bailey TC, Fraser VJ, Spitznagel EL, and Dunagan WC. Risk factors for a positive tuberculin skin test among employees of an urban, midwestern teaching hospital. *Annals of Internal Medicine* 122:580–585, 1995.

Ball R and Van Wey M. Tuberculosis skin test conversion among health care workers at a military medical center. *Military Medicine* 162:338–343, 1997.

Bangsberg DR, Crowley K, Moss A, Dobkin JF, McGregor C, and Neu HC. Reduction in tuberculin skin-test conversions among medical house staff associated with improved tuberculosis infection control practices. *Infection Control and Hospital Epidemiology* 18:566–570, 1997.

Barnhart S, Sheppard L, Beaudet N, Stover B, and Balmes J. Tuberculosis in health care settings and the estimated benefits of engineering controls and respiratory protections. *Journal of Occupational and Environmental Medicine* 39(9):849–854, 1997.

Beck-Sague C, Dooley SW, Hutton MD, Otten J, Breeden A, Crawford JT, et al. Hospital outbreak of multidrug-resistant *Mycobacterium tuberculosis* infections. Factors in transmission to staff and HIV-infected patients. *Journal of the American Medical Association* 268(10):1280–1286, 1992.

Behrman AJ and Shofer FS. Tuberculosis exposure and control in an urban emergency department. *Annals of Emergency Medicine* 31(3):370–375, 1998.

Bergmire-Sweat D, Barnett BJ, Harris SL, Taylor JP, Mazurek GH, and Reddy V. Tuberculosis outbreak in a Texas prison, 1994. *Epidemiology and Infection* 117:485–492, 1996.

BLS (Bureau of Labor Statistics). Unemployment Rates for States: Annual Average Rankings. Year: 1998. 2000a. (http://stats.bls.gov/laus/astrk98.htm. accessed November 1, 2000).

BLS. Unemployment Rates for States: Annual Average Rankings. Year: 1999. 2000b. (http://stats.bls.gov/laus.lauastrk.htm, accessed November 1, 2000).

Blumberg, HM. Tuberculosis and infection control: What now? *Infection Control and Hospital Epidemiology* 18(8):538–541, 1997.

Blumberg, HM. One hospital's experience. Presentation at the workshop Tuberculosis Control in the 21st Century. Sponsored by the American Thoracic Society, the American College of Chest Physicians, and the Infectious Disease Society of America, Arlington, Virginia, December 10–12, 1999.

Blumberg, HM. Tuberculosis infection control. In *Tuberculosis: A Comprehensive International Approach*. Reichman LB and Hershfeld ES, eds. New York: Marcel Dekker, Inc., 2000.

Blumberg HM and Bock N. *Georgia TB Reference Guide.* Atlanta: Georgia TB Prevention Coalition, July 1999.

Blumberg HM, Watkins DL, Berschling JD, Antle A, Moore P, White N, et al. Preventing the nosocomial transmission of tuberculosis. *Annals of Internal Medicine* 122:658–663, 1995.

Blumberg HM, Moore P, Blanchard DK, and Ray SM. Transmission of *Mycobacterium tuberculosis* among health care workers infected with human immunodeficiency virus. *Clinical Infectious Diseases* 22(3):597–598, 1996.

Blumberg HM, Sotir M, Erwin M, Bachman R, and Shulman JA. Risk of house staff tuberculin skin test conversion in an area with a high incidence of tuberculosis. *Clinical Infectious Diseases* 27:826–833, 1998.

Blumberg HM, White N, Parrott P, Gordon W, Hunter M, and Ray S. False-positive tuberculin skin test results among health care workers. *Journal of the American Medical Association* 283:2793, 2000.

Bock NN, McGowan JE Jr, Ahn J, Tapia J, and Blumberg HM. Clinical predictors of tuberculosis as a guide for a respiratory isolation policy. *American Journal of Respiratory and Critical Care Medicine* 154:1468–1472, 1996.

Bock NN, Metzger BS, Tapia JR, and Blumberg HM. A tuberculin screening and isoniazid preventive therapy program in an inner-city population. *American Journal of Respiratory and Critical Care Medicine* 159:295–300, 1999.

Boudreau AY, Baron SL, Steenland NK, Van Gilder TJ, Decker JA, Galson SK, and Seitz T. Occupational risk of Mycobacterium tuberculosis infection in hospital workers. *American Journal of Industrial Medicine* 32:528–534, 1997.

Brennen C, Muder RR, and Muraca PW. Occult endemic tuberculosis in a chronic care facility. *Infection Control and Hospital Epidemiology* (9)12:548–552, 1988.

Brock NN, Reeves M, LaMarre M, and DeVoe B. Tuberculosis case detection in a state prison system. *Public Health Reports* 113(4):359–364, 1998.

Brown V, Bishop C, Rutala WA, and Webber DJ. HEPA respirators and tuberculosis in hospital workers. Letter to the editor. *New England Journal of Medicine* 331(24): 1659, 1994.

Camins BC, Bock N, Watkins DL, and Blumberg HM. Acceptance of isoniazid preventive therapy by health care workers after tuberculin skin test conversion. *Journal of American Medicine* 275(13):1013–1015, 1996.

Campbell R, Sneller V-P, Khoury N, Hinton B, DeSouza L, Smith S, et al. Probable transmission of multidrug-resistant tuberculosis in a correctional facility—California. *Morbidity and Mortality Weekly Report* 42:48–51, 1993.

Cantwell MF, McKenna MT, McCray E, and Onorato IM. Tuberculosis and race/ethnicity in the United States: Impact of socioeconomic status. *American Journal of Respiratory Critical Care Medicine* 157(4, Part 1)1016–1020, 1998.

Casper C, Singh SP, Rave S, Daley CL, Schecter GS, Riley LW, Kreiswirth BN, and Small PM. The transcontinental transmission of tuberculosis: A molecular epidemiological assessment. *American Journal of Public Health* 86(4):551–553, 1996.

CDC (Centers for Disease Control, U.S. Department of Health and Human Services). *Guidelines for the Prevention of Tuberculosis in Hospitals.* U.S. Department of Health and Human Services Publication no. (CDC) 82-8371. Atlanta: Centers for Disease Control, 1982.

CDC. Diagnostic standards/classification of TB. *Morbidity and Mortality Weekly Report* 142(3):725–735, 1990a. (http://aepo-xdv-www.epo.cdc.gov/wonder/prevguid/p0000425/- p0000425.htm, accessed May 9, 2000)

CDC. Guidelines for preventing the transmission of tuberculosis in health-care settings with special emphasis on HIV-related issues. *Morbidity and Mortality Weekly Report* 39(RR-17):1–29, 1990b.

CDC. Prevention and control of tuberculosis in facilities providing long-term care to the elderly. *Morbidity and Mortality Weekly Report* 39(RR-10):7–20, 1990c (http://www.cdc.gov/epo/mmwr/preview/mmwrhtml/00001711.htm, accessed May 1, 2000).

CDC. Anergy skin testing and preventive therapy for HIV-infected persons: Revised recommendations. *Morbidity and Mortality Weekly Report* 46:1–10, 1991 (http://www.cdc.gov/epo/mmwr/preview/mmwrhtml/00049386.htm, accessed May 9, 2000).

CDC. Prevention and control of tuberculosis among homeless persons. *Morbidity and Mortality Weekly Report* 41(RR-5):001, 1992a (http://www.cdc.gov/epo/mmwr/preview/mmwrhtml/00019922.htm. accessed May 1, 2000).

CDC. Prevention and control of tuberculosis in migrant farm workers. *Morbidity and Mortality Weekly Report* 41 (RR-10):, 1992b (http://www.cdc.gov/epo/mmwr/preview/mmwrhtml/00032773.htm, accessed May 1, 2000).

CDC. Prevention and control of tuberculosis in U.S. communities with at-risk minority populations. *Morbidity and Mortality Weekly Report* 41 (RR-5):001, 1992c (http://www.- cdc.gov/epo/mmwr/preview/mmwrhtml/00019899.htm, accessed May 1, 2000).

CDC. Draft guidelines for preventing the transmission of tuberculosis in health-care facilities, 2nd ed. Notice of comment period. *Federal Register* 58:52810–52854, 1993.

CDC. Expanded tuberculosis surveillance and tuberculosis morbidity—United States, 1993. *Morbidity and Mortality Weekly Report* 43:361–366, 1994a.

CDC. Guidelines for preventing the transmission of Mycobacterium tuberculosis in health-care facilities, 1994. *Morbidity and Mortality Weekly Report* 43(RR-13):1–132, 1994b (http://www.cdc.gov/epo/mmwr/preview/mmwrhtml/00035909.htm, accessed April 10, 2000).

CDC. Proportionate mortality from pulmonary tuberculosis associated with occupations. *Morbidity and Mortality Weekly Report* 44:14–19, 1995a.

CDC. Screening for tuberculosis and tuberculosis infection in high-risk populations. *Morbidity and Mortality Weekly Report* 44(RR-11):19–34, 1995b (http://www.cdc.gov/-epo/mmwr/preview/mmwrhtml/00038873.htm, accessed May 1, 2000).

CDC. *Guidelines: Improving the Quality.* Atlanta: Centers for Disease Control and Prevention, 1996a.

CDC. Prevention and control of tuberculosis in correctional facilities. *Morbidity and Mortality Weekly Report* 45(RR-8):1–27, 1996b (http://www.cdc.gov/epo/mmwr/preview/mmwrhtml/00042214.htm, accessed April 10, 2000).

CDC. The Role of BCG Vaccine in the Prevention and Control of Tuberculosis in the United States: A Joint Statement by the Advisory Council for the Elimination of Tuberculosis and the Advisory Committee on Immunization Practices. *Mortality and Morbidity Weekly Report* 45(RR-4);1-18, April 26, 1996c.

CDC. Anergy skin testing and preventive therapy for HIV-infected persons: Revised recommendations. *Morbidity and Mortality Weekly Report* 46(No. RR-15):1–10, 1997.

CDC. Prevention and treatment of tuberculosis among patients infected with human immunodeficiency virus: Principles of therapy and revised recommendations. *Morbidity and Mortality Weekly Report* 47(RR-20):1–51, 1998a (http://www.cdc.gov/epo/mmwr/- preview/mmwrhtml/00055357.htm, accessed May 9, 2000).

CDC. Recommendations for prevention and control of tuberculosis among foreign-born persons. *Morbidity and Mortality Weekly Report* 47 (RR-16), 1998b. (http://www.cdc.gov/epo/mmwr/preview/mmwrhtml/00054855.htm, accessed May 9, 2000).

CDC. Achievements in public health, 1900–1999: Improvements in workplace safety—United States, 1900–1999. *Morbidity and Mortality Weekly Report* 48(22):461–469, 1999a. (http://www.cdc.gov/epo/mmwr/preview/mmwrhtml/mm4822a1.htm, accessed June 22, 2000).

CDC. *Reported Tuberculosis in the United States, 1998.* 1999b (http://www.cdc.gov/-nchstp/tb/surv/surv98/surv98.htm, accessed May 12, 2000).

CDC. Self-study modules on tuberculosis. 1999c last updated April 23, 1999; (http://www.cdc.gov/phtn/tbmodules/modules1-5/Default.htm, accessed May 9, 2000).

CDC. Ten great public health achievements—United States, 1900–1999. *Morbidity and Mortality Weekly Report* 48(12):241–243, 1999d (http://www.cdc.gov/epo/mmwr/preview/mmwrhtml/00056796.htm, accessed June 22, 2000).

CDC. *Core Curriculum on Tuberculosis: What Every Clinician Should Know,* 4th ed., 2000a last reviewed April 5, 2000, (http://www.cdc.gov/nchstp/tb/pubs/corecurr/default.htm, accessed May 9, 2000).

CDC. *Reported Tuberculosis in the United States, 1999.* 2000b (http://www.cdc.gov/-nchstp/tb/surv/surv99/surv99.htm, accessed May 9, 2000).

CDC. Updated guidelines for the use of rifabutin or rifampin for the treatment and prevention of tuberculosis among HIV-infected patients taking protease inhibitors or nonnucleoside reverse transcriptase inhibitors. *Morbidity and Mortality Weekly Report* 49(9):185–189, 2000c (http://www.cdc.gov/epo/mmwr/preview/mmwrhtml/mm4909-a4.htm, accessed November 1, 2000).

Chaparas SD, Vandiviere HM, Melvin I, Koch G, and Becker C. Tuberculin test. Variability with the Mantoux procedure. *American Review of Respiratory Diseases* 132(1):175–177, 1985.

Chaulk CP, Moore-Rice K, Rizzo R, and Chaisson RE. Eleven years of community-based directly observed therapy for tuberculosis. *Journal of the American Medical Association* 274(12):945–951, 1995.

Coffey CC, Campbell DL, and Ziqing Z. Simulated workplace performance of N95 respirators. *American Industrial Hygiene Association Journal* 60:618–624, 1999.

Cohen, BS. Industrial hygiene measurement and control. In *Environmental and Occupational Medicine*, 2nd ed., William NR, ed. New York: Little, Brown Company, pp. 1389–1404, 1992.

Cohn DL, Catlin BJ, Peterson KL, Judson FN, and Sbarbaro JA. A 62-dose, 6-month therapy for pulmonary and extrapulmonary tuberculosis: A twice-weekly, directly observed, and cost-effective regimen. *Annals of Internal Medicine* 112(6):407-15, 1990.

Comstock, GW. Epidemiology of tuberculosis. in *Tuberculosis: A Comprehensive International Approach* 2nd ed., Reichman LB and Hershfield ES, eds. New York: Marcel Dekker, Inc., 2000.

Comstock GW and Edwards PQ. The competing risks of tuberculosis and hepatitis for adult tuberculin reactors. *American Review of Respiratory Diseases* 111(5):573–577, 1975.

Combs DL, O'Brien RJ, and Geiter LJ. USPHS tuberculosis short-course chemotherapy trial 21: effectiveness, toxicity, and acceptability. The report of final results. *Annals of Internal Medicine* 112:397-406, 1990.

Curtis AB, McCray E, and Onorato IM. Tuberculosis among health care workers in United States, 1994–1998. Presentation (by AB Curtis) at the workshop Tuberculosis Control in the 21st Century. Sponsored by the American Thoracic Society, the American College of Chest Physicians, and the Infectious Disease Society of America, Arlington, Virginia, December 10–12, 1999.

Curtis AB, Ridzon R, Novick LF, Driscoll J, Blair D, Oxtoby M, et al. Analysis of *Mycobacterium tuberculosis* transmission patterns in a homeless shelter outbreak. *International Journal of Tuberculosis and Lung Disease* 4:308–313, 2000.

Daniel BL and Daniel TM. Graphic representation of numerically calculated predictive values: An easily comprehended method of evaluating diagnostic tests. *Medical Decision Making* 13:355–358, 1993.

Daniel, T. *Captain of Death: The Story of Tuberculosis.* Rochester, NY: University of Rochester Press, 1997.

Daniel, TM. *Pioneers of Medicine and Their Impact on Tuberculosis.* Rochester, NY: University of Rochester Press, 2000.

Daniel TM and Debanne SM. Estimation of the annual risk of tuberculous infection for white men in the United States. *Journal of Infectious Disease* 175:1535–1537, 1997.

Dankner WM and Davis CE. *Mycobacterium bovis* is a significant cause of tuberculosis in children residing along the United States-Mexico border in the Baja California region. *Pediatrics* 105(6):E79, 2000.

DeJoy DM, Murphy LR, Gershon RRM. Safety Climate in Health Care Settings. *Advances in Industrial Ergonomics and Safety* 8:923–929, 1995.

Densen P, Clark RA, and Nauseef WM. Granulocytic phagocytes. In *Principles and Practices of Infectious Diseases*, 4th ed., Vol. 1., Mandell G, Bennett J, and Dolin R, eds. New York: Churchill Livingstone, 1995.

162 TUBERCULOSIS IN THE WORKPLACE

DeRiemer K, Daley CL, and Reingold AL. Preventing tuberculosis among HIV-infected persons: A survey of physicians' knowledge and practices. *Preventive Medicine* 28(4):437–444, 1999.

DiStasio AJ 2d and Trump DH. The investigation of a tuberculosis outbreak in the closed environment of a U.S. navy ship, 1987. *Military Medicine* 155:347–351, 1990.

DOL (U.S. Department of Labor). Fiscal year 2001 budget. Washington, D.C.: U.S. Department of Labor, 2000 (http://www.dol.gov/dol/_sec/public/budget/osha2001.htm, accessed July 10, 2000).

DOL, OSHA (Occupational Safety and Health Administration). *Enforcement Policy and Procedures for Occupational Exposure to Tuberculosis.* Washington, D.C.: Occupational Safety and Health Administration, October 18, 1993.

DOL, OSHA. Occupational exposure to tuberculosis. *Federal Register* 62(201):54159–54309, 1997.

Dooley SW and Tapper M. Epidemiology of nosocomial tuberculosis. In *Prevention and Control of Nosocomial Infections*, 3rd ed., Wenzel RP, ed. Baltimore: Williams & Wilkins, pp. 357–394, 1997.

Dye C, Scheele S, Dolin P, Pathania V, and Raviglione MC. Consensus statement. Global burden of tuberculosis: Estimated incidence, prevalence, and mortality by country. WHO global surveillance and monitoring project. *Journal of the American Medical Association* 282:677–686, 1999.

Edlin BR, Tokars JI, Grieco MH, Crawford JT, Williams J, Sordillo EM et al. An outbreak of multidrug resistant tuberculosis among hospitalized patients with the aquired immunodeficiency syndrome. *New England Journal of Medicine* 326(23):1514–1521, 1992.

Engel A and Roberts J. *Tuberculin Skin Test Reaction Among Adults 25-74 Years, 1971–1972.* DHEW publication; no (HRA) 77–1649. Washington, D.C.: U.S. Department of Health, Education and Welfare, 1977.

Etkind SC and Veen J. Contact follow-up in high- and low-prevalence countries. In *Tuberculosis: A Comprehensive International Approach*, 2nd ed., Reichman LB and Hershfield, ES, eds. New York: Marcel Dekker, Inc., 2000.

Evans ME, Perkins DJ, and Simmons GD. Tuberculosis management practices in Kentucky: Comparison with national guidelines. *Southern Medical Journal* 92(4):375–379, 1999.

Evenson W. Occupational exposure to *Mycobacterium tuberculosis*. Legal issues in workers' compensation. *AAOHN Journal* 47(8):373–380, 1999.

Fella P, Rivera P, Hale M, Squires K, and Sepkowitz K. Dramatic decrease in tuberculin skin test conversion rate among employees at a hospital in New York City. *American Journal of Infection Control* 23(6):352–356, 1995.

Fennelly KP and Nardell EA. The relative efficacy of respirators and room ventilation in preventing occupational tuberculosis. *Infection Control and Hospital Epidemiology* 19(10):754–759, 1998.

Fischl MA, Uttamchandani RB, Caikos GL, Poblete RB, Reyes RR, Boota A, et al. An outbreak of tuberculosis caused by multiple-drug-resistant tubercle bacilli among patients with HIV infection. *Annals of Internal Medicine* 117:177–183, 1992.

Fraser VJ, Kilo CM, Bailey TC, Medoff G, and Dunagan WC. Screening of physicians for tuberculosis. *Infection Control and Hospital Epidemiology* 15(2):95–100, 1994.

French AL, Welbel SF, Dietrich SE, Mosher LB, Breall PS, Paul WS, et al. Use of DNA fingerprinting to assess tuberculosis infection control. *Annals of Internal Medicine* 129(11):856–861, 1998.

Fridkin SK, Manangan L, Bolyard E, and Jarvis WR. SHEA-CDC TB Survey, Part I: Efficacy of TB infection control programs at member hospitals, 1989–1992. *Infection Control and Hospital Epidemiology* 16:129–134, 1995a.

Fridkin SK, Manangan L, Bolyard E, and Jarvis WR. SHEA-CDC TB Survey, Part II: Efficacy of TB infection control programs at member hospitals, 1992. *Infection Control and Hospital Epidemiology* 16:135–140, 1995b.

Fujiwara PI, Simone PM, and Munsiff SS. Treatment of tuberculosis. In *Tuberculosis: A Comprenhensive International Approach,* 2nd ed., Reichman LB and Hershfield ES. eds. New York: Marcel Dekker, Inc., 2000.

Fuss EP, Israel E, Baruch N, and Roghmann M. Improved tuberculosis infection control practices in Maryland acute care hospitals. *American Journal of Infection Control* 28:133–137, 2000.

Gangadharam PRJ and Jenkins PA, eds. *Mycobacteria: I Basic Aspects.* New York: Chapman & Hall Medical Microbiology Series, International Publishing Series, 1998.

Garcia Rodriguez LA, Ruigomez A, and Jick H. A review of epidemiologic research on drug-induced acute liver injury using the general practice research data base in the United Kingdom. *Pharmacotherapy* 4:721–728, 1997.

Garrett DO, Dooley SW, Snider DE Jr, and Jarvis WR. Mycobacterium tuberculosis. In *Infection Control and Hospital Epidemiology,* 2nd ed., Mayhall CG, ed. Philadelphia: Lippincott Williams & Wilkins, pp. 477–503, 1999.

Geiter L. Defining tuberculosis elimination in the United States? Background paper prepared for the Institute of Medicine Committee on the Elimination of Tuberculosis in the United States, Washington, D.C., June 1999.

Gershon R, Vlahov D, Felknor S. Compliance with universal precautions among health care workers at three regional hospitals. *American Journal of Infection Control* 23:225–236, 1995a.

Gershon RRM, Vlahov D, Farzadegan H, Alter M. Occupational risk of HIV, HVC and HCV among funeral service practitioners in Maryland. *Infection Control and Hospital Epidemiology* 16(4):194–197, 1995b.

Gershon R, Vlahov D, Escamilla-Cejudo JA, Badawi M, McDiarmid M, Karkashian C, et al. Tuberculosis risk in funeral home employees. *Journal of Occupational Environmental Medicine* 40(5):497–503, 1998.

Gigerenzer G. The psychology of good judgment: Frequency formats and simple algorithms. *Medical Decision Making* 16:270–280, 1996.

Haas DW and Des Prez RM. Mycobacterium tuberculosis. In *Principles and Practices of Infectious Diseases,* 4th ed., Vol 2, Mandell G, Bennett J, and Dolin R, eds. New York: Churchill Livingstone, 1995.

Hammett TM, Harmon P, and Maruschak LM. *Issues and Practices: 1996–1997 Update: HIV/ AIDS, STDs, and TB in Correctional Facilities.* Washington, DC: U.S. Department of Justice, July 1999.

Hannum D, Cycan K, Jones L, Stewart M, Morris S, Markowitz SM, et al. The effect of respirator training on the ability of healthcare workers to pass a qualitative fit test. *Infection Control and Hospital Epidemiology* 17(10):636–640, 1996.

HCFA (Health Care Financing Administration, U.S. Department of Health and Human Services). In *Medicare Carriers Manual,* Part 3. Chapter II, Coverage and limitations, Section 2100.2. Washington, D.C.: Health Care Financing Administration, 1999 (http://www.hcfa.gov/pubforms/14_car/3b2051.htm#_1_14, accessed September 3, 2000).

Hernandez J and Baca D. Effect of tuberculosis on milk production in dairy cows. *Journal of the American Veterinary Medical Association* 213(6):851–854, 1998.

Hoch DE and Wilcox KR Jr. Transmission of multidrug-resistant tuberculosis from an HIV-positive client in a residential substance-abuse treatment facility—Michigan. *Morbidity and Mortality Weekly Report* 40:129–131, 1991.

Hoover, M. State faces TB fears—Health officials meet with prison workers. *York Dispatch/ Sunday News,* September 12, 2000. (Reported in *TB-Related News and Journal Items—* Week of September 11, 2000, *CDC HIV/STD/TB Prevention News Update,* September 15, 2000, (http://www.cdcnpin.org/news/prevnews.htm, accessed).

Howell JT, Scheel WJ, Pryor VL, Tavris DR, Calder RA, and Wilder MH. *Mycobacterium tuberculosis* transmission in a health clinic—Florida, 1988. *Morbidity and Mortality Weekly Report* 38(15):256–258, 263–264, 1989.

Hutton MD, Cauthen GM, and Bloch AB. Results of a 29-state survey of tuberculosis in nursing homes and correctional facilities. *Public Health Reports* 108:305–314, 1993.

Hux JE, Naylor CD. Communicating the benefits of chronic preventive therapy: Does the format of efficacy data determine patients' preferences for therapeutic outcomes? *Medical Decision Making* 15:152–157, 1995.

Ijaz K, White E, McGriff E, Hedden S, Vester W, Ramsey S, et al. Unrecognized fatal tuberculosis in a nursing home with subsequent spread to the community (abstract). Meeting of the North American Chapter of the International Union Against Tuberculosis and Lung Disease, Chicago, February 23–27, 1999.

IOM (Institute of Medicine). *Guidelines for Clinical Practice: From Development to Use.* Field MJ and Lohr KN, eds. Washington D.C.: National Academy Press, 1992.

IOM. *Ending Neglect: The Elimination of Tuberculosis in the United States.* Geiter L, ed. Washington D.C.: National Academy Press, 2000.

Iseman MD. Management of multidrug-resistant tuberculosis. *Chemotherapy.* Suppl. 2 45:3–11, 1999a.

Iseman MD. Treatment and implications of multidrug-resistant tuberculosis for the 21st century. *Chemotherapy.* Suppl. 2 45:34–40, 1999b.

Jeffress C. Statement by the Assistant Secretary for Occupational Safety and Health before the Subcommittee on Labor, Health and Human Services, and Education, House Appropriations Committee. Washington, D.C.: March 22, 2000 (http://www.dol.gov/dol/-_sec/public/budget/osha000323.htm, accessed July 10, 2000).

Jereb JA, Klevens RM, Privett TD, Smith PJ, Crawford JT, Sharp VL, et al. Tuberculosis in health care workers at a hospital with an outbreak of multidrug-resistant *Mycobacterium tuberculosis. Archives of Internal Medicine* 155(8):854–859, 1995.

Jones TF, Craig AS, Valway SE, Woodley CL, and Schaffner W. Transmission of tuberculosis in a jail. *Annals of Internal Medicine* 131:557–563, 1999.

Kahn HA and Sempos CT. *Statistical Methods in Epidemiology* New York: Oxford University Press, 1989.

Kakesako GI. State sends 16 female inmates from Kailua to Oklahoma. *Honolulu Star-Bulletin,* November 10, 1998 (http://starbulletin.com/test/adtest/news/story4.html, accessed August 14, 2000).

Kao AS, Ashford DA, McNeil MM, Warren NG, and Good RC. Descriptive profile of tuberculin skin testing programs and laboratory-acquired tuberculous infections in public health laboratories. *Journal of Clinical Microbiology* 35:1847–1851, 1997.

Kendig EL Jr, Kirkpatrick BV, Carter WH, Hill FA, Caldwell K, and Entwistle M. Underreading of the tuberculin skin test reaction. *Chest* 113:1175-1177, 1998.

Kenyon TA, Valway SE, Ihle WW, Onorato IM, and Castro KG. Transmission of multidrug-resistant Mycobacterium tuberculosis during a long airplane flight. *New England Journal of Medicine* 11;334(15):933–938, 1996.

Kenyon TA, Ridzon R, Luskin-Hawk R, Schultz C, Paul WS, Valway SE, et al. A nosocomial outbreak of multidrug-resistant tuberculosis. *Annals of Internal Medicine* 127(1):32–36, 1997.

Knirsch CA, Jain NL, Pablos-Mendez A, Friedman C, and Hripcsak G. Respiratory isolation of tuberculosis patients using clinical guidelines and an automated clinical decision support system. *Infectious Control and Hospital Epidemiology* 19:94–100, 1998.

Kohn MR, Arden MR, Vasilakis J, and Shenker IR. Directly observed preventive therapy. Turning the tide against tuberculosis. *Archives of Pediatric and Adolescent Medicine* 150:727–729, 1996.

Labor Coalition to Fight TB in the Workplace. Letter to the Honorable Robert B. Reich, Secretary of Labor August 25, 1993.

Lai KK, Fontecchio SA, Kelley AL, and Melvin ZS. Knowledge of the transmission of tuberculosis and infection control measures for tuberculosis among healthcare workers. *Infection Control and Hospital Epidemiology* 17:168–170, 1996.

Lang M. Error exposes yorkers to rare TB. *York Dispatch/Sunday News*, July 14, 2000. (Reported in *TB-Related News and Journal Items—Week of July 17, CDC HIV/STD/TB Prevention News Update*, July, 21, 2000, http://www.cdcnpin.org/news/prevnews.htm, accessed).

Larsen N, Larson CE, Sotir MJ, White N, Bock NN, Blumberg HM. Risk of tuberculin skin test conversion among employees at a public inner-city hospital in a high incidence area. *The 9th Annual Meeting of the Society for Healthcare Epidemiology of America,* San Francisco, April 1999.

Lauzardo M, Duncan H, Hale Y, and Lee P. Transmission of *Mycobacterium tuberculosis* to a funeral director during routine embalming. *American Journal of Respiratory and Critical Care Medicine* 161:A299, 2000 (abstract) (http://www.hopkinsid.edu/ats_2000/- ats_3.html, accessed August 15, 2000).

Lebo L and Scolforo M. Third TB case at prison—OSHA inspection reveals violation, brings fine over tuberculosis procedures—Guards Concerned, *York Dispatch/Sunday News*, September 3, 2000. (Reported in *TB-Related News and Journal Items—Week of September 4, 2000, CDC HIV/STD/TB Prevention News Update*, September 8, 2000, http://www.cdcnpin.org/news/prevnews.htm, accessed September 8, 2000).

LoBue P and Catanzaro A. Healthcare worker compliance with nosocomial tuberculosis control policies. *Infection Control and Hospital Epidemiology* 20:623–624, 1999.

Lorvick J, Thompson S, Edlin BR, Kral AH, Lifson AR, and Watters JK. Incentives and accessibility: A pilot study to promote adherence to TB prophylaxis in a high-risk community. *Journal of Urban Health* 76:461–467, 1999.

Louther J, Rivera P, Feldman J, Villa N, DeHovitz J, and Sepkowitz KA. Risk of tuberculin conversion according to occupation among health care workers at a New York City hospital. *American Journal of Respiratory and Critical Care Medicine* 156:201–205, 1997.

Maloney SA, Pearson ML, Gordon MT, Del Castillo R, Boyle JF, and Jarvis WR. Efficacy of control measures in preventing nosocomial transmission of multidrug-resistant tuberculosis to patients and health care workers. *Annals of Internal Medicine* 122: 90–95, 1995.

Manangan LP, Perrotta DM, Banerjee SN, Hack D, Simonds D, and Jarvis WR. Status of tuberculosis infection control programs at Texas hospitals, 1989 through 1991. *American Journal of Infection Control* 25(3):229–235, 1997.

Manangan LP, Simonds DN, Pugliese G, Kroc K, Banerjee SN, Rudnick JR, et al. Are U.S. hospitals making progress in implementing guidelines for prevention of *Mycobacterium tuberculosis* transmission? *Archives of Internal Medicine* 158:1440–1444, 1998.

Manangan LP, Collazo ER, Tokars J, Paul S, and Jarvis WR. Trends in compliance with the guidelines for preventing the transmission of Mycobacterium tuberculosis among New Jersey hospitals, 1989 to 1996. *Infection Control and Hospital Epidemiology* 20:337–340, 1999.

Manangan LP, Bennett CL, Tablan N, Simonds DN, Pugliese G, Collazo E, et al. Nosocomial tuberculosis prevention measures among two groups of US hospitals, 1992 to 1996. *Chest* 117:380–384, 2000.

Mangura BT and Galanowsky KE. Case management: The key to a successful tuberculosis-control program. In *Tuberculosis: A Comprehensive International Approach*, 2nd ed., Reichman LB and Hershfield ES, eds. New York: Marcel Dekker, Inc., 2000.

Mazur DJ, Hickam DH. Treatment preferences of patients and physicians: Influences of summary data when framing effects are controlled. *Medical Decision Making* 10:2–5, 1990.

McAuley J. Presentation at public meeting conducted by the Institute of Medicine Committee on Regulating Occupational Exposure to Tuberculosis, Washington, D.C., August 7, 2000.

McCaffrey DP. *OSHA and the Politics of Health Regulation* New York: Plenum Press, 1982.

McCray E. Prospective surveillance for TST conversions among health care workers (HCWs) using StaffTRAK-TB. Presentation to the Institute of Medicine Committee on the Elimination of Tuberculosis, Washington, D.C., June 1999a.

McCray E. Prospective surveillance for TST conversions among health care workers. Presentation at the workshop Tuberculosis Control in the 21st Century. Sponsored by the American Thoracic Society, the American College of Chest Physicians, and the Infectious Disease Society of America, Arlington, Virginia, December 10–12, 1999b.

McDiarmid M, Gamponia MJ, Ryan MA, Hirshon JM, Gillen NA, and Cox M. Tuberculosis in the workplace: OSHA's compliance experience. *Infection Control and Hospital Epidemiology* 17:159–164, 1996.

McKay R. An evaluation of a qualitative fit-test agent (Bitrex) to detect exhalation valve leakage in full face piece respirators (abstract 281). Presented at 2000 American Industrial Hygiene Conference and Exposition, Orlando, Florida, May 20–25, 2000.

McKay RT and Davies E. Capability of respirator wearers to detect aerosolized qualitative fit test agents (sweetener and Bitrex) with known fixed leaks. *Applied Occupational and Environmental Hygiene* 15(6):479–484, 2000.

Mendeloff J. *Regulating Safety: An Economic and Political Analysis of Occupational Safety and Health Policy.* Cambridge: The MIT Press, 1978.

Mendeloff J. *The Dilemma of Toxic Substance Regulation: How Overregulation Causes Underregulation.* Cambridge: The MIT Press, 1988.

Menzies D, Fanning A, Yuan L, and Fitzgerald M. Tuberculosis among health care workers. *New England Journal of Medicine* 332:92–98, 1995.

Menzies D, Fanning A, Yuan L, FitzGerald JM, the Canadian Collaborative Group in Nosocomial Transmission of TB. Hospital Ventilation and Risk for Tuberculous Infection in Canadian Health Care Workers. *Annals of Internal Medicine* 133:779–789, 2000. (http://www.annals.org/issues/v133n10/full/200011210-00010.html, accessed November 30, 2000).

Mikol EX, Horton R, Lincoln NS, and Stokes AM. Incidence of pulmonary tuberculosis among employees of tuberculosis hospitals. *American Review of Tuberculosis* 66:16–27, 1953.

Mintz BW. *OSHA History, Law and Policy.* [Washington D.C.]: The Bureau of National Affairs, 1984.

Moran GJ, Fuchs MA, Jarvis WR, and Talan DA. Tuberculosis infection-control practices in United States emergency departments. *Annals of Emergency Medicine* 26:283–289, 1995.

Moss AR, Hahn JA, Tulsky JP, Daley CL, Small PM, and Hopewell PC. Tuberculosis in the homeless. A prospective study. *American Journal of Respiratory Critical Care Medicine* 162(2 Pt 1):460–464, 2000.

Munger R, Anderson K, Leahy R, Allard J, and Kobayashi JM. Epidemiologic notes and reports tuberculosis in a nursing care facility—Washington. *Morbidity and Mortality Weekly Report* 32:121–122, 128, 1983 (http://www.cdc.gov/epo/mmwr/preview/- mmwrhtml/00001267.htm, accessed August 14, 2000).

Narain JP, Lofgren JP, Warren E, and Stead WW. Epidemic tuberculosis in a nursing home: A retrospective cohort study. *Journal of American Geriatric Society* 33(4):258–263, 1985.

Nardell EA. Tuberculosis. In *Saunders Infection Control Reference Service*. Abrutyn E, Goldman D and Schedder W eds. [Philadelphia, Pennsylvania: W.B. Saunders Company], pp. 195–200, 1997.

Nardell EA and Piessens WF. Transmission of tuberculosis. in *Tuberculosis: A Comprehensive International Approach*, 2nd ed., Reichman LB and Hershfield ES, eds. New York: Marcel Dekker, Inc., 2000.

NCCHC (National Commission on Correctional Health Care). *Standards for Health Services in Jails* Chicago: National Commission on Correctional Health Care, 1992.

NCCHC. *Management of Tuberculosis in Correctional Facilities* Chicago: National Commission on Correctional Health Care, 1996 (http://www.ncchc.org/statements/tb-.html, accessed August 14, 2000.)

NIJ (National Institute of Justice). Tuberculosis in correctional facilities 1994–95. NIJ Research in Brief. Washington, DC: U.S. Department of Justice, July 1996 (http://www.ncjrs.org/txtfiles/corrfac.txt, accessed August 12, 2000).

NIJ. 1996–1997 Update: HIV/AIDS, STDs, and TB in correctional facilities. Issues and practices services Washington, D.C.: U.S. Department of Justice, July 1999 (http://www.ojp.usdoj.gov/nij/pubs-sum/176344.htm, accessed August 12, 2000).

NIOSH (National Institute of Occupational Safety and Health, Centers for Disease Control and Prevention). *Protect Yourself Against Tuberculosis—A Respiratory Protection Guide for HealthCare Workers*, DHHS (NIOSH) Publication No. 96-102, December 1995.

NIOSH. *NIOSH Guide to the Selection and Use of Particulate Respirators Certified Under 42 CFR 84*, DHHS (NIOSH) Publication No. 96-101, January 1996.

NIOSH. *TB Respiratory Protection Program in Health Care Facilities—Administrator's Guide*, DHHA (NIOSH) Publication No. 99-143, September, 1999.

Nolan CM, Elarth AM, Barr H, Saeed AM, and Risser DR. An outbreak of tuberculosis in a shelter for homeless men. A description of its evolution and control. *American Review of Respiratory Diseases* 143(2):257–261, 1991.

Nolan CM, Roll L, Goldberg SV, and Elarth AM. Directly observed isoniazid preventive therapy for released jail inmates. *American Journal of Respiratory Critical Care Medicine* 155(2):583–586, 1997.

Nolan CM, Goldberg SV, and Buskin SE. Hepatoxicity associated with isoniazid preventive therapy: A 7-year survey from a public health tuberculosis clinic. *Journal of the American Medical Association* 281:1014–1018, 1999.

NRC (National Research Council). *Risk Assessment in the Federal Government: Managing the Process*. Washington, D.C.: National Academy Press, 1983.

NRC. *Understanding Risk: Informing Decisions in Democratic Society*. Stern PC and Fineberg HV, eds. Washington, D.C.: National Academy Press, 1996.

OSHA (Occupational Safety and Health Administration, U.S. Department of Labor). OSHA Directives, CPL 2.106 Enforcement Procedures and Scheduling for Occupational Exposure to Tuberculosis. February 9, 1996 (http://www.osha-slc.gov/OshDoc/Directive_data/CPL_2_106.html, accessed November 1, 2000).

OSHA, Region 6. OSHA issues willful citations to two INS facilities in Houston for tuberculosis exposure. News Release. Washington, D.C.: Occupational Safety and Health Administration, May 8, 2000 (http://www.osha.gov/media/oshnews/may00/reg6-20000508.html, accessed

OSHSPA (Occupational Safety and Health State Plan Association). *Grassroots Worker Protection: How State Programs Help to Ensure Safe and Healthful Workplaces.* 1999 Annual Report. Washington, D.C.: Occupational Safety and Health State Plan Association 1999. (http://www.osha-slc.gov/fso/osp/oshspa/grassroots_worker_ protection99/index.html, accessed July 10, 2000).

Osterholm MT, Hedberg CW, and MacDonald KL. Epidemiology of infectious diseases. In *Principles and Practices of Infectious Diseases,* 4th ed., Vol. 1, Mandell G, Bennett J, and Dolin R, eds. New York: Churchill Livingstone, 1995.

OTA (Office of Technology Assessment). *The Continuing Challenge of Tuberculosis.* Washington, D.C.: U.S. Government Printing Office, 1993 (http://www.wws.princeton.edu/~ota/ns20/year_f.html, accessed).

Ozuah PO, Burton W, Lerro KA, Rosenstock J, and Mulvihill M. Assessing the validity of tuberculin skin test readings by trained professionals and patients. *Chest* 116:104–106, 1999.

Page J and O'Brian MW. *Bitter Wages.* New York: Grossman Publishers, 1973.

Palmer MV, Whipple DL, Payeur JB, Alt DP, Esch KJ, Bruning-Fann CS, et al. Naturally occurring tuberculosis in white-tailed deer. *Journal of the American Veterinary Medical Association* 15;216(12):1921–1924, 2000.

Panlilio L and Curtis A. Lessons learned at the CDC. Presentation to Institute of Medicine Committee on Regulating Occupational Exposure to Tuberculosis, Washington, D.C., August 2000.

Patterson CH. The joint commission/OSHA educational partnership. *Journal of Healthcare Safety, Compliance & Infection Control* 3(10):447, 1999.

Pearson ML, Jereb JA, Frieden TR, Crawford JT, Davis BJ, Dooley SW, et al. Nosocomial transmission of multidrug-resistant *Mycobacterium tuberculosis.* A risk to patients and health care workers. *Annals of Internal Medicine* 1;117(3):191–196, 1992.

Pelletier AR, DiFerdinando GT Jr, Greenberg AJ, Sosin DM, Jones WD Jr, Bloch AB, et al. Tuberculosis in a correctional facility. *Archives of Internal Medicine* 153(23):2692–2695, 1993.

Perez-Stable EJ and Slutkin G. A demonstration of lack of variability among six tuberculin skin test readers. *American Journal of Public Health* 75(11):1341–1343, 1985.

Pierce JR, Sims SL, and Holman GH. Transmission of tuberculosis to hospital workers by a patient with AIDS. *Chest* 101:581–582, 1992.

Pillai SD, Widmer KW, Ivey LJ, Coker KC, Newman E, Lingsweiler S, et al. Failure to identify non-bovine reservoirs of *Mycobacterium bovis* in a region with a history of infected dairy-cattle herds. *Preventive Veterinary Medicine* 43(1):53–62, 2000.

Prendergast T, Hwang B, Alexander R, Charron T, Lopez E, Culton J, et al. Tuberculosis outbreaks in prison housing units for HIV-infected inmates—California, 1995–1996. *Morbidity and Mortality Weekly Report* 48:79–82, 1999.

Price LE, Rutala WA, and Samsa GP. Tuberculosis in hospital personnel. *Infection Control* 8:97–101, 1987.

Pugliese G. Discussion of the presentation "Lessons learned at CDC" by Curtis A and L Panlilio L. Workshop of the Institute of Medicine Committee on Regulating Occupational Exposure to Tuberculosis Washington, D.C., August 8, 2000.

Puisis M, Feinglass J, Lidow E, and Mansour M. Radiographic screening for tuberculosis in a large urban county jail. *Public Health Reports* 111(4):330–334, 1996.

Ramirez JA, Anderson P, Herp S, and Raff MJ. Increased rate of tuberculin skin test conversion among workers at a university hospital. *Infection Control and Hospital Epidemiology* 13(10):579–581, 1992.

Ramphal-Naley L, Kirkhorn S, Lohman WH, and Zelterman D. Tuberculosis in physicians: Compliance with surveillance and treatment. *American Journal of Infection Control* 24(4):243–253, 1996.

Ransohoff DF, Harris RP. Lessons from the mammography screening controversy: Can we improve the debate? *Annals of Internal Medicine* 127(11):1029–1034, 1997.

Rao SN, Mookerjee AL, Obasanjo OO, and Chaisson RE. Errors in the treatment of tuberculosis in Baltimore. *Chest* 117(3):734–737, 2000.

Reich R. U.S. Secretary of Labor Robert Reich urges Senate lawmakers to undertake OSHA reform. *Health Facilities Management* 7(7):27, 1994.

Reichman LB, Hershfield ES. *Tuberculosis: A Comprehensive International Approach,* 2nd ed., New York: Marcel Dekker, Inc., 2000.

Reuters Health. CDC to revise guidelines for prevention of TB transmission in health care facilities. October 25, 2000 (*Reported in TB-Related News and Journal Items – Week of October 23, 2000 CDC HIV Prevention News Update,* October 27, 2000 http://www.cdcpin.org/news/prevnews.htm, accessed October 27, 2000).

Rieder HL, Kelly GD, Bloch AB, Cauthen GM, and Snider DE Jr. Tuberculosis diagnosed at death in the United States. *Chest* 100:678–681, 1991.

Robinson JC. *Toils and Toxics: Workplace Struggles and Political Strategies for Occupational Health.* Berkeley: University of California Press, 1991.

Rothstein M. *Occupational Safety and Health Law.* St. Paul, Minnesota: West Publishing Company, 1998.

Salpeter SR. Fatal isoniazid-induced hepatitis. Its risk during chemoprophylaxis. *Western Journal of Medicine* 159:560–564, 1993.

Schluger NW, Huberman R, Holzman R, Rom WN, and Cohen DI. Screening for infection and disease as a tuberculosis control measure among indigents in New York City, 1994–1997. *International Journal of Tuberculosis and Lung Disease* 3:281–286, 1999.

Schmitt SM, Fitzgerald SD, Cooley TM, Bruning-Fann CS, Sullivan L, Berry D, et al. Bovine tuberculosis in free-ranging white-tailed deer from Michigan. *Journal of Wildlife Diseases* 33(4):749–758, 1997.

Schwartz LM, Woloshin S, Black WC, Welch HG. The role of numeracy in understanding the benefit of screening mammography. *Annals of Internal Medicine* 127:966–972, 1997.

Scott B, Schmid M, and Nettleman MD. Early identification and isolation of inpatients at high risk for tuberculosis. *Archives of Internal Medicine* 154:326–330, 1994.

Sepkowitz KA. Tuberculosis and the health care workers: A historical perspective. *Annals of Internal Medicine* 120:71–79, 1994.

Sepkowitz KA. AIDS, tuberculosis, and the health care worker. *Clinical Infectious Diseases* 20(2):232–242, 1995.

Sepkowitz KA, Fella P, Rivera P, Villa N, and DeHovitz J. Prevalence of PPD positivity among new employees at a hospital in New York City. *Infection Control and Hospital Epidemiology* 16(6):344–347, 1995.

Sinkowitz RL, Fridkin SK, Managan L, Wenger PN, and Jarvis WR. Status of tuberculosis infection control programs at United States hospitals, 1989 to 1992. *American Journal of Infection Control* 24:226–234, 1996.

Slovis BS, Plitman JD, and Haas DW. The case against anergy testing as a routine adjunct to tuberculin skin testing. *Journal of the American Medical Association* 19;283(15):2003–2007, 2000.

Sotir MJ, Khan A, Bock NN, and Blumberg HM. Risk factors for tuberculin skin test (TST) positivity and conversion among employees at a public inner-city hospital in a high incidence area (abstract). *Journal of Investigative Medicine* 45:64A, 1997.

Sotir MJ, Parrott P, Metchock B, Bock NN, McGowan JE Jr, Ray SM, et al. Tuberculosis in the inner city: impact of a continuing epidemic in the 1990s. *Clinical Infectious Disease* 29(5):1138–1144, 1999.

Spradling S, McLaughlin S, Drociuk D, Ridzon R, Pozsik C, and Onorato I. Transmission of Mycobacterium tuberculosis among inmates in an HIV-dedicated prison dormitory (Abstract). Presentation for the XIII International AIDS Conference, Durban, South Africa, July 9–14, 2000.

Starke J. Pediatric tuberculosis Presentation to the Institute of Medicine Committee on Regulating Occupational Exposure to Tuberculosis, Washington, D.C., August 7, 2000.

Stead WW. Tuberculosis among elderly persons: An outbreak in a nursing home. *Annals of Internal Medicine* 94:606–610, 1981.

Stead WW. Tuberculosis as an endemic and nosocomial infection among the elderly in nursing homes. *New England Journal of Medicine* 6:312(23):1483–1487, 1985.

Steenland K, Levine AJ, Sieber K, Schulte P, and Aziz D. Incidence of tuberculous infection among New York State prison employees. *American Journal of Public Health* 87: 2012–2014, 1997.

Steimke EH, Tenholder MF, McCormick MI, and Rissing JP. Tuberculosis surveillance: Lessons from a cluster of skin test conversions. *American Journal of Infection Control* 22(4):236–241, 1994.

Sterling TR, Pope DS, Bishai WR, Harrington S, Gershon RR, and Chaisson RE. Transmission of *Mycobacterium tuberculosis* from a cadaver to an embalmer. *New England Journal of Medicine* 342:246–248, 2000a.

Sterling TR, Stanley RL, Thompson D, Brubach GA, Madison A, Harrington S, et al. HIV-related tuberculosis in a transgender network—Baltimore, Maryland and New York City area, 1998–2000. *Morbidity and Mortality Weekly Report* 49(15):317–320, 2000b.

Stricof RL, DiFerdinando GTJ, Osten WM, and Novick LF. Tuberculosis control in New York City hospitals. *American Journal of Infection Control* 26:270–276, 1998.

Stroud LA, Tokars JI, Grieco MH, Crawford JT, Culver DH, Edlin BR, et al. Evaluation of infection control measures in preventing nosocomial transmission of multidrug-resistant *Mycobacterium tuberculosis* in a New York City hospital. *Infection Control and Hospital Epidemiology* 16(3):141–147, 1995.

Sutton PM, Nicas M, Reinisch F, and Harrison RJ. Evaluating the control of tuberculosis among health care workers: Adherence to CDC guidelines of three urban hospitals in California. *Infection Control and Hospital Epidemiology* 19 (7):487–493, 1998.

Sutton PM, Nicas M, and Harrison RJ. Tuberculosis isolation: Comparison of written procedures and actual practices in three California hospitals. *Infection Control and Hospital Epidemiology* 21(1):28–32, 2000.

Tabet SR, Goldbaum GM, Hooton TM, Eisenach KD, Cave MD, and Nolan CM. Restriction fragment length polymorphism analysis detecting a community-based tuberculosis outbreak among persons infected with human immunodeficiency virus. *Journal of Infectious Diseases* 169(1):189–192, 1994.

Templeton GL, Illing LA, Young L. Cave D, Stead WW, and Bates JH. The risk for transmission of Mycobacterium tuberculosis at the bedside and during autopsy. *Annals of Internal Medicine* 122:922–925, 1995.

Tenover FC, Crawford JT, Huebner RE, Geiter LJ, Horsburgh CR Jr, and Good RC. The resurgence of tuberculosis: Is your laboratory ready? *Journal of Clinical Microbiology* 31(4):767–770, 1993.

Tokars JI, Rudnick JR, Kroc K, Manangan L, Pugliese G, Huebner RE, et al. U.S. hospital mycobacteriology laboratories: status and comparison with state public health department laboratories. *Journal of Clinical Microbiology* 34:680–685, 1996.

Trump DH, Hyams KC, Cross ER, and Struewing JP. Tuberculosis infection among young adults entering the US navy in 1990. *Archives of Internal Medicine* 153:211–216, 1993.

Tulsky JP, White MC, Dawson C, Hoynes TM, Goldenson J, and Schecter G. Screening for tuberculosis in jail and clinic follow-up after release. *American Journal of Public Health* 88(2)223–226, 1998.

Tulsky JP, Pilote L, Hahn JA, Zolopa AJ, Burke M, Chesney M, et al. Adherence to isoniazid prophylaxis in the homeless: A randomized controlled trial. *Archives of Internal Medicine* 160:697–702, 2000.

USPSTF (U.S. Preventive Services Task Force). Guide to Clinical Preventive Services: Second Edition. Washington D.C.: U.S. Department of Health and Human Services, 1996.

Ussery XT, Bierman JA, Valway SE, Seitz TA, DiFerdinando GT Jr, and Ostroff SM. Transmission of multidrug-resistant *Mycobacterium tuberculosis* among persons exposed in a medical examiner's office, New York. *Infection Control and Hospital Epidemiology* 16:160–165, 1995.

Van Drunen N, Bonnicksen G, and Pfeiffer AJ. A survey of tuberculosis control programs in seventeen Minnesota hospitals: Implications for policy development. *American Journal of Infection Control* 24:235–242, 1996.

Villarino ME, Burman W, Wang YC, Lundergan L, Catanzaro A, Bock N, et al. Comparable specificity of 2 commercial tuberculin reagents in persons at low risk for tuberculosis infections. *Journal of the American Medical Association* 281(2):169–171, 1999.

Wenger PN, Otten J, Breeden A, Orfas D, Beck-Sague CM, and Jarvis WR. Control of nosocomial transmission of multidrug-resistant *Mycobacterium tuberculosis* among healthcare workers and HIV-infected patients. *The Lancet* 345:235–240, 1995.

WHO (World Health Organization). *Groups at Risk: WHO Report on the Tuberculosis Epidemic 1996*. Geneva 1996: World Health Organization, (http://www.who.int/gtb/-publications/tbrep_96/index.htm, accessed June 12, 2000).

WHO. *Guidelines for the Prevention of Tuberculosis in Health Care Facilities in Resource-Limited Settings*. Geneva: World Health Organization, 1999.

WHO. *Global Tuberculosis Control: WHO Report 2000*. Geneva: World Health Organization, 2000a. (http://www.who.int/gtb/publications/globrep00/index.html, accessed September 25, 2000).

WHO. *Tuberculosis*. Fact Sheet No. 104. Geneva: World Health Organization, April 2000b. (http://www.who.int/inf-fs/en/fact104.html, accessed June 12, 2000).

Woeltje KF, L'Ecuyer PB, Seiler S, and Fraser VJ. Varied approaches to tuberculosis control in a multihospital system. *Infection Control and Hospital Epidemiology* 18:548–553, 1997.

Woods GL, Harris SL, and Solomon D. Tuberculosis knowledge and beliefs among prison inmates and lay employees. *Journal of Correctional Health Care* 4:1–9, 1997.

The York (Pennsylvania) Dispatch. INS, County owe answers on TB. July 24, 2000 *TB-Related News and Journal Items—Week of July 17*, Weekly email news listing compiled by John Seggerson, Atlanta: Centers for Disease Control and Prevention, July 28, 2000.

Zaza S, Blumberg HM, Beck-Sague C, Haas WH, Woodley CL, Pineda M, et al. Nosocomial transmission of *Mycobacterium tuberculosis*: Role of health care workers in outbreak propagation. *Journal of Infectious Diseases* 172(6):1542–1549, 1995.

A

Study Origins and Activities

In November 1999, the U.S. Congress directed the Secretary of Health and Human Services to contract with the National Academy of Sciences (NAS) for a study of the Occupational Safety and Health Administration's (OSHA's) rule making related to occupational exposure to tuberculosis (P.L. 106-113, Conference Report 196-749). The report was requested within 14 months of the legislation. The study was neither to delay issuing of the final rule nor to be delayed pending the rule's publication. (OSHA released the standard after the committee completed its work.)

The agreement between the U.S. Department of Health and Human Services (DHHS) and the Institute of Medicine (IOM; the health policy arm of NAS) allowed the study to began officially on April 1, 2000. To undertake the requested study, the IOM appointed an 11-member committee of experts that met in April, August, and September 2000.

The legislative conference language listed three sets of questions. First, are health care workers at a greater risk of infection, disease, and mortality due to tuberculosis than individuals in the general community within which they reside? If so, what is the excess risk due to occupational exposure? Second, can the occupationally acquired risk be quantified for different work environments, different job classifications, etc., as a result of implementation of the 1994 guidelines of the Centers for Disease Control and Prevention (CDC) for the prevention of tuberculosis transmission at the work site or the implementation of specific parts of the CDC guidelines? Third, what effect will the implementation of OSHA's proposed tuberculosis standard have on minimizing or eliminating the risk of infection, disease, and mortality due to tuberculosis?

For clarity in presenting its analysis, the committee slightly edited the questions as follows. (1) Are health care and selected other categories of workers at greater risk of infection, disease, and mortality due to tuberculosis than others in the community within which they reside? If so, what is the excess risk due to occupational exposure? Can the risk be quantified for different work environments and different job classifications? (2) What is known about the implementation and effects of CDC guidelines to control worker exposure to tuberculosis in hospitals, correctional facilities, and other work settings? (3) Given what is known about the CDC guidelines, what will be the likely effects on tuberculosis infection, disease, or mortality of an OSHA rule to protect workers from occupational exposure to tuberculosis?

Although the revised questions broadened the scope of the committee's work beyond health care workers, most of the information identified by the committee focused on health care workers, mainly hospital employees. The committee arranged for five background papers that appear as Appendixes B, C, D, E, and G in this report. It also conducted a 1-day workshop and a half-day public meeting to solicit oral and written statements from interested organizations. Both these meetings were open to the public. The agendas are listed below.

INSTITUTE OF MEDICINE
COMMITTEE ON REGULATING OCCUPATIONAL EXPOSURE TO TUBERCULOSIS
Public Meeting
Lecture Room, National Academy of Sciences
2101 Constitution Avenue NW, Washington, DC.
Monday, August 7, 2000

AGENDA

1:00 pm   Welcome and Overview of Meeting
           Walter Hierholzer, M.D., Committee Chair
1:10   Panel 1
           Service Employees International Union, AFL-CIO
               William Borwegen, M.P.H.
               Occupational Health and Safety Director
           American Federation of State, County, and Municipal Employees
               James August, M.P.H.
               Assistant Director for Research and Health Services

American Nurses Association
    Karen A. Worthington, M.S., R.N., COHN-S
    Senior Occupational Safety and Health Nurse Specialist
New York State Public Employees Federation
    Jonathan Rosen, M.S., C.I.H.
    Director, Occupational Safety and Health Department
2:00   Panel 2
American Hospital Association
    Roslyne D. W. Schulman, M.H.A., M.B.A.
    Senior Associate Director, Policy Development
    Gina Pugliese, R.N., M.S.
    Director, Premier Safety Institute
American Association of Homes and Services for the Aged
    Linda Bunning, R.N., N.H.A.
    Director of Residential Services, Presbyterian Homes, Inc.
American Academy of Pediatrics
    Jeffrey R. Starke, M.D.
    Member, AAP Committee on Infectious Diseases
    Baylor College of Medicine
American Public Health Association Occupational Health
and Safety Section
    Melissa A. Mc Diarmid, M.D., M.P.H.
    Professor of Medicine
    Director, Occupational Health Project, University of Maryland
3:00   Break
3:20   Panel 3
National Tuberculosis Controllers Association
    Betty L. Gore, R.N., M.S.N., C.I.C.
    Nurse Consultant, Tuberculosis Control Program
    South Carolina Department of Health and Environment
California Department of Health
    Robert Harrison, M.D.
    California Department of Health Services
    Chief, Occupational Health Surveillance and Evaluation Program
American Society for Microbiology
    Mary Gilchrist, Ph.D.
    Director, University Hygienic Laboratory, University of Iowa
Cook County Department of Corrections
    James McAuley, M.D.
    Medical Director, Cermak Health Services

4:10   Panel 4
              Veterans Administration
                  Gary Roselle, M.D.
                  National Program Director for Infectious Diseases
                  Chief, Medical Services, Cincinnati VA Medical Center
              American College of Occupational Medicine
                  John Balbus, M.D.
                  Center for Risk Science and Public Health, George Washington
                  University Medical Center
              American Thoracic Society
                  Edward Nardell, M.D.
                  Associate Professor of Medicine, Harvard Medical School
                  Tuberculosis Control Officer, Massachusetts Department of
                  Health
              Society for Healthcare Epidemiology of America
                  Patrick Brennan, M.D.
                  Hospital Epidemiologist, University of Pennsylvania
                  Association for Professionals in Infection Control
              Rachel Stricof, M.T., M.P.H.
                  Epidemiologist, New York State Department of Health
5:10   Public Comment Period
              Adjourn

                      INSTITUTE OF MEDICINE
          WORKSHOP ON REGULATING OCCUPATIONAL
                  EXPOSURE TO TUBERCULOSIS
          Lecture Room, National Academy of Sciences
          2101 Constitution Avenue NW, Washington, DC.
                   Tuesday, August 8, 2000

                            AGENDA

8:30 am   Welcome, Workshop Objectives
                  Walter Hierholzer, M.D., Committee Chair
                  Professor Emeritus of Internal Medicine, Infectious Diseases
                  and Epidemiology, Yale University
8:40–9:40   Occupational Exposure to Tuberculosis: Evidence Review
                  Thomas Daniel, M.D.
                  Professor Emeritus of Medicine and International Health
                  Case Western Reserve University
              Discussant:
                  George Comstock, M.D., Dr. P.H.
                  Professor of Epidemiology
                  Johns Hopkins University

9:40–10:40   Strengths and Limitations of Tuberculin Skin Testing:
             Evidence Review
                   John Bass, Jr., M.D.
                   Chair, Department of Medicine
                   University of South Alabama
             Discussant:
                   C. Fordham von Reyn
                   Professor of Medicine
                   Section Chief, Infectious Disease Section
                   Dartmouth, Hitchcock Medical Center
10:40–11:00 Break
11:00–12:15 Personal Respirators and Tuberculosis Control: Evidence
             Review
                   Phillip Harber, M.D.
                   Professor, Department of Family Medicine
                   Chief, Occupational and Environmental Medicine
                   University of California, Los Angeles
             Discussants:
                   Lisa Brosseau, Ph.D.
                   Associate Professor, Division of Environmental &
                   Occupational Health, University of Minnesota
                   Barry Farr, M.D.
                   Professor of Internal Medicine, University of Virginia
12:15pm   Lunch in Refectory (tickets in meeting folder)
1:30–3:30   1994 CDC Guidelines: Preventing Transmission of
             Tuberculosis in Health-Care Facilities
             Effects of the CDC Guidelines: Evidence Review
                   Keith Woeltje, M.D., Ph.D.
                   Assistant Professor, Section of Infectious Diseases,
                   Department of Medicine, Medical College of Georgia
             Lessons Learned at the CDC
                   Amy Curtis, Ph.D.
                   Epidemiologist, CDC Division of TB Elimination
             and
                   Lisa Panlilio, M.D.
                   Medical Epidemiologist, CDC Hospital Infections Program
             Discussants:
                   Gina Pugliese, R.N.
                   Director, Premier Safety Institute, Premier Health System
                   James August, M.P.H.
                   Assistant Director for Research and Health
                   American Federation of State, County, and Municipal
                   Employees

3:30–3:50   Break
3:50–4:30   Ethical Issues in Regulating Workplace Exposure to TB
                Ronald Bayer, Ph.D.
                Professor of Public Health, Columbia University
4:30   Public Comment and Continued Discussion
5:00   Adjourn

B

The Tuberculin Skin Test

John B. Bass, Jr., M.D. [*]

About 8 years after announcing the discovery of the tubercle bacillus, Robert Koch announced that he had discovered a cure for the disease.[1] He had prepared a concentrated filtrate from cultures of *Mycobacterium tuberculosis* which had been killed by heat, and he found that this material would protect guinea pigs from experimental tuberculosis. He called this material tuberculin and reported that a series of graduated injections starting with a dilute solution resulted in the cure of selected humans with tuberculosis. His work was hailed in the editorial pages of *The Lancet*[2] and the *Journal of the American Medical Association*,[3] but skeptics were plentiful and included such figures as Billroth, Virchow, and Sir Arthur Conan Doyle. The skepticism of the detractors was quickly confirmed, and Koch's "cure" for tuberculosis was abandoned as a therapeutic maneuver. Despite its failure as a therapeutic substance, tuberculin rapidly became an important diagnostic test. Patients who received tuberculin in an attempt to cure them had generalized systemic reactions including fever, muscle aches, and abdominal discomfort with nausea and vomiting. People without tuberculosis did not develop this violent reaction and a number of investigators suggested the use of tuberculin as a diagnostic test. Local application of tuberculin avoided the serious systemic reactions and provided a local method of determining hypersensitivity to the substance. Methods of local application included a cutaneous scratch (Von Pirquet), a percutaneous patch (Moro), and conjunctival application (Calmette). Intracutaneous injection of tuberculin was described by Mantoux, and his method became widespread because of the reproducibility of the results.

---

[*]Chair, Department of Medicine, University of South Alabama, Mobile.

TUBERCULINS

Koch's original preparation of tuberculin was a relatively crude extraction from heat-killed cultures of *M. tuberculosis*.[4] His material contained a large number of carbohydrate and protein antigens as well as antigens from the beef broth used as a culture medium. Old tuberculin (O.T.) is still produced using methods similar to Koch's original description, although antigens from the beef broth are no longer present. For many years tuberculins were manufactured without much attempt at standardization. Green described this situation:

> It would surely simplify life for manufacture's if O.T. were plainly described as "any witches" brew derived by evaporation of any unspecified fluid medium in which any unspecified strain of mammalian *M. tuberculosis* had been grown, provided its potency matched that of another witches' brew kept in Copenhagen and called international standard, or any allegedly equivalent sub-standard thereof, when tested on an unspecified number of guinea-pigs without worrying too much about statistical analysis of results.[5]

In the 1930s Florence Seibert prepared trichloroacetic acid and ammonium sulfate precipitates of OT and called the material purified protein derivative (PPD).[6] PPD contains a number of antigenic components, most of which are low- and medium-weight proteins. PPD has less carbohydrate antigens than OT and results in fewer nonspecific immediate hypersensitivity reactions. In 1941, Seibert and Glenn[7] prepared a large batch of PPD (PPD-S) that has served as the standard reference material in the United States. The supply of PPD-S is currently becoming exhausted, and a replacement standard is being developed. Other improvements in tuberculin testing include the addition of Tween, a detergent that prevents adsorption of tuberculin to glass and plastic syringes[8,9] and a U.S. Food and Drug Administration requirement that all PPD lots in the United States demonstrate equal potency to PPD-S by bioassay.[10] Despite this demonstration of equal potency, there have been a number of reports suggesting an increase in false-positive reactions in skin testing programs that switched from Tubersol (Connaught, Swiftwater, PA) to Aplisol (Parke-Davis, Morris Plains, NJ).

"Tuberculins" and "PPDs" have been prepared from other mycobacterial species and have provided useful epidemiologic information,[11] but have not been demonstrated to have efficacy as diagnostic tests.

IMMUNE RESPONSE TO TUBERCULIN

Following infection with *M. tuberculosis* there is a sensitization and proliferation of T lymphocytes specific for antigens contained in tuberculin. In the Mantoux method of tuberculin testing, these T lymphocytes accumulate at the site of injection and result in palpable induration. This response requires 24 to 48 hours and has been termed delayed-type hypersensitivity. Delayed hypersensitivity develops 2-10 weeks after initial infection and persists for many years, although reactivity may wane with advancing age.

Dose of Tuberculin

In the early 1900s, tuberculin testing consisted of a series of graduated doses of tuberculin. Any reaction to any dose was considered a positive test, and testing was used largely to eliminate tuberculosis as a diagnostic possibility in sick patients. In the 1920s and 1930s, the decreasing prevalence of tuberculosis resulted in decreased transmission of the infection to younger age groups and tuberculin was suggested as a method of diagnosing the infected state rather than the disease. The use of a series of skin tests with graduated doses of tuberculin was impractical, and in 1941, Furcolow and colleagues[12] reported a dose of 0.0001 mg discriminated patients with tuberculosis from others with the greatest accuracy. This amount of tuberculin was five times the usual starting dose with the graduated regimen and was said to contain 5 tuberculin units (TUs). This 5-TU dose has become the standard for tuberculin testing in the United States. Newly manufactured batches of tuberculin are currently bioassayed, and the 5-TU standard is the amount of material which produces results equal to those produced by 0.0001 mg of PPD-S. Other doses of tuberculin, such as "first strength" (1 TU) and "second strength" (250 TU) represent the smallest and largest doses of tuberculin that were administered in the abandoned graduated tuberculin testing method. These doses have been commercially available in the past, but they are not standardized by bioassay and have no use in diagnostic tuberculin testing programs.

Reading the Tuberculin Test

Although induration is generally accompanied by erythema, results using erythema are less precise and repeatable than those measuring induration, and measurement of induration is the standard. The injection is usually administered on the volar surface of the forearm, and induration is measured 48 to 72 hours following administration. Variation in tests administered simultaneously to both forearms averages about 15 percent and variability in measuring induration among experienced observers is similar. Although interobserver variability may be decreased by using the ballpoint pen method of Sokal,[13] most studies are based on palpation by experienced observers. Even with experienced observers, there is a tendency for clustering around predetermined cut-points and this can be avoided by reading the tests using unmarked calipers. Interpretation of results using methods other than the Mantoux method is problematic, and multiple puncture devices appear to be less sensitive and specific than the Mantoux method. Specificity becomes increasingly important as the prior probability of infection becomes low and the Mantoux method is suggested as the standard.

OPERATING CHARACTERISTICS OF THE TUBERCULIN TEST

Despite the fact that PPD is a relatively crude material and results are dependent on the variability in immunologic reactivity in recipients of the test, the operating characteristics of the tuberculin test appear to be superior to those of many other tests which are commonly used in clinical medicine. Despite the superior operating characteristics, the positive predictive value of the test is probably poor whenever the prior probability of infection is less than 1 percent.[14,15] Unfortunately for the test, but fortunately for the individuals involved, this situation applies to almost all medical occupations currently. This difficulty was recognized as early as 1960: "There may be nostalgia for the days when all tuberculin reactions meant tuberculous infection, and no nonsense"[16]

Sensitivity

In the absence of an independent means of determining whether or not a person is infected with *M. tuberculosis,* the sensitivity of the tuberculin test in detecting latent infection cannot be determined with absolute accuracy. Most estimates of sensitivity have been derived from testing in patients with known tuberculosis. The sensitivity of tuberculin testing in patients presenting with newly diagnosed pulmonary tuberculosis is approximately 80 percent.[17,18] The 20 percent false-negative rate is due to a combination of specific immunosuppression of delayed hypersensitivity from cytokines plus overwhelming acute illness and poor nutrition. After such patients have received several weeks of therapy and nutrition, the sensitivity of tuberculin testing is approximately 95 percent. This correlates well with older studies in the prechemotherapeutic area which showed a 96 percent sensitivity in relatively stable patients in tuberculosis hospitals. Patients who are critically ill with tuberculosis (especially those with disseminated tuberculosis and tuberculous meningitis) may have false-negative rates exceeding 50 percent. T-cell depletion from infection with human immunodeficiency virus also commonly causes false-negative tuberculin reactions. Anergy testing with several other delayed hypersensitivity antigens will not detect all of these false-negative reactions,[18] and the recommendation to use anergy testing clinically in such circumstances has been deleted from the latest American Thoracic Society/Centers for Disease Control and Prevention recommendations.[19]

Although the sensitivity of tuberculin testing cannot be accurately determined in subjects without tuberculosis, a reasonable assumption is that the sensitivity is approximately that seen in patients with tuberculosis who have received adequate treatment and is approximately 95 percent. There are hypothetical reasons that the test might be more or less sensitive in people without disease. It is possible that people infected with *M. tuberculosis* without disease have better immunity to the infection and might be more likely to react to tuberculin. It is also possible that people who are infected without disease have a smaller antigenic burden and might be less reactive to tuberculin. The likelihood that either of these hypotheses is of major importance is small, and the sensitivity of the tuberculin test in latent tuberculosis infection is assumed to be approximately 95 percent.

Specificity

Just as with the sensitivity, the lack of an independent method of determining infection means that the specificity cannot be determined with complete accuracy. The major reasons for false-positive tests in uninfected persons are thought to be cross-reactions in persons who have been vaccinated with bacille Calmette-Guérin (BCG)[20] or persons who have environmental exposure to other mycobacteria.[21] Prior BCG vaccination is generally known, but environmental exposure to other mycobacteria varies widely geographically and is difficult to estimate.

The large scale skin-testing surveys in the past have shown a great deal of geographic variability in skin testing results.[11] In areas of the country where environmental mycobacteria are uncommon, the distribution of skin-test reactions approximates that shown in Figure B-1. This distribution is similar to results obtained in skin testing of patients with active tuberculosis, and the presumption is that there are few false-positive tests in such a population. At the other end of the spectrum, areas of the country with likely exposures to environmental mycobacteria more closely resemble the distributions seen in Figure B-2. In such a population there is no clear-cut unimodal distribution of positive results and many more false-positive tests are present. In such a population, false-positive results can be minimized and the specificity of the test can be improved by progressively increasing the cutoff point for determination of positivity. In the United States there is a tendency for results to resemble those shown in Figure B-2 in the eastern and southern parts of the country. However, considerable variability occurs even within a single state, and the U.S. population is much more diverse and mobile than it was when these results were obtained.

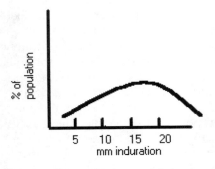

FIGURE B-1. Distribution of skin test reactions in a population with little cross sections.

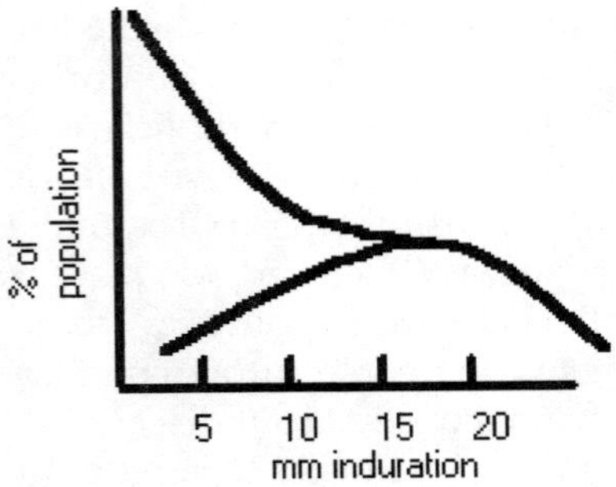

FIGURE B-2. Distribution of skin test reactions in a population with many cross sections. A hypothetical population of true positives is superimposed.

A large number of recent studies of serial skin testing programs in hospitals and other medical facilities have shown a clustering of yearly conversion rates around 0.5–1 percent in institutions without obvious exposure to undiagnosed and untreated cases of tuberculosis.[22,23] Although it is unproveable, it seems a reasonable assumption that these rates of conversion represent the false-positive rate of serial tuberculin testing and that the specificity of the test is 99 to 99.5 percent. The specificity is likely to be somewhat less than this in areas of the country where exposure to other mycobacteria is common.

Table B-1 shows the influence of prior probability or prevalence of infection on the positive predictive value of a tuberculin test for varying levels of specificity. The two columns on the right give the range of the positive predictive value for any given prevalence of infection for a specificity of 99 to 99.5 percent. The column with a specificity of 95 percent may represent a "worse-case" scenario in areas where cross-reactions to other mycobacteria are very common. To put these prevalences in perspective, 100 years ago about 90 percent of all adults were infected with *M. tuberculosis*. This was when the tuberculin test was introduced, and at that time it had a very high positive predictive value. Many nations around the globe continue to have infection rates of 25 to 50 percent and people from these countries commonly immigrate to the United States. Close contacts to active cases of tuberculosis may also have a 25 to 50 percent likelihood of being infected. Tuberculin testing targeted toward such populations is warranted.[19] The general adult population of the United States at this time has an infection rate approximately 5 to 10 percent and in this group the predictive value of a positive test begins to fall. Baseline transmission of tuberculosis infection in the United States has been estimated to be 0.05 percent per person a year. Testing of the

TABLE B-1. Predictive Value of a Positive Tuberculin Test

Prevalence of Infection (%)	Predictive Value (%) at Indicated Specificity		
	0.95	0.99	0.995
90	99	99	99
50	95	99	99
20	86	97	98
10	67	91	95
5	50	83	90
2	29	67	80
1	16	49	67
.1	3	10	17
.05	.9	4.8	9

general population of the country on a yearly basis to detect this transmission would have a positive predictive value of less than 10 percent (see Table B-1).

THE BOOSTER PHENOMENON

Although skin testing with tuberculin does not induce enough immunologic challenge to induce a positive reaction on subsequent tests, waned delayed hypersensitivity reactions from remote infections with *M. tuberculosis* and cross-reactions to antigens from other mycobacteria can be boosted or enhanced.[24] Such boosting generally occurs within 1 week and may persist for a year or more. Boosted reactions are particularly common in people who have received BCG vaccination,[20] people with environmental exposure to other mycobacteria, and people from countries with a high prevalence of tuberculosis. False conversions due to boosting are particularly common in these populations when the second skin test is placed in a serial skin testing program.[25] In order to detect this phenomenon, it is recommended that serial skin testing programs use an initial two-step test in which a second skin test is placed approximately 1-week after the first if there is no reaction to the first and that significant reactions to the second test are considered boosted reactions rather than conversions. There is a suggestion that boosted reactions may continue to occur subsequent to the second test in persons who have been vaccinated with BCG and persons from high-prevalence countries, but no practical method of detecting these late boosters is available.

Implications of Operating Characteristics of Tuberculin Test for Serial Skin Testing in Medical Populations

In considering serial tuberculin testing, the values in Table B-1 will represent incidence rather than prevalence, and this incidence is the likelihood of true transmission of *M. tuberculosis* infection in the interval between skin tests. The influence of serial skin testing on the specificity of the test is unknown. To the extent that false-positive results are random biologic events, the false-positive rate will remain relatively constant regardless of the interval between tests, and the number of people in a given population with false-positive test results will gradually grow over time in inverse proportion to the testing interval. Thus, frequent testing will gradually result in the accumulation of a large proportion of the population with false-positive results regardless of the incidence of true transmission of infection.

If false-positive results are not true random biologic events but, rather, reflect individual immunologic responsiveness to tuberculin, persons predisposed to such false-positive results may be removed from a serially tested population and the specificity of the test may improve with time. Most authors have concluded that serial skin testing programs tend to overestimate the incidence of new tuberculosis infection in the populations being tested,[26,27] and it seems likely that false-positive results are random biologic events which will be magnified as the interval between serial tests is decreased.

In the absence of documented nosocomial epidemics of tuberculosis, almost all estimates of hospital transmission of tuberculosis infection are less than 1 percent yearly. If the previous estimates of specificity are accepted, the predictive value of positive tuberculin test done at yearly intervals in such populations will be less than 50 percent. If the assumption that the false-positive rate is a random biologic event is correct, this positive predictive value would be further reduced by testing at 6- or 3-month intervals.

The major value of a serial skin testing program is to alert the system that an abnormally high rate of tuberculosis transmission is occurring.[28,29,30,31,32] Table B-2 shows the range of actual transmission of infection based on the observed rate of skin test conversion assuming a 99 to 99.5 percent specificity. Skin test conversion rates below 1 percent probably reflect very low actual transmission and the majority of skin test conversions are probably false-positive reactions. Conversion rates above 2 percent probably represent actual transmission of infection.

Implications of Decreased Positive-Predictive Value for Tuberculin Test on a Tuberculosis Program

Almost all information concerning interventions in tuberculosis infection without disease are based on studies in populations with a high prevalence of tuberculosis infection and thus a high positive predictive value of the tuberculin skin test. A good example is preventive therapy. Estimates of efficacy and efficiency of preventive therapy are based on

TABLE B-2. Range of Actual Transmission Rates for Observed Skin Test Conversion Rate

Conversion Rate	Actual Transmission Rate (%)
0.5	~0
1	0–0.5
2	0.5–1
5	4–4.5

data from populations where a positive tuberculin reaction had a very high likelihood of indicating true infection.

If we apply these interventions to populations with a lesser likelihood of being truly infected, two phenomena will occur. The first is that the effectiveness of the intervention will appear to be increased. As the number of persons with false-positive reactions increases, the likelihood of true infection in the population decreases, and the likelihood of disease developing subsequent to the intervention decreases in like proportion. Second, the true effectiveness of the intervention actually decreases. As the proportion of people with the condition to be prevented decreases, there is less to prevent and the number of cases actually prevented falls. This actual decrease in true benefit results in a rise in the cost-benefit and risk-benefit ratios.

REFERENCES

1. Koch R. Über bacteriologische Forschung. *Deutsche Medizinische Wochnschrift* 1890; 16:756 (translated in *Lancet* 1890; 2:673).
2. Editorial. The nature of Dr. Koch's liquid. *Lancet* 1890; 2:1233.
3. Editorial. Koch and his critics. *Journal of the American Medical Association* 1890; 15:902.
4. Koch R. Fortsetzung der Mittheilungen über ein Heilmittel gegen Tuberculose. *Deutsche Medizinische Wochnschrift* 1891; 17:101 (translated in *Lancet* 1891; 1:168).
5. Green H.H. Discussion on tuberculins in human and veterinary medicine. *Proceedings of the Royal Society of Medicine* 1951; 44:1045.
6. Seibert F.B. The isolation and properties of the purified protein derivative of tuberculin. *American Review of Tuberculosis* 1934; 30:713.
7. Seibert F.B. and Glenn J.T. Tuberculin purified protein derivative: preparation and analyses of a large quantity for standard. *American Review of Tuberculosis* 1941; 44:9.
8. Landi S., Held H.R., Houschild A.H.W., et al. Adsorption of tuberculin PPD to glass and plastic surfaces. *Bulletin of the World Health Organization* 1966; 35:593–602.
9. Zack M.B. and Fulkerson L.L. Clinical reliability of stabilized and nonstabilized tuberculin PPD. *American Review of Respiratory Diseases* 1970; 102:91–93.
10. Sbarbaro J.A. Skin test antigens: an evaluation whose time has come. *American Review of Respiratory Diseases* 1978; 118:1–5.
11. Edwards L.B., Acquaviva F.A., Livesay V.T., Cross F.W., and Palmer C.E. An atlas of sensitivity to tuberculin, PPD-B, and histoplasmin in the United States. *American Review of Respiratory Diseases* 1969; 99:1–132.
12. Furcolow M.L., Hewell B., Nelson W.E., and Palmer C.E. Quantitative studies of the tuberculin reaction. I. Titration of tuberculin sensitivity and its relation to tuberculous infection. *Public Health Reports* 1941; 56:1082.

13. Sokal J.E. Measurement of delayed skin-test responses. *New England Journal of Medicine* 1975; 293:501–502.

14. Bass J.B. The tuberculin test. IN: Reichman L.B., Hershfield E.S. (eds.). *Tuberculosis: A Comprehensive International Approach*. Marcel Dekker, New York, 1993.

15. Huebner R.E., Schein M.F., and Bass J.B. The tuberculin skin test. *Clinical Infectious Diseases* 1993; 17:968–975.

16. Edwards P.Q. and Edwards L.B. Story of the tuberculin test. *American Review of Respiratory Diseases* 1960; 81:1–49.

17. Holden M., Dubin M.R., and Diamond P.H. Frequency of negative intermediate-strength tuberculin sensitivity in patients with active tuberculosis. *New England Journal of Medicine* 1971; 285:1506–1509.

18. Nash D.R. and Douglass J.E. A comparison between positive and negative reactors and an evaluation of 5 TU and 250 TU skin test doses. *Chest* 1980; 77:32–37.

19. ATS/CDCP (American Thoracic Society/Centers for Disease Control and Prevention). Targeted tuberculin testing and treatment of latent tuberculosis infection. *American Journal of Respiratory and Critical Care Medicine* 2000; 161:S221–S247.

20. Sepulveda R.L., Ferrer X, Latrach C., and Sorensen R.U. The influence of Calmette-Guérin bacillus immunization on the booster effect of tuberculin testing in healthy young adults. *American Review of Respiratory Diseases* 1990; 142:24–28.

21. Daniel T.M. and Janicki B.W. Mycobacterial antigens: a review of their isolation, chemistry, and immunological properties. *Microbiological Review* 1978; 42:84–113.

22. Bowden K.M. and McDiarmid M.A. Occupationally acquired tuberculosis: what's known. *Journal of Occupational Medicine* 1994; 36:320–325.

23. Aitken M.L., Anderson K.M., and Albert R.K. Is the tuberculosis screening program of hospital employees still required? *American Review of Respiratory Diseases* 1987; 136:805–807.

24. Thompson N.J., Glassroth J.L., Snider D.E., Jr., and Farer L.S. The booster phenomenon in serial tuberculin testing. *American Review of Respiratory Diseases* 1979; 119:587–597.

25. Bass J.B., Jr., and Serio R.A. The use of repeat skin tests to eliminate the booster phenomenon in serial tuberculin testing. *American Review of Respiratory Diseases* 1981; 123:394–396.

26. Bass J.B., Sanders R.V., and Kirkpatrick M.B. Choosing an appropriate cutting point for conversion in annual tuberculin skin testing. *American Review of Respiratory Diseases* 1985; 132:379–381.

27. De March-Ayuela P. Choosing an appropriate criteria for true or false conversion in serial tuberculin testing. *American Review of Respiratory Diseases* 1990; 141:815–820.

28. Louther J., Rivera P., Feldman J., Villa N., DeHovitz J., and Sepkowitz K.A. Risk of tuberculin conversion according to occupation among health care workers at a New York City hospital. *American Journal of Respiratory and Critical Care Medicine* 1997; 156:201–205.

29. Fella P., Rivera P., Hale M., Squires K., and Sepkowitz K. Dramatic decrase in tuberculin skin test conversion rate among employees at a hospital in New York City. *American Journal of Infection Control* 1995; 23:352–356.

30. Sotir M.J., Khan A., Bock N.N., and Blumberg H.M. Risk factors for tuberculin skin test (TST) positivity and conversion among employees at a public inner-city hospital in a high incidence area. *Journal of Investigative Medicine* 1997; 45:64A.

31. Blumberg H.M., Sotir M., Erwin M., Bachman R., and Shulman J.A. Risk of house staff tuberculin skin test conversion in an area with a high incidence of tuberculosis. *Clinical and Infectious Diseases* 1998; 27:826–833.

32. Boudreau A.Y., Baron S.L., Steenland N.K., Van Gilder T.J., Decker J.A., Galson S.K., Seitz T. Occupational risk of *Mycobacterium tuberculosis* infection in hospital workers. *American Journal of Industrial Medicine*. 1997; 32:528–534.

C

The Occupational Tuberculosis Risk of Health Care Workers

Thomas M. Daniel, M.D. [*]

SUMMARY AND CONCLUSIONS

A review of published literature has been undertaken in response to a commission from the Institute of Medicine Committee on Regulating Occupational Exposure to Tuberculosis. The charge of this commission was to prepare a review paper addressing the question of whether health care workers (and workers at other sites covered by the proposed regulations of the Occupational Safety and Health Administration [OSHA]) are at a greater risk of infection, disease, and mortality due to tuberculosis than the general community within which they reside. This paper focuses principally on the risk of infection, with only limited comments on the risks of disease and mortality. In conducting this review, the author faced limitations imposed by the quality of the published data and by the lack of published information relevant to some of the aspects of the charge. In particular, much of the quantitative data presented here can be taken as no more than approximate. Nevertheless, certain conclusions have been drawn by the author.

Health care workers are at risk of contracting tuberculous infection in the workplace. This risk has been declining in recent decades. In those health care facilities where modern infection control measures are in place, it now approaches the level of risk incurred by health care workers in the communities in which they reside. That it has declined and continues to

[*]Professor Emeritus of Medicine and International Health, Case Western Reserve University, Cleveland, Ohio.

decline means that it has been higher than the baseline community risk, and it will not be possible to assume that there is no excess risk until no further decline is observed.

A large portion of the current and recent risk to health care workers of tuberculous infection is the result of exposure to unsuspected cases of infectious tuberculosis or to exposure in circumstances of poor ventilation. In some outbreaks from unsuspected sources, exposed employee infection rates have been as high as 50 percent. When effective infection control procedures are in place, unsuspected contagious cases of tuberculosis may provide nearly all of the occupational tuberculosis risk.

The risk to health care workers of tuberculous infection varies with job category. In general, health care workers in contact with patients are at higher risk than those with no patient contact. Noncontact employees often have a higher incidence of infection than contact employees, but this is due to community exposure risk. Job situations of exceptionally high risk are those involving the generation of respiratory aerosols from patients, including bronchoscopy, endotracheal suctioning and intubation, cough and sputum induction, and the administration of irritation medications (e.g., pentamidine) by aerosol.

The risk to health care workers of tuberculous infection varies in the United States with geographic locale. The incidence of tuberculosis varies greatly with location in the United States. Coastal urban cities bear the greatest tuberculosis burden and rural Midwest and mountain state regions the least. Health care facilities in these various regions care for numbers of patients with tuberculosis that vary substantially in parallel with variations in incidence.

The risk to health care workers of tuberculous infection varies in the United States with demography and ethnicity. In general, individuals of African-American, Hispanic, and Asian heritage have a higher incidence of tuberculous infection than do persons of European extraction. Foreign-born Americans bring with them much of the tuberculous infection risk of the countries of their origins. The risk of tuberculous infection varies greatly with socioeconomic status, most of the infection risk being incurred by those who are less affluent. For health care workers, these variations in population tuberculosis incidence have two important consequences. First of all, the tuberculous infection risk in the community in which health care workers reside and in which they usually spend more time than they do in their job setting is correlated with these ethnic and demographic variables. Second, the population served by the health care facility will influence the amount of potential tuberculosis exposure of the employees.

The occupational tuberculosis risk to American health care workers can be quantified only in approximate terms. The magnitude of the tuberculosis risk to American health care workers at the current time in those facilities where recent Centers for Disease Control and Prevention (CDC) guidelines for infection control have been implemented is usually not substantially greater than the risk incurred by these individuals in the communities in which they reside.

The risk to infected health care workers of progression to tuberculous disease (tuberculosis) is lower than often stated; the risk of mortality for immunocompetent individuals harboring drug-susceptible organisms is negligible. The risks of tuberculous disease and mortality in *Mycobacterium tuberculosis*-infected health care workers is probably no higher than that of individuals in the general population. Overall, the risk of tuberculosis in individuals who become infected as adults is probably of the order of 5 percent. Nearly all of the tuberculosis mortality in the United States today is accounted for by individuals who fail to be diagnosed or treated in timely fashion, who are immunocompromised (usually by human immunodeficiency virus [HIV] infection), or who suffer from multidrug-resistant tuberculosis.

INTRODUCTION

In an era of recently resurgent tuberculosis and accompanying concern about the occupational tuberculosis risk of health care workers, the Institute of Medicine has been asked by the U.S. Congress to study the magnitude of this occupational risk and the potential impact on it of a newly proposed rule regulating the environment in which care of tuberculosis patients is conducted. At the present time, health care workers account for about 3 percent of the cases of tuberculosis reported in the United States (1).

Charge to the Reviewer

This paper reviews the published medical literature relevant to the occupational tuberculosis risks of American health care workers. It was commissioned by the Institute of Medicine Committee on Regulating Occupational Exposure to Tuberculosis. The charge of this committee was to prepare a state-of-the-art literature review addressing the following questions:

> Are health care workers (and workers at other sites covered by the proposed OSHA regulations) at a greater risk of infection, disease, and mortality due to tuberculosis than the general community within which they reside? If so, what is the excess risk due to occupational exposure? Can the occupationally acquired risk be quantified for different work environments and different job classifications?

Determinants of Tuberculosis Risks

Consideration of the occupational tuberculosis risk of health care workers must be done in two parts: the risk of infection and the risk of disease. The determinants of these risks are multiple. Exposure is a major determinant of infection risk, and it may be related to the work place, although it must be realized that health care workers may also face exposure in the communities in which they reside. Individual factors such as age, immune status, and genetic composition (possibly including race) are also important, especially for the risk of disease. These factors are not per se related to the workplace, but that does not mean they are not operative in the workplace.

Published Literature Reviews

There have been a number of well-done literature reviews of the occupational tuberculosis risk to health care workers published during the past decade (2–9). In general, these reviews emphasize the risk of tuberculous infection and do not deal with the subsequent risk of disease. Nor do they provide much information permitting one to compare the workplace risk to that incurred in the community in which health care workers reside. These reviews have documented that tuberculin conversion rates for American health care workers in the recent past were as high as 4–5 percent/year in many urban areas and perhaps twice that in some areas of New York City and for certain job situations with high exposures to aerosols of respiratory secretions. In nonurban areas, they were generally lower than 0.2 percent/year. With the implementation of enhanced infection control measures recommended by such advisory groups as CDC during the past decade, these rates have dropped to below 1 percent generally. However, outbreaks continue to occur from unrecognized sources, and with these outbreaks the tuberculin conversion rates among exposed employees may be as high as 50 percent.

METHODS

Literature Review

This paper is based on a review of published literature. Searching was done using PubMed (MedLine) with a variety of topics relevant to tuberculosis and health care workers. Additional publications were selected from the bibliographies of published reports. Identified papers were then retrieved using the resources of the Health Sciences Library and Allen Memorial Library of Case Western Reserve University. Finally, a number of relevant papers were already present in the author's personal library and reprint collection.

Data presented in this paper have been converted, when possible, from the form in which they were originally presented to percent per year. In a few reports, the original data are given as per 100 person-years, and this more precise form has been retained. In many instances, no time interval was given, and in these cases percent is used. Because many of these conversions to percentages are based on small absolute numbers, the actual numbers are given in those cases to allow the reader to note this fact.

Annual Risk of Tuberculous Infection

The annual risk of infection (ARI) with *M. tuberculosis*, the tubercle bacillus, is central to any consideration of the occupational tuberculosis risk of health care workers. Ideally, one would like to know this figure not only for employees but also for the community in which they reside. Data upon which the ARI for American populations can be calculated are generally lacking, however, and many of the reports of infections in health care workers do not provide relevant time intervals. In this review, ARI is expressed as percent per year, the usage of most workers who have dealt with this subject.

It is acknowledged that the term "annual risk" as it is used here is imprecise—annual probablilty or likelihood would be more accurate terms—but its use is widely established in the published literature on this subject, and it is used here for consistency with that literature. It is also true that such calculations on an annual basis ignore the fact that the pool of individuals considered may change during a year. However, data are almost always lacking in the studies reviewed here for estimation of the more accurate use of person-years at risk. Errors thus introduced are small at low levels of risk and do not affect the conclusions drawn in this review.

Two types of ARI are reported here: (a) calculated annual risks, when the data permit such direct calculation, and (b) estimated annual risks based on tuberculosis incidence when direct calculation is not possible.

Calculated Annual Risk of Infection

If one accepts the development of tuberculin hypersensitivity as a reliable index of primary tuberculous infection, then it is a straightforward task to calculate the ARI with *M. tuberculosis* expressed as percent per year from serial skin testing data. The algebraic formula for this calculation is

$$ARI = [1 - (Q_b/Q_a)^{1/(b-a)}] * 100,$$

where Q is $1 - P$, P is the probability of being infected at a given age or year a or b, a is the initial age or year of observation, and b is the second year or age of observation (10). In the text of the present review paper, ARI thus calculated is referred to as the "calculated ARI."

Estimated Annual Risk of Infection

Styblo has observed that there is an empiric and relatively constant relationship between the incidence of smear-positive tuberculosis and the annual risk of infection (11). He estimated that the ratio between this incidence and the ARI ranged between 50 and 60 in a variety of populations, pricipally those of high tuberculosis prevalence. Daniel and Debanne reasoned that this relationship could be used in reverse to estimate ARI when good case reporting was available but tuberculin skin test data were absent. They tested this hypothesis using data from white male U.S. naval recruits and found that in this population the ratio of incidence of tuberculosis of all forms to ARI was approximately 150 (10). The disparity between this figure and the lower figure of Styblo may result in part from the use of low-incidence populations, but the largest reason for the difference rests with the use by Daniel and Debanne of rates for all forms of tuberculosis, whereas Styblo considered only single-sputum smear-positive, pulmonary tuberculosis. In the current review paper estimation of ARIs is based on a ratio of 150, and ARI thus derived is referred to as the "estimated ARI." While this method is imprecise, it is often the only means available to judge ARI in American populations.

Limitations of This Study

In doing this review, three limitations were deliberately imposed. First, papers published prior to 1970 were used only to a limited degree and then only to provide historical context. Second, limited use was made of reports of outbreaks, for these accounts are usually anecdotal in character. Third, most papers describing studies done in other countries were excluded because both health care occupational sites and attitudes toward occupational risks in most other countries differ substantially from those in the United States.

A major limitation in this review and in the entire body of knowledge that it approaches rests with the definitions of tuberculous infection and of tuberculous disease. This subject is separately addressed in a paper authored by John B. Bass Jr., and is included in this report as Appendix B.

RISK OF TUBERCULOUS INFECTION

Risk in the U.S. General Population

If one is to examine the occupational risk of tuberculous infection among health care workers in relation to the communities in which they reside, then it is first important to try to determine the annual risk of infection in the general American public. Tuberculin testing data upon which such a determination can be based are limited. The last systematic attempt to estimate the prevalence of tuberculin reactivity in the United States was that of the National Health Survey of 1971–72, which concluded that in American adults aged 25 to 74 years the prevalence of tuberculin reactivity was 21.5 percent (12). A reasonable estimate for the current date for Americans of all ages might be 5 to 10 percent, and perhaps 10 percent in adults.

Tuberculous infection is not uniformly distributed among Americans, and it is important to stratify any assessment of the general population risk so that infection in health care workers can be compared with that in the appropriate reference community. For example, tuberculosis is much more common in urban areas than in rural areas, and even in the cities of middle America it is not as frequent as in this country's coastal cities. Many demographic factors correlate with tuberculosis incidence in America. Health care workers are employed, while nearly 60 percent of tuberculosis in the United States occurs among the unemployed (1). Importantly for this consideration, a substantial number of health care workers are foreign-born, one-third of them coming from the Philippines; among other employed persons, one-quarter come from Mexico (A. Curtis, personal communication of material presented to a workshop held in December 1999). The importance of this difference rests with the difference in tuberculosis in the countries of origin for these groups. Based on recent World Health Organization estimates, the current incidence of sputum smear-positive tuberculosis in the Philippines is 260/100,000, and that in Mexico is 58/100,000 (13).

Calculated ARI with *M. tuberculosis* in Selected American Populations

There are relatively few tuberculin surveys available from which one can calculate the ARI in American populations and none in recent years. Moreover, those surveys that have been conducted have often been flawed by the use of poorly standardized tuberculin testing techniques and by poor characterization of the populations studied, especially with respect to demographic characteristics. The use of tuberculins other than purified protein derivative (PPD) at 5 tuberculin units may lead to an overestimation of the actual prevalence of tuberculin reactivity. Data from 12 selected surveys conducted in the United States during the middle half of the 1990s are presented in Table C-1. These studies rarely involved serial testing or testing of more than one age group. In that situation, the calculation of ARI for Table C-1 was done from birth, assuming a reactor rate of zero at birth, a maneuver admittedly flawed because it assumes the risk to be uniform throughout life. The error thus introduced has the potential for underestimating the adult risk relevant to health care workers.

TABLE C-1. Tuberculin Surveys in the United States and ARI with *M. tuberculosis* Calculated from Them

Year of Study	Population (Reference)	Tuberculin*	Calculated ARI (%/year)
1930	New York City, schoolchildren (17)	OT, 10 TU	11.14
1957	Pamlico County, GA, general population (18)	PPD-S, 5 TU	0.25
1957–60	Chicago nursing students (19)	OT, 2 TU	0.75
1958–65	White naval recruits (20)	PPD-S, 5 TU	0.14
1963	Pennsylvania high school students (21)	PPD, 5 TU	0.19
1964–65	Air force recruits (14)	Tine test	0.16
1965–69	First grade children in United States (21)	Probably PPD-S	0.08–0.05
1964–67	CDC surveys at selected sites (22)	PPD, 5 TU	0.16
1971–72	National health survey (HANES) (12)	PPD-S, 5 TU	0.58
1973–74	New York City Board of Education employees (16)	PPD, 5 TU	0.23
1975–79	CDC–reported data from selected sites (1)	Variable	0.20–0.15
1980–81	New York City school children (23)	PPD, 5 TU	0.45

*Tuberculins used for skin testing have included old tuberculin (OT), a crude preparation, and purified protein derivative (PPD), a somewhat purified preparation made from OT. PPD has been made by many manufacturers. PPD-S refers to a single large batch of PPD prepared by Florence Seibert, of which half was deposited as the reference standard against which all other PPDs are standardized and half was given to the U.S. Public Health Service for use in research studies. Tine tests use OT. The dose of tuberculin used for testing is expressed in tuberculin units (TU), which are based upon bioequivalent standardization with PPD-S. The usual dose, for which the largest amount of validation data are available, is 5 TU.

It is evident that ARIs are larger in urban populations—specifically, New York City—than elsewhere. Unfortunately, the available data often are not sufficient to make generalizations with respect to geography nor with respect to such demographic factors as ethnicity or socioeconomic status. Two studies of military recruits allow one to examine race and ethnicity (14, 15). The annual risks of infection calculated from these studies are shown in Table C-2. Data from a single study in New York City school board employees allow one to examine race and ethnicity in the urban setting (16). The calculated ARIs from this study are shown in Table C-3. The ARI calculated for African American and Hispanic military recruits for 1990 was approximately six times that for whites. For Asian recruits the calculated ARI was approximately 36 times that for whites. For New York City, calculation from the 1973 data yielded an ARI for African Americans 8.6 times those in whites and for Puerto Ricans 6.5 times those in whites.

TABLE C-2. ARIs Calculated for U.S. Military Recruits in 1965 (14) and 1990 (15)

Racial/Ethnic Group as Characterized by Study Author	Calculated ARI, 1965 (30) (%/year)	Calculated ARI, 1990 (35) (%/year)
White	0.16	0.04
Black	0.56	0.25
Puerto Rican	1.12	0.26
American Indian	0.92	
Asian		1.45

TABLE C-3. ARIs Calculated for New York City in 1962 (20) and 1973 (16)

Racial/Ethnic Group as Characterized by Study Author	Calculated ARI, 1962 (20) (%/year)	Calculated ARI, 1973 (16) (%/year)
White	0.2	0.08
Black		0.69
Puerto Rican		0.52

Estimated ARI with *M. Tuberculosis* in Selected American Populations

As noted previously, it is possible to estimate the ARI from reported case rates. However, one must be cautious about the precision of these estimates. Having expressed this concern about their use, estimated ARIs are presented for various American populations in Tables C-4, C-5, and C-6.

TABLE C-4. ARI in 1998 Estimated by Method of Daniel and Debanne (10) for Various Demographic and Racial Segments of the U.S. Population, 25- to 44-Year-Old Age Cohort

Population Group	Tuberculosis Case Rate per 100,000, 1998[*]	Estimated ARI (%/year)
United States total	6.8	0.05
White, not Hispanic, male	3.1	0.02
White, not Hispanic, female	1.5	0.01
Black, not Hispanic, male	23.5	0.16
Black, not Hispanic, female	12.7	0.08
Hispanic male	17.1	0.11
Hispanic female	9.9	0.07
Asian/Pacific Islander, male	42.8	0.29
Asian/Pacific Islander, female	30.9	0.21

[*]Tuberculosis case rates for 1998 are CDC-reported data (1).

TABLE C-5. ARI in 1998 Estimated by Method of Daniel and Debanne (10) for Selected American Cities, All Ages

City	Tuberculosis Case Rate per 100,000, 1998*	Estimated ARI (%/year)
Atlanta, GA	8.9	0.06
Baltimore, MD	7.6	0.05
Greensboro, NC	5.6	0.04
Los Angeles, CA	14.9	0.10
Miami, FL	13.4	0.09
New York, NY	19.1	0.13
Newark, NJ	10.7	0.07
Philadelphia, PA	5.8	0.04
St. Louis, MO	4.3	0.03
Salt Lake City, UT	3.3	0.02
San Francisco, CA	18.2	0.12
Seattle, WA	5.9	0.04

*Tuberculosis case rates for 1998 are CDC-reported data (1).

Summary of Risk of Tuberculous Infection in the General U.S. Population

In general, the ARI in American populations has been declining during the past century and is now very low, although it may have increased in New York City and certain other urban areas with the recent resurgence of tuberculosis. The risk is much lower in rural areas and cities in the Midwest and mountain states than it is in major coastal cities, where most of the infectious cases of tuberculosis occur. The risk in America's

TABLE C-6. ARI Estimated by Method of Daniel and Debanne (10) for Selected Demographic Groups Ages 16–64 Years as Reported for 1984–85 by McKenna and Colleagues (24)

Demographic Group	Tuberculosis Case Rate per 100,000	Estimated ARI (%/year)
Total	8.4	0.06
Not Hispanic, white	3.6	0.02
Not Hispanic, black	35.1	0.23
Hispanic	20.2	0.13
Asian	56.1	0.37
Male	11.8	0.08
Female	5.1	0.03
Currently employed	4.9	0.03
Previously employed	11.6	0.08
Unemployed	337.2	2.25
U.S.-born	7.2	0.05
Foreign-born	29.2	0.19

ethnic minority populations is much higher than it is in Americans of European extraction—of the order of 0.1 to 0.2 percent/year as opposed to 0.01 to 0.02 percent/year. For unemployed individuals, the group from which more than half of American tuberculosis cases are reported, the annual risk of infection probably exceeds 2.0 percent/year. Tuberculosis among foreign-born individuals now accounts for about 40 percent of new cases each year in the United States. Foreign-born individuals bring with them their infection histories from the countries in which they originate, many of them high-tuberculosis-incidence countries. The ARI in foreign-born persons in the United States is probably about 0.2 percent/year. Considering the country as a whole, 0.05 percent is probably a reasonable estimate of the ARI.

Risk in Hospital-Based Health Care Workers

Until the 1950s, when effective chemotherapy heralded the closing of most tuberculosis sanatoria and categorical tuberculosis hospital services, the occupational risk of tuberculous infection was generally accepted by all health care workers. Indeed, primary tuberculous infection was welcomed by many because of the immunity to subsequent infection that accompanied it. Numerous studies showed student nurses to be at especially high risk, and medical students fared little better.

Following the widespread introduction of isoniazid in 1953, tuberculosis sanatoria saw a dramatic fall in their patient censuses, with much shortened hospital stays, and they began to close their doors. The May 1969 issue of the *Bulletin of the National Tuberculosis and Respiratory Disease Association* announced on its cover and above the first page of every article it contained, "The General Hospital is the logical place" (25). The contents of this publication are largely devoted to reassuring health care workers that there is little risk to them, although it stated that "good ventilation without recirculation of air is essential for rooms or wards used for tuberculous patients." Unfortunately, such ventilation was not widely available in many hospitals at that time.

During the 1970s and 1980s, the decades following these changes in the venue of care of tuberculous patients, a number of outbreaks of tuberculous infection among health care workers were reported and the first attempts at systematic study of nosocomial transmission of tuberculous infection were undertaken. Most of these studies are not relevant to the current situation, but a few are worth noting because their conclusions remain important.

In 1975, Ruben, Norden, and Schuster evaluated the tuberculosis screening program for employees of a Pittsburgh hospital (26). This study is of particular note because it was among the first to look at patient contact in relation to infection. Employees considered to work in patient contact had a tuberculin test conversion rate of 3.2 percent; employees working in noncontact jobs had a conversion rate of 7.8 percent. Thus, nonhospital sources of infection were considered to be more likely than hospital sources for the acquisition of infection.

In contrast with the high infection rates in the Pittsburgh experience, Vogeler and Burke found that an annual tuberculin testing program among the employees of a hospital in Salt Lake City discovered only seven converters among 2,900 to 3,400 employees tested in each year between 1972 and 1977 (27). During the 5-year period, converter rates ranged from zero to 0.49 percent/year, with an overall rate of 0.11 percent. This study illustrated the geographic variability of the risk of tuberculous infection for health care workers. The Pittsburgh hospital admitted approximately 30 to 40 cases of tuberculosis annually during the study period; the Salt Lake City hospital admitted 9 or 10.

Berman and colleagues studied tuberculin skin test conversions among the employees of a hospital in Baltimore during a 5-year period from 1971 to 1976 (28). During that time, 58 patients had cultures positive for *M. tuberculosis*; an unknown number of patients with negative cultures or for whom no cultures were done may have also been hospitalized. The results of this illuminating study are summarized by job category and demography in Table C-7. It is apparent that the risk of infection was much greater in maintenance, engineering, housekeeping, and laundry employees than in nursing employees. It is also apparent that risk of infection correlated strongly with race and economic status. These observations led to the conclusion that the source of tuberculous infection for most of the employees who converted their tuberculin skin tests was in the communities in which they resided rather than in the hospital.

Aitken, Anderson, and Albert conducted a prospective study of tuberculin skin test conversions among employees at all 114 hospitals in the

TABLE C-7. Tuberculin Skin Test Conversions and Calculated ARI for Employees of a Baltimore Hospital, 1971–1976 (28)

Job or Demographic Category	Number Tested	Converters	Percent	ARI (percent/year)
Nursing	733	36	4.9	.98
Maintenance, engineering, housekeeping	231	34	14.7	3.13
Laundry	32	11	34.4	8.08
Pathology	105	3	2.9	0.58
Radiology	86	2	2.3	0.47
White	1,045	38	3.6	0.74
Nonwhite	759	96	12.7	2.67
Highest economic quintile	645	36	5.6	1.14
Lowest economic quintile	151	24	15.9	3.40

state of Washington from January 1982 through December 1984 (29). During these 3 years the tuberculosis incidence in Washington was 7.1/100,000 in 1982, 5.6/100,000 in 1983, and 4.8/100,000 in 1984; national case rates for these years were 11.0/100,000 in 1982, 10.2/100,000 in 1983, and 9.4/100,000 in 1984 (1). In this survey 124,869 skin tests were completed and 110 skin test conversions were documented (excluding 19 additional converters identified by health department contact investigations). Overall, the conversion rate was 0.09 percent (calculated ARI = 0.03 percent/year). For hospitals with no cases of tuberculosis admitted during the study interval the rate was 0.07 percent (calculated ARI = 0.02 percent/year), and for hospitals to which cases of tuberculosis were admitted the rate was 0.091 percent (calculated ARI = 0.03 percent/year) in those hospitals with sputum smear-positive cases and 0.094 percent (calculated ARI = 0.03 percent/year) for those with smear-negative, culture-positive cases. In larger urban hospitals the rate was 0.11 percent (calculated ARI = 0.04 percent/year) and for small hospitals the rate was 0.08 percent (calculated ARI = 0.03 percent/year). There were no significant differences among these rates. The authors estimated that the tuberculin test conversion rate in the general population of Washington at that time was between 0.008 and 0.11 percent/year. They concluded that hospital employees were at no greater risk than the general public.

From these studies certain generalizations can be made about occupational tuberculosis in the 1970s and 1980s. First, it is evident that the risk of tuberculous infection was much greater in hospitals located in such cities as Baltimore than in those represented by Salt Lake City. This almost certainly reflected the tuberculosis incidence in those communities. Next, the evidence presented here indirectly, but not directly, implicates the communities in which health care workers resided as the major source of tuberculous infection. That does not mean that occupation-related infection did not occur; rather, it means that the risk in the community was often as great as or greater than the risk in the workplace. Finally, that risk related to employment was probably greatest for certain hazardous work activities, such as bronchoscopy and other aerosol-generating procedures.

Beginning in the mid-1980s and extending into the early to mid-1990s, the United States witnessed an unprecedented resurgence of tuberculosis. Borne on a tide of AIDS, homelessness, and immigration, tuberculosis rates increased in most major urban areas of the Northeast, southern Florida, and California, as well as along the Mexican-American border. In other areas of the country, notably the less densely populated central portions of the continental United States, tuberculosis case rates did not increase and continued to decline. In many of the areas of resurgence, this emerging epidemic was accompanied by increasing rates of drug resistance, including multidrug resistance. Public health agencies responded with a variety of measures, including well-reasoned guidelines intended to decrease nosocomial tuberculous infections. Today, case rates are again falling nationally.

Recent Risk for Health Care Workers in Urban Locations of High Tuberculosis Incidence

Much of the recent information available comes from studies performed in the wake of outbreaks, and selection bias is inevitably introduced into such situations. The bias introduced by studying the problem in such a situation will tend to overstate the risk. On the other hand, the mere fact that a study is being conducted will tend to increase employee compliance with isolation procedures, thus reducing the risk. These biases must be remembered in drawing conclusions or making generalizations.

There have been two recent reports from St. Clare's Hospital and Health Center in New York City (30,31). This hospital cares for many patients with tuberculosis and for many HIV-infected patients. It was the original focal point of an outbreak of multidrug-resistant strain W of *M. tuberculosis* in New York. During the period 1991 to 1994, 56 to 118 new cases of tuberculosis were diagnosed annually at that hospital (the reports do not give data on the secular trend). During the same time period, tuberculin skin test information was available for 1,303 employees, 711 of whom were initially tuberculin skin test negative. The conversion rates for these 711 employees grouped by occupation are shown in Table C-8 for the years 1991–1992 and 1993–1994. The rates in Table C-8 are expressed per 100 person-years, a reasonable approximation of the annual risk of infection expressed as percent. When adjusted for age, bacille Calmette-Guérin (BCG) vaccination status, country of birth, gender, and the tuberculosis incidence in the postal code zone of residence, the differences in occupational category remained significant in a multivariate

TABLE C-8. Tuberculin Conversion Rates Among Employees of St. Clare's Hospital in New York City by Occupation Comparing 1991–1992 and 1993–1994 (30)

	Conversion Rate[a]		
Occupation	Total, 1991–1994	1991–1992	1993–1994
Laboratory	4.4	6.3	2.3
Physician or nurse	5.0	7.2	3.0
Social service	4.8	8.1	2.2
Housekeeping	9.2	11.7	6.7
Finance	2.5	3.0	1.9
Total	5.2	7.2	3.3

[a]Conversion rates are expressed as number of conversions per 100 person-years.

analysis. When conversion rates were examined at 6-month intervals, the rate fell from 20.7 percent during the first 6 months of the 1991 observation period to 5.8 percent during the last 6 months of 1993 (31). During that time, negative-pressure isolation rooms, ultraviolet lights, and personal respirators were all introduced at St. Clare's Hospital.

Maloney and coworkers studied the impact of enhanced infection control measures on nosocomial transmission of tuberculosis infection at the Cabrini Medical Center in New York City following an outbreak of multidrug-resistant tuberculosis at that facility in 1991 (32). Employee tuberculin rates were determined for an 18-month period prior to the institution of enhanced infection control measures and a 12-month period subsequent to the changes in infection control. The findings of their study are summarized in Table C-9, along with annual risks of infection calculated from their data. Overall, the annual risks of infection were higher in personnel working in contact with patients and, considering the small number of conversions documented in the noncontact group, were not changed by the implementation of infection control measures. However, conversion rates decreased following the infection control intervention on medical and HIV wards admitting patients with tuberculosis. This did not happen elsewhere in the hospital. In this study, there was no evidence of residence postal code clustering of employee conversions, nor were demographic or racial characteristics identified that contributed to the infection risk.

TABLE C-9. Tuberculin Conversions and Calculated ARI for Employees at Cabrini Medical Center, New York City, Before and After Interventions Made to Improve Infection Control (32)

Employee Category	Pre-intervention Conversions	18 months ARI (%/year)	Post-intervention Conversions	12 months ARI (%/year)
Working in patient contact	22/342 (6.4)	4.3	14/296 (4.7)	4.7
Not working in patient contact	4/409 (1.0)	0.7	8/354 (2.3)	2.3
Working on ward admitting TB patients	15/90 (16.7)	11.5	4/78 (5.1)	5.1
Working on ward not admitting tuberculosis patients	7/254 (2.8)	1.9	9/228 (4.0)	4.0

NOTE: The preintervention period included an outbreak. Note that the time intervals for the pre- and postintervention periods differ, meaning that the conversions as expressed as percentages by the authors are not directly comparable. Data from Maloney and coworkers. Conversion rates are number of skin test conversions/number of employees tested (percent).

Blumberg, Sotir, and colleagues studied nosocomial transmission of tuberculosis infection and skin test conversions among employees at Grady Hospital in Atlanta, Georgia, a public hospital admitting about 200 tuberculous patients annually during the first half of the 1990s before and after implementation of intensified infection control measures (33,34). Six-month conversion rates fell from 118/3,579 (3.3 percent; calculated ARI = 6.49 percent/year) in the first 6 months of 1992 to 23/5,153 (0.4 percent; calculated ARI = 0.89 percent/year) during the first 6 months of 1994. During the latter period, the conversion rate was not related to job status but was positively correlated with black race and low economic status. Subsequently, Blumberg and associates studied tuberculin skin test conversions among house staff in the Emory University Affiliated Hospitals Training Program (35). These interns and residents spend approximately half of their training time at Grady Hospital. As noted above, expanded infection control measures were implemented at Grady Hospital in 1992, and tuberculin test conversion rates were compared for the 6-month period at the initiation of these measures with the rates for the subsequent 4.5 years. The rate fell from 6.0 per 100 person-years to 1.1 per 100 person-years (p <0.001). Rates were significantly higher for house officers in medicine and obstetrics/gynecology than for those other clinical departments. Graduates of foreign medical schools had higher conversion rates than American graduates. As at St. Clare's Hospital and the Cabrini Medical Center in New York, the implementation of control measures was thought to have had an impact on transmission of infection to the health care workers at Grady Hospital.

An important study of tuberculosis in New York City health care workers was conducted using restriction fragment length polymorphism (RFLP) DNA fingerprinting techniques (36). In 1992–1994 among six New York City hospitals where no recognized nosocomial outbreaks of tuberculosis occurred, isolates from 20 cases of tuberculosis occurring in health care workers were available for typing. Of the 20, 8 were nurses or nurses aides, 7 were physicians, and the remaining 5 were not in patient contact positions. The tuberculous health care workers from whom the fingerprinted organisms were isolated did not differ from those from 181 non-health care workers similarly studied with respect to age, sex, country of birth, race, and HIV infection status. The fingerprinting technique allowed the identification of clusters of patients all infected with the same strain of *M. tuberculosis*. Overall, 87 of 201 isolates fingerprinted in New York during the period of the study were clustered, indicating that they represented recent transmission of currently circulating strains. Among health care workers, clustered strains were found in six of the seven physicians and in eight of the nine HIV-infected workers (all occupations). This suggests that physicians and HIV-infected persons were particularly susceptible to occupational infection.

In a single tuberculin test survey of 91 patient transport and house-keeping hospital employees in Philadelphia, patient contact was not related to tuberculin skin test positivity (37). Foreign birth was, with a relative risk of 0.4 (U.S. birth to foreign birth) for employees with patient contact and 0.8 for employees without patient contact.

At a large military medical center in Bethesda, Maryland, the ARI with *M. tuberculosis* was found to range from 0.4 to 2.6 percent for most occupational categories. It was not significantly different for those in patient contact and non-patient contact positions (38). However, the rate was 15.6 percent for respiratory therapists.

Boudreau and others studied the occupational tuberculosis infection risk at Jackson Memorial Hospital in Miami, Florida (39). They compared infection rates for 248 initially tuberculin skin test negative employees who worked exclusively on hospital divisions from which the laboratory had received respiratory specimens positive for *M. tuberculosis* (exposed employees) with the rates for 355 employees who worked on divisions from which no such cultures had been received (unexposed employees). The cumulative risk among exposed employees was 14.5 percent; among unexposed employees it was 1.4 percent. The risk in exposed employees did not vary with job classification within the patient care division setting. Ward clerks had a risk similar to that of nurses. On the other hand, risk decreased coincident with the implementation of infection control measures from 6.2 percent (13/209) in 1989 to 0.6 percent (1/158) in 1992, at which time there was no difference between the risk in exposed and unexposed employees.

In Table C-10 the calculated annual risks of infection are listed for five hospitals in the studies described above. These five studies are the only ones among those described that this author feels are adequate to permit this calculation, and even then the resulting ARIs can be taken as only approximate. The 8- to 10-fold disparity between Barnes Hospital in St. Louis and the two New York City hospitals is obvious. The ARIs for Grady Hospital and the military medical center are intermediate between these extremes. These differences may reflect both the tuberculosis exposure risk due to larger number of tuberculosis admissions and also greater community risk. There are also substantial differences in risk related to occupation in those studies for which data are available.

The importance of job category for the risk in health care workers exposed to aerosols is made clear by the ARI of 17.1 percent/year in respiratory therapists at the military medical center. With respect to risk by occupation, it should be noted that there is a consensus among infectious disease experts that there is no risk from fomites or dust, although the latter may contain tubercle bacilli (even when ground, dust contains few respirable particles). Thus, any risk among laundry workers, for example, is generally not thought to be occupational.

TABLE C-10. ARI with *M. tuberculosis* for Various Populations of Hospital-Based Health Care Workers (HCWs) as Calculated Directly from Reported Several Selected Surveillance Studies with Sufficient Data to Permit This Calculation

Health Care Worker Group (reference)	Year	Calculated ARI of HCWs (%/year)
Barnes Hospital, St. Louis (40)	1989–1991	0.4
Cabrini Medical Center, New York (32)	1991	
Wards admitting tuberculosis patients		5.1
Other wards		4.0
St. Clare's Hospital, New York (30,31)	1993–1994	3.3
Laboratory		2.3
Physicians and nurses		3.0
Social service		2.2
Housekeeping		6.7
Finance		1.9
Grady Memorial Hospital, Atlanta (33)	1994	0.9
House officers (35)	1993–1997	1.1
Military medical center, Bethesda (38)	1994–1995	1.2
Respiratory therapy		17.1
Maintenance, engineering		2.6
Food service		2.6
Nursing technicians		2.3
Laboratory		2.1
Custodial		1.8
Practical nurses		1.8
Physicians		0.9
Registered nurses		0.4

NOTE: When applicable, all risks were calculated for periods following the implementation of current infection control measures.

Recent Risk for Health Care Workers in Locations of Low Tuberculosis Incidence

Since the United States is not homogeneous with respect to the incidence of tuberculosis, it is reasonable to expect that the risk to health care workers in areas of low incidence will be lower than the risks cited above in areas of higher incidence. Bailey and colleagues studied tuberculous infection among employees at Barnes Hospital, a 1,000-bed hospital in St. Louis, between January 1989 and July 1991 (40). At that time the new case rate in Missouri was 5/100,000/year and in St. Louis it was 11/100,000/year. A total of 11.3 percent of employees were initially skin test positive. During the study period 0.93 percent of the initially tuberculin skin test negative employees converted to positivity, for an calculated annual risk of infection of 0.37 percent. The risk of infection was not correlated with occupational exposure; it was correlated with minority group status, residence in a postal code zone of low income status, and residence in a postal zone of high tuberculosis incidence. While the same group of investigators reported an 8.6 percent conversion rate among physicians at Barnes Hospital, the latter finding is difficult to evaluate because prior tuberculin nonreactive status was based solely on the physician's report of a prior test at an unspecified time (41).

Among 2,500 to 3,800 employees tested annually between 1986 and 1994 at a pediatric hospital in Cincinnati, Ohio, the tuberculin skin test conversion rates ranged from 0.03 percent to 0.28 percent per year (42). There was no correlation with occupational exposure, and an apparent cluster of five infections occurred. In a survey of 17 Minnesota hospitals, the tuberculin reactor rate among employees was 0.3 percent in 1989–1991 (43).

Managan and coworkers compared tuberculin skin test conversion rates by questionnaire survey in two groups of hospitals: 38 hospitals admitting patients with *Pneumocystis carinii* pneumonia (PCP) in high-HIV-infection-incidence areas and 136 randomly selected hospitals without significant numbers of PCP patients that admitted more than six tuberculosis patients annually (44). During 1992, the tuberculosis infection rate among employees of the hospitals with PCP patients was 1.2 percent. If fell during the following 5 years to 0.43 percent, a change attributed to the institution of better infection control measures. The comparable tuberculosis infection rates in the non-PCP hospitals were 0.43 percent initially and 0.26 percent finally. In the hospitals with PCP patients with low tuberculosis case loads, the rate of conversion actually increased, although the numbers were small, and this suggested to the authors that the risk of tuberculosis infection was principally in the community rather than in the workplace.

Summary of Risk in Hospital-Based Health Care Workers

Although the limitations of the available data must be recognized, certain conclusions seem reasonable. First of all, there does appear to be a risk of tuberculous infection incurred by health care workers in the workplace that in some job circumstances may be greater than that incurred in the community. Aerosol-generating procedures are particularly hazardous to exposed employees. Second, the risk varies geographically, as it does in the general population. Next, it also varies with the ethnic and demographic compositions of the employees. Finally, the workplace risk has been decreasing in recent years. Quantitatively, the studies described above would suggest recent occupational tuberculous infection risks of about 0.5 to 1.0 percent/year for hospitals in low-tuberculosis-incidence areas and about 1.0 to 5.0 percent/year for hospitals in high-incidence areas, with these risks falling steadily and influenced by implementation of appropriate infection control measures.

Risk in Other Than Hospital-Based Health Care Workers

The rule proposed by OSHA would cover individuals providing services not only in hospitals but also in other situations including nursing homes, correctional facilities, immigration detainment facilities, law enforcement facilities, hospices, substance abuse treatment centers, homeless shelters, medical examiners' offices, home heath care providers, emergency medical services personnel, research and clinical laboratories culturing tubercle bacilli and processing infectious specimens, ventilation system workers serving buildings housing tuberculous patients, social service workers, personnel service agencies providing workers to covered facilities, and attorneys visiting known or suspected infectious tuberculous patients (45). While it is logical to believe that contact of uninfected persons with infectious tuberculosis patients may occur in these situations, published data that support this hypothesis are lacking in many and sparse in others of these cases. Much of what has been reported is in the form of descriptions of outbreaks for which no denominator exists, so that the risk cannot be quantified.

Risk in Nursing Homes and Similar Chronic Care Facilities

In 1995, about 1.5 million Americans, 89 percent of them age 65 or older, about 5 percent of the elderly population, resided in nursing homes, and they contributed 7.7 percent of the tuberculosis cases nationally in individuals older than 64 years (46, 47, 48). The age-specific case rate for these persons is 1.8 times that for older persons not in nursing homes.

Stead reported an outbreak of tuberculosis in an Arkansas nursing home in 1978, with the index case being an elderly man thought to have bronchogenic carcinoma whose disease had not been adequately investigated (49). He was a gregarious individual who had many contacts throughout the home. Among 138 previously tuberculin-negative employees, 21 (15 percent) converted their skin tests and one developed active tuberculosis. In 1980 an outbreak of tuberculosis occurred in a Washington State nursing home after an elderly long-time resident was found to have sputum smear-positive tuberculosis (50). Upon investigation, 11 other cases of active tuberculosis were identified in the same facility. A skin testing survey found that 38 of 87 employees (44 percent) had newly positive tuberculin reactions. The air in this facility moved from patient rooms through dining and activity areas into two exhaust vents in the corridor. In both of these outbreaks, the diagnosis of the index case was not suspected for a substantial period of time.

In 1987 Price and Rutala published the results of a questionnaire survey of 12 long-term-care facilities in North Carolina; 101 skin test conversions occurred among 9,545 (1.1 percent) employees during the years

1981 through 1984 (51). The mean time interval was 5 years (calculated ARI = 0.21 percent/year). During the study period, annual conversion rates varied from 0.4 to 1.9 percent, with no apparent secular trend. Tuberculin conversion rates in the institutions's patients were similar. There was wide variability in the skin testing techniques used, and these figures can be considered only approximate.

Risk in Correctional Facilities: Prisons and Jails

Studies in prisons and jails must be considered with the understanding that, among other variables, prisons typically house long-term inmates and jails detain many people for very short periods. The spread of multidrug-resistant tuberculosis among prisoners in New York City and State jails and prisons provoked great concern for the employees of those institutions. For example, in 1988 and 1989, one-quarter of the 205 tuberculosis cases in Nassau County, New York, were associated with a jail (52). Although inmates were screened on admission, there was no screening or infection control program for employees. Statewide, the incidence of active tuberculosis among New York prison inmates increased from 15/100,000/year in 1976 to 139/100,000/year in 1993 (53). Nationally, inmates of correctional facilities contribute just under 2 percent of the tuberculosis case load (48). The age-adjusted case rate for adult inmates is 3.9 times higher than that for the general population.

A system-wide annual tuberculin skin testing program for New York State prison employees was instituted in 1991–1992, and Steenland and coworkers reported on the conversions found at a 1-year follow-up (53). Overall, the conversion rate was 1.9 percent among 24,487 employees. Rates ranged from 1.4 percent in prisons with no known tuberculous inmates to 2.6 percent in prisons with more than the median number of tuberculous prisoners.

Transmission of tuberculous infection from inmates to correctional facility personnel has been documented in several published reports from California penal systems. Two of 11 prison infirmary employees converted their tuberculin skin test after contact with an infected prisoner in 1990–1991 (54). In two other outbreaks, employee tuberculin test conversions occurred in 9 of 319 (2.8 percent) and in 11 of 223 (4.9 percent) employees (55). In all cases, the conversions occurred within 2 years of a previously negative test. In a 1981 outbreak, one employee developed active tuberculosis (56). No information on employee skin test conversions was reported.

A 1994 outbreak of tuberculosis in a Texas prison housing a number of mentally retarded prisoners centered on a classroom used for education of these inmates (57). RFLP analysis demonstrated clustering of the patients. The report does not provide information allowing an assessment of the infection risk to prison workers, but an instructor was among those who developed active tuberculosis.

Jones and colleagues studied the transmission of tuberculosis in a city jail in Memphis, Tennessee, where inmates were housed for a median of 1 day, often returning several times to the same facility, commonly housed in rooms holding up to 36 inmates (58). During a 3-year period beginning in January 1995, 38 inmates were recognized as tuberculous, and five guards developed tuberculosis. RFLP fingerprinting demonstrated that one strain of *M. tuberculosis* was responsible for the disease in 16 of 24 inmates for whom results were available and two of the five guards. Tuberculin testing of guards revealed a conversion rate of 2.7 percent in an unknown time period and of 1.2 percent during a subsequent 1-year interval.

Two studies of tuberculosis in prisons are of particular interest because they give some insights into the risk of tuberculous infection in relation to that in the community. In a study of 28 contact investigations in New York City correctional facilities, Johnsen noted that the tuberculin conversion rate among inmates exposed to sputum smear-positive prisoners with tuberculosis was 6.6 percent (59). On the other hand, when the investigation revealed that a putative index case did not, in fact, have tuberculosis, the conversion rate was 5.5 percent, not significantly different from the rate among those exposed to documented cases of tuberculosis. Johnsen suggested that some of the conversions were confounded by booster effects.

Erdil and Stahl reported preemployment tuberculin reactor rates for the Connecticut Department of Corrections for 1991 and 1992 (60). Because they reported age cohort-specific data, it is possible to calculate the actual annual risk of infection that these individuals brought with them to the workplace from the communities in which they resided. In this respect, this report is nearly unique and of considerable importance. For the 25- to 40-year-old age range, the calculated annual risk of infection was 0.18 percent/year. This rate is relatively high when compared to that for the adult U.S. population as a whole, but it is similar to the 0.20 percent/year estimated ARI for black males.

Risk in Homeless Shelters

That tuberculosis is a problem among the urban homeless is well known, having been widely publicized in the lay press. In New York City, 68 percent of tuberculosis patients discharged from Harlem Hospital in 1988 were homeless (61), and 30 percent of all tuberculosis cases in 1991 were homeless (62). The shelters where these individuals spend their nights are often in substandard buildings with limited ventilation, and the sleeping conditions are generally crowded, thus facilitating the spread of airborne infections among the clients. Using both drug sensitivity patterns and mycobacterial phage typing, Nardell and colleagues convincingly demonstrated transmission of tuberculosis among the clients of a homeless shelter in Boston in 1983 (63). An outbreak of tuberculosis in a poorly ventilated shelter for homeless men in Seattle, Washington, in 1987 was described by Nolan and coworkers (64). In San Francisco, a study conducted in 1993 and 1994 demonstrated by RFLP analysis that the *M. tuberculosis* isolates from 24 of 34 homeless tuberculosis patients belonged to six clusters, thus providing strong evidence for transmission of infection among these homeless individuals (65).

Despite the well-recognized risks of transmission of tuberculous infection in homeless shelters, there are almost no data concerning infection rates in the staff of these facilities. In fact, many of the workers at these shelters are drawn from the clients themselves, and they tend to be transient, often unavailable for repeated skin testing, and frequently tuberculin-positive. In the only published report giving information on infections among staff found in the author's literature search, Curtis and colleagues from CDC studied an outbreak occurring in a homeless shelter for men in Syracuse, New York, in 1987 and 1988 (66). Seventy percent of the clients and staff of the shelter were tuberculin-positive. Tuberculin skin test conversions were documented in two of eight previously tuberculin-negative staff members. Perhaps reflective of much of the generally transient nature of shelter staffs, 52 additional staff members who may have been exposed were not available for skin testing.

Risk in Other Nonhospital Health Care Situations

Layton and coworkers studied a single-room-occupancy hotel used to shelter homeless persons with AIDS (67). Sixteen cases of tuberculosis were found among 116 persons surveyed; 8 of them were compliant with antituberculous therapy, 4 noncompliant, and 4 not under treatment. None of 11 employees had tuberculosis, and the authors found "[no] evidence of recent tuberculous infection" in them, although no skin test data were reported. These employees worked in a small lobby area that was reasonably well ventilated and not conducive to socializing with the residents (P. Kellner, personal communication).

Pierce, Sims, and Holman reported that 11 of 65 (17 percent) of workers in a residential hospice for AIDS patients converted their tuberculin skin tests after a patient with tuberculosis spent 29 days in the facility prior to being recognized as having tuberculosis (68). Information about the HIV infection status of the employees was not given, nor was information about ventilation in the facility. A tuberculin test conversion was documented in one employee of a residential substance abuse facility in Michigan where a client was found to have multidrug-resistant tuberculosis in 1989 (69).

Data relating to ambulatory facilities and their employees are sparse. An outbreak of tuberculous infection occurred among health care workers in a Palm Beach County, Florida, clinic in 1988 (70). Of 30 previously skin test-negative employees, 17 became tuberculin-positive. The clinic ventilation system provided greater than 90 percent recirculation of air with less than one-half fresh air changes per hour. In a nonoutbreak setting, 766 tuberculin-negative health care workers in 16 urban ambulatory care units caring for HIV-infected patients, six of which were located in greater New York City, participated in a prospective tuberculin skin testing study in 1992 and 1993 (71). The conversion rate in these individuals was 1.6 per 100 person-years.

Prezant and colleagues studied prospectively a cohort of New York City prehospital health care workers consisting of nearly 200 emergency medical technicians and paramedics who had been stably employed in their positions for at least 15 years (72). Documented tuberculin skin test conversions occurred in one worker in 1993, none in 1994, one in 1995, and three in 1996. Overall, the calculated annual risk of infection for this small group was 0.6 percent/year.

A single report described a survey of 56 American clinical microbiology laboratories processing samples for culture of mycobacteria (73). Fourteen tuberculin skin test conversions were noted, but neither the time interval nor the number of persons at risk were given, so that no conclusions can be drawn from this report.

Transmission of tuberculous infection from cadavers is well known, and autopsy rooms have been considered especially hazardous. Much of the past tuberculous infection risk for medical students cited previously was attributed to participation in autopsies. In a county medical examiner's office in New York State 2 of 15 morgue assistants converted their tuberculin skin tests during a 15-month period (calculated ARI = 10.8 percent/year) (74). This facility performed autopsies on deceased inmates from a nearby prison, and eight autopsies had been performed on tuberculous individuals during that time. In a further autopsy risk, prosector's wart occurs as a result of direct percutaneous inoculation of M. tuberculosis; there are no data on its frequency.

Recently transmission of M. tuberculosis has been documented and much publicized in funeral homes. Gershon and coworkers surveyed 864 funeral home workers who were attending a convention of the National Funeral Directors Association (75). Of them, 101 (11.7 percent) were tuberculin skin test positive. Reactivity correlated positively with older age, male gender, and nonwhite race. After controlling for these factors, reactivity was twice as frequent among embalmers as other funeral home employees.

Sterling and colleagues reported the first episode of documented transmission of tuberculous infection from a cadaver to an embalmer (76).

In this case, the deceased individual had had AIDS and partially treated tuberculosis. A sputum culture was positive on the day of death. Close family members were exposed but not infected. The mortuary employee who embalmed the body subsequently developed tuberculosis, and the organism was shown by RFLP typing to be identical to that of the cadaver. Aerosolization from the airway during the embalming process was suggested as a possible means of transmission. One other case of well-documented transmission of *M. tuberculosis* during embalming, again with identical strains of tubercle bacilli as determined by RFLP typing, has recently been reported in abstract form (77).

Summary of Risk in Other Than Hospital Based Health Care Workers

The data are too few to permit any generalizations about the magnitude of the occupational tuberculosis risk for health care workers in non-hospital situations. There probably is a risk, and it probably varies with the incidence of tuberculosis in the populations served by the facilities. Although data in this regard are scarce, ventilation, recognition of cases of tuberculosis, and isolation procedures may be less adequate in non-hospital settings than in hospital settings. It is also possible that workers in these settings may have community-based infection risks that differ from those of hospital employees. Table C-11 summarizes the annual risks of infection calculated from three studies deemed adequate to support this calculation.

Risk Assessment by the Occupational Safety and Health Administration

OSHA has proposed a rule to enforce infection control measures on all facilities employing health care workers (45). As part of its proposal OSHA

TABLE C-11. ARI with *M. tuberculosis* for Three Populations of Nonhospital-Based Health Care Workers (HCWs) as Calculated Directly from Reported Surveillance Studies with Sufficient Data to Permit This Calculation

Health Care Setting (Reference)	Year	Calculated ARI of HCWs (%/year)
Nursing homes, North Carolina (51)	1980–1985	0.21
Prisons, New York State (53)	1991–1992	
Exposed workers		2.6
Nonexposed workers		1.4
Prisons, New York City (59)	1990	
Exposed workers		6.6
Nonexposed workers		5.5

conducted a risk assessment using some of the data cited above. For its estimation of the annual risk of infection in general populations, OSHA developed a model based on relating risk of infection to incidence of disease. Estimates of the prevalence of tuberculous infection in the United States were also provided to OSHA by Dr. Christopher Murray of Harvard University. OSHA concluded that the overall annual rate of infection in the general population of the United States varied by state, from a low of 0.0194 percent/year to 0.3542 percent/year, and chose a population size-weighted average of 0.146 percent/year for the country as a whole.

As its database for estimating the annual rate of tuberculous infection in health care workers, OSHA used information published and obtained directly from the state of Washington (29, 45), the state of North Carolina (45, 78), and Jackson Memorial Hospital in Miami, Florida (39, 45, 79). Using these data, OSHA estimated that the occupational risk in Washington was 1.5 times, that in North Carolina was 5 times, and that at Jackson Memorial Hospital 9 times that for the general population of the surrounding state, region, or community. Similar estimates were made for workers in nonhospital settings. For Washington State the occupational risk for employees of long-term-care facilities was judged to be 11 times that for the general population and for home health care workers it was 2 times that for the general population. OSHA's risk estimate for the population of the United States as a whole in 1994 is about three times that of 0.05%/year considered by the author to be his best estimate of the national rate.

Risk Assessment in Relation to Job Category in Studies by the Centers for Disease Control and Prevention

The most careful attempts to assess the occupational tuberculosis risk of health care workers in relation to their workplaces and the communities in which they reside are studies conducted by the Division of Tuberculosis Elimination of CDC. These investigations include some of the only prospective studies of the problem. They are also notable because they all included initial two-step tuberculin skin testing to minimize confounding booster effects. Some of them have not yet been published, but abstracts were kindly made available to me by their authors, who gave me permission to cite them.

Panlilio and Burwen followed 1,961 initially tuberculin-negative health care workers in Boston and New York City at 6-month intervals beginning in April 1994 and reporting their results in abstract form in May 1996 (80). Overall, 30 (1.5 percent) conversions were documented. Conversion was correlated with foreign birth, Asian race, and recent entry into the United States. The authors concluded that it was difficult to determine the source of infections in their subjects.

In a national questionnaire survey of 1,494 hospitals Sinkowitz and coworkers found conversion rates based on reports from these hospitals of 0.6 to 0.7 percent/year for 1989 through 1992 (81). Bronchoscopy was associated with a high conversion rate of 3.7 percent/year among personnel. Respiratory therapists were also at high risk, with a rate of 1.0 percent/year. The main body of this report focused on compliance with CDC infection control guidelines, and demographic data on the employees were not included.

In 1995, McCray, Curtis, Onorato, and colleagues initiated a prospective study of health care workers in 32 facilities caring for patients with tuberculosis in six states, New York City, San Francisco, and San Diego (E. McCray and A.B. Curtis, personal communications of data presented at a December 1999 workshop). The sites included nine hospitals, seven health departments, five correctional institutions, two long-term-care facilities, and nine others. All were sites at which care for tuberculosis patients occurred, many in areas with relatively high tuberculosis case rates. During the next 3 years, a skin test conversion rate of 0.8 percent (112/13,597) was observed (calculated ARI = 0.28 percent/year). The rate was highest in New York City at 2.4 percent (calculated ARI = 0.81 percent/year), but no conversions were observed among health care workers in Oregon, Colorado, and Florida. Conversions occurred with about equal frequency in correctional facilities (1.0 percent), health departments (0.9 percent), hospitals (0.8 percent), and long-term-care facilities (1.1 percent). Outreach workers had a risk approximately 2.5 times that of those in other occupations. Foreign birth and Asian or black race were independent predictors of risk, and after adjusting for these variables, no specific occupational risk remained. Some of the annual risks of infection that can be calculated from this study are shown in Table C-12.

TABLE C-12. Calculated Annual Risks of Infection Derived from Tuberculin Skin Test Conversion Data for Selected Groups of Health Care Workers (E. McCray and A.B. Curtis, personal communication)

Health Care Worker Group, Work Sites and Categories, Racial and Demographic Categories	Calculated Annual Risk of Tuberculous Infection (%/year)
Administrative/clerical	0.6
Nurses	0.5
Outreach worker	2.4
Doctor/physician's assistant	0.6
Not Hispanic, white	0.3
Not Hispanic, Black	1.0
Asian	1.4
Hispanic	0.8
U.S.-born	0.4
Foreign-born	2.0

In reviewing their data, McCray and colleagues concluded that the risk of new tuberculous infection for most health care workers was not substantially greater in the workplace than in the community in which they resided. The annual risks calculated from the data of McCray and colleagues are higher than those estimated and previously presented in this report for general populations. Their data were based on prospectively collected and currently reported information available in more specific categories with better demographic stratification than the data used for the author's estimations of ARIs. However, there may be a selection bias introduced by the choice of sites for the study of McCray and colleagues.

The CDC data suggest that the tuberculosis risks of health care workers closely parallel those for the communities in which they reside. This does not mean that transmission of tuberculosis infection does not occur in the health care-related workplace. It simply means that the occupational risk is not great compared with the community risk.

RISKS OF TUBERCULOUS DISEASE AND MORTALITY IN *M. TUBERCULOSIS*-INFECTED HEALTH CARE WORKERS

There are no studies available allowing one to estimate the risks of tuberculous disease and mortality in *M. tuberculosis*-infected health care workers per se. One must generalize from what is known about these risks in the general population. This risk has frequently been stated to be about 10 percent over the life of the infected individual, but the available data suggest that it is closer to 5 percent, with about half of the risk occurring in the first 1 to 3 years after infection. In fact, the risk of tuberculosis for infected health care workers should be less than that for other persons because they work in circumstances that are optimal for monitoring of tuberculin test conversion, for implementation of therapy of latent infection, and for education and orientation concerning the importance of this form of therapy. Isoniazid treatment of latent tuberculous infection has been shown to reduce the risk of disease by about 60 percent (82). Similarly, the mortality risk should be low because health care workers should have prompt access to detection and therapy of disease. In considering these risks, it is important to distinguish between those in immunocompetent persons and those in immunocompromised individuals.

Risk for Immunocompetent Health Care Workers

Longitudinal Surveillance of Tuberculin Skin Test Reactors Not Treated for Latent Infection

J. Arthur Myers and coworkers traced University of Minnesota medical students who were tuberculin-positive at medical school entry or who converted their tuberculin reactions while students in the classes of 1930 to 1953 (83). Among 1,480 such students, 1,353 were alive at the time of follow-up in 1953; none of the decedents had tuberculosis at the time of death. In total, there were 39,205 person-years of follow-up. There were 92 cases of clinical tuberculosis in these individuals, or a rate of 6.2 percent (92/1,480). It is possible that this rate is low because of the short period of follow-up of recent reactors. Myers and colleagues used tuberculin skin testing techniques with high doses of old tuberculin. While Minnesota is a geographic region where nonspecific reactivity is rare, it is also possible, although not likely, that the number of reactors was overstated, again leading to underestimation of the risk.

In a parallel study covering the same time period, Myers and colleagues surveyed the graduates of three Minnesota nursing schools (84). Follow-up information was obtained on 2,880 of 3,192 graduates (90.2%). Of nursing students who either were tuberculin reactors on nursing school entry or who became tuberculin positive during their nursing studies, 5.2 percent (33/637) developed clinical tuberculosis. As with the earlier studies, the caveats about possible underestimation of the risk apply. In both the medical and nursing student populations, the risk was greater for students who converted in school than for those who were infected prior to entry. This observation is consonant with others that suggest that the primary school years may be years of infection with a relatively low risk of subsequent disease in comparison with the risk from infection during the years of young adulthood.

A longitudinal study of tuberculin reactors in Britain from 1933 to 1944 (Prophit study) has been recently reanalyzed by Sepkowitz (85). Nearly 1,500 medical students and more than 3,000 nurses were followed for a decade. Among medical students, the rates were 1.0/100 person-years for females and 0.6/100 person-years for males. Nurses were classified as high and low exposure depending on their current work status. In the high-exposure group, the tuberculosis incidence was 1.5/100 person-years, and in the low exposure group it was 0.7/100 person-years. The higher attack rate among high-exposure nurses was thought by Sepkowitz to indicate exogenous reinfection as a source of some of the disease. As in the studies of Myers and colleagues, old tuberculin was used for skin testing.

In her postal survey of physicians who graduated from California medical schools prior to 1975, Barrett-Connor found that 5.0 percent (100/1,988) of doctors who had been tuberculin-positive on medical school entry or who converted their tuberculin tests later developed tuberculosis (86).

Lydia B. Edwards and colleagues obtained follow-up information as of the end of 1969 for 823,199 (85 percent of those tested) naval recruits tuberculin tested with 5 tuberculin units of PPD between 1958 and 1967

(87). Tuberculosis developed in 0.4 percent (111/28,478) of individuals initially tuberculin positive with reactions of 10 millimeters or greater. Tuberculosis developed in 0.03 percent (272/794,721) of those with initial tuberculin reactions smaller than 10 millimeters. The morbidity for men 10 percent underweight was three times that for men 10 percent overweight.

Horwitz, Wilbek, and Erickson followed more than 626,000 persons aged 15 to 44 years in Denmark who were tuberculin tested in 1950–1952 for 12 years (88). Their results were age stratified and are shown in Table C-13. It is clear that the risk was greatest in the postpubertal years and decreased later in adulthood.

Studies of Control Subjects in BCG Vaccination Trials

Useful data can be obtained from follow-up of the tuberculin-positive individuals excluded from BCG vaccination trials. In general, this information is excellent because the tuberculin skin testing was usually done by skilled, specifically trained individuals, the studies were done prospectively, and great effort was put into data management. For the purposes of this review, many of them have the disadvantage of having been conducted in children with follow-up through the adolescent and postpubertal years. Studies done in high-tuberculosis-prevalence, developing countries have not been considered here, as they are unlikely to represent the risks to American health care workers.

Sol Roy Rosenthal and coworkers gave BCG vaccine to student nurses in Chicago during the 1940s and early 1950s (19). Among initially tuberculin-positive students followed for 12 years, tuberculosis developed in 0.7 percent (3/420).

The British Medical Research Council conducted a trial of BCG vaccination among more than 58,000 schoolchildren in 1950–1952 and reported results of a 15-year follow-up of 54,239 of them (89). Including as tuberculin positive both those who reacted to 3 tuberculin units of PPD and those

TABLE C-13. Tuberculosis Developing in Tuberculin Reactors by Age Group in Denmark (88)

Age at Initial Tuberculin Testing (years)	Number Tuberculin Positive	Number Developing Tuberculosis	Twelve-Year Incidence of Tuberculosis (%)
15–24	45,850	219	0.48
25–34	116,375	327	0.28
35–44	103,263	201	0.19
Total	162,225	546	0.34

who reacted only to 100 units, tuberculosis developed in 1.2 percent (406/ 33,518). Follow-up surveillance was conducted at 2.5-year intervals. The incidence in the first interval was nearly double that in ensuing follow-up periods.

Comstock reported 18-year follow-up data on a 1946 tuberculin survey and BCG vaccination program in Muscogee County, Georgia (90). Among 1,492 individuals positive for reactivity to 5 tuberculin units of PPD, 24 (1.6 percent) had developed tuberculosis. In a larger trial conducted in Muskogee County about 10 years later, Comstock and colleagues observed more than 22,000 individuals of all ages who reacted to PPD with more than 10 millimeters of induration for 20 years (91; G.W. Comstock, personal communication). Overall, 207 of the reactors (0.94 percent) developed tuberculosis. The average annual rate was 0.73 percent. Thirty-eight pecent of the cases developed during the first 5 years of observation.

Perhaps the most useful data on the occurrence of tuberculosis in tuberculin skin test reactors excluded from BCG vaccination trials comes from the report of Comstock, Livesay, and Woolpert that includes data from the Puerto Rican trial (92). Using case registers from both Puerto Rico and New York City, they traced more than 80,000 individuals with a mean follow-up of 18.9 years. They reported data by several demographic characteristics, which are presented in Table C-14. Not surprisingly, tuberculosis occurred much more frequently among urban than rural residents. It occurred more frequently in females than males and substantially more frequently in young children.

TABLE C-14. Tuberculosis Occurring in Nonvaccinated Puerto Ricans Identified in a BCG Trial, Initially Reacting to 1 or 10 Tuberculin Units of PPD with ≥6 millimeters of Induration (92)

Demographic Category	Number of PPD-Positive Persons	Number of Tuberculosis Cases	Percent
Total	82,269	1,400	1.7
Urban residence	47,021	844	1.8
Rural residence	35,248	56	0.2
White	67,184	1,152	1.7
Black	15,085	248	1.6
Male	43,100	674	1.6
Female	39,169	726	1.9
Age 1–6 years	3,906	119	3.0
Age 7–12 years	35,869	520	1.4
Age 13–18 years	42,494	761	1.8

Studies of Control Subjects in Trials of Treatment of Latent Tuberculous Infection

The U.S. Public Health Service trials of isoniazid treatment of latent tuberculous infection provide useful 10-year follow-up information for the untreated, control groups (82). A variety of studies were conducted, of which those with household contacts and inmates of mental hospitals are probably the most relevant to health care workers. Overall, tuberculous infection marked by a PPD reaction of ≥10 millimeters occurred in 2.9 percent of infected household contacts and 1.2 percent of infected mental hospital inmates. Approximately one-third of cases developed during the first year of observation. Attack rates were higher in adults (essentially at the overall levels cited above) than children, and at least in the household contact group, the adult rate did not change through age 55.

A small study of a shipboard outbreak in the Dutch navy was cited by Ferrebee in her review (82). Tuberculosis developed in 12 of 128 seamen (9.4 percent) not given isoniazid in a trial of the effectiveness of this therapy, a figure much higher than that reported in any other investigation. This study, although small, is of interest because it reflects results in employed individuals. Shipboard exposures have been found to be more intense and have higher attack rates than those in other situations, and the population was probably skewed toward the young-adult age group that has the highest risk.

In an editorial dealing with the use of isoniazid for the treatment of latent tuberculous infections in young adults, George Comstock and Phyllis Edwards used published and unpublished data from both BCG trials and isoniazid chemotherapy trials to estimate the lifetime risk of tuberculosis among tuberculin skin test reactors (93). They noted that the risk declined with passing years. Lumping together their estimates of lifetime tuberculosis risks for tuberculin-positive black and white males and females, their estimates were approximately 3.5 to 4.5 percent at age 25, 3.1 to 3.6 percent at age 35, 2.6 to 3.0 percent at age 45, 2.0 to 2.5 percent at age 55, and 1.2 to 1.6 percent at age 65.

Impact of HIV Infection

HIV infection, even before the onset of frank AIDS, increases the risk of tuberculosis in infected individuals. In fact, tuberculosis is one of the major intercurrent infections of dually infected persons, and tuberculosis often occurs at a time when immune function is relatively well preserved.

Setting aside some excellent studies done in Africa as perhaps not applicable to American health care workers, the 2-year prospective study of Selwyn and colleagues conducted in a New York City methadone clinic in 1985–1987 provided what has been widely quoted and generally accepted as a measure of the risk of tuberculosis in dually infected persons (94). He found a tuberculosis risk of 7.9/100 person-years in PPD-positive, HIV-infected addicts and a risk of 0.3/100 person-years in PPD-negative, HIV-seropositive individuals. Isoniazid treatment of latent tuberculous infection was offered to all tuberculin-positive addicts, but the rate of compliance was low.

In a second study in 1987–1990, Selwyn and collaborators documented patient compliance with isoniazid treatment and also used a battery of delayed hypersensitivity antigens to assess skin test anergy (95). Among 25 persons who did not complete isoniazid, the tuberculosis incidence was 9.7/100 person-years. No cases occurred among those who completed treatment of latent infection. Among anergic individuals, the incidence was 6.6/100 person-years.

Useful information on the risk of tuberculosis in HIV-infected persons exposed to tuberculosis comes from two outbreak studies. Di Perri and coworkers described an outbreak of tuberculosis among AIDS patients in a hospital in Italy at which no patient with tuberculosis had been hospitalized during the previous 3 years (96). Ventilation included air recirculation. An individual with initially unsuspected tuberculosis was admitted, and an outbreak ensued. Among 18 exposed HIV-infected individuals, tuberculosis developed in eight, seven of them within 60 days.

Daley and colleagues described an outbreak in a congregate living facility for AIDS patients in San Francisco (97). A person with unrecognized tuberculosis was admitted to the facility; the diagnosis was made 6 weeks later after 3 weeks of progressive respiratory symptoms. Eleven of 30 exposed residents developed tuberculosis within the next 6 months, and organisms isolated from them were all of the same RFLP type as the organism from the index case. These two outbreaks demonstrate the enormous impact of HIV infection on susceptibility to tuberculosis.

In sum, one should probably accept a 10 percent annual risk of disease among tuberculin-positive persons who become HIV infected and a 35 to 45 percent early disease risk among AIDS patients who acquire infection with *M. tuberculosis*. Appropriate treatment of latent infection in both groups should reduce these risks.

Risk of Mortality Among American Health Care Workers with Tuberculosis

Clinical trials of antituberculosis therapeutic regimens conducted in the United States and elsewhere beginning the 1950s demonstrated low mortality rates among adequately treated individuals. The only modern American data come from United States Public Health Service trial number 21, a multicentered national trial of modern drug treatment regimens. Nine deaths occurred among 1,451 participants, 0.6 percent (98). HIV status of the participants in this trial was not determined as part of the study and was generally unknown. One of the nine persons who died was known to be receiving treatment for AIDS at the time of death, however. Of the other eight, at least six were noncompliant or did not complete prescribed therapy because of drug toxicity. Moreover, the causes of death reported in this trial were taken from death certificates, which may not have reflected the true cause (L. Geiter, personal communication, December 2000).

A large portion of individuals dying of tuberculosis have the diagnosis made at the time of death and hence do not receive therapy. Rieder and his colleagues examined this aspect of tuberculosis mortality in the United States for the years 1985 through 1988, a time period preceding the major explosion of both AIDS and multidrug-resistant tuberculosis in America (99).

Overall, 5.1 percent of tuberculosis diagnosed nationwide in those years was recognized at the time of death. During those years, there were a total of 7,210 tuberculosis deaths in the United States (1). Rieder and coworkers identified 4,373 diagnoses made at death. This represents 60.7 percent of the total deaths due to tuberculosis for those years.

Tuberculosis is not evenly distributed among Americans (1). About 23 or 24 percent occurs in individuals over the age of 65; presumably most of them are no longer in the work force. Nearly 60 percent occurs among the unemployed. Six percent of patients are inmates of correctional facilities; 6 percent are homeless; and 3 percent are residents of long-term-care facilities. Reduced access to health care among the homeless and the unemployed can be presumed to increase their risk of being diagnosed and treated late or not at all and, in turn, their risk of death from untreated tuberculosis.

HIV infection and drug resistance increase the mortality risk. During the decade prior to the HIV epidemic, Goble and colleagues at a national referral hospital noted a rate of mortality of 20.1 percent (27/134) among patients with tuberculosis due to organisms resistant to both isoniazid and rifampin (100). Data from 466 patients with a culture positive for *M. tuberculosis* in New York City in April 1991 were assembled by Frieden and collaborators (62). Follow-up of these patients was achieved until death or for 14 months. The case fatality rate for patients with multidrug-resistant organisms who were HIV infected was 80 percent; for HIV-uninfected individuals it was 47 percent.

In summary, the risk for immunocompetent individuals in the United States of dying from appropriately treated tuberculosis due to drug-susceptible organisms is vanishingly small. For health care workers it should be smaller than for the general population because they should have the advantages of more rapid diagnosis and institution of appropriate therapy and should not come from the malnourished, often homeless population that contributes substantially to national tuberculosis mortality.

Summary of Risks of Tuberculous Disease and Mortality Among *M. tuberculosis*-Infected Health Care Workers

In the surveillance studies cited above the methods of tuberculin skin testing, the completeness of follow-up, and the definitions of tuberculin positivity and of tuberculosis varied, and the rigor of examination for tuberculosis may also be open to challenge. Yet certain generalizations seem justified.

First, the attack rates among tuberculin reactors is substantially lower than the oft-stated 10 percent. Even if risks observed during the first few years after infection are projected forward in linear fashion, it is hard to envision a cumulative risk as high as 10 percent. The lifetime risk estimates by Comstock and Edwards (93) suggest that perhaps 3 percent should be chosen; other studies suggest a rate closer to 5 percent.

Next, although the risk cannot be converted to annual risk in any of them, it is apparent from these studies that the risk diminishes with the passage of time. In those studies in which age-specific data are presented, the risk among adults is greatest in the young adult, postpubertal years. This is the age when many individuals enter the health care workforce, but it is not representative of the many older health care workers.

The disease risk is dramatically increased in immunocompromised individuals. The risk of tuberculosis in infected persons is substantially reduced by appropriate treatment of latent infection, and health care workers should be ideally situated for the use of such treatment. Tuberculosis mortality risk in immunocompetent health care workers with tuberculosis not due to multidrug-resistant organisms is probably close to zero.

ACKNOWLEDGMENTS

This review could not have been accomplished without the help of others whom the author wishes to acknowledge. The reference librarians at the Health Sciences and Allen Memorial Libraries of Case Western Reserve University were helpful in finding many of the articles reviewed here, including obtaining a few by interlibrary loan. Marilyn Field, Elizabeth Epstein, and Cara Christie of the Institute of Medicine were helpful in supplying additional background material. Amy Curtis and Eugene McCray at CDC kindly gave me permission to cite some of their unpublished work. Finally, I am grateful to the members and staff of the Institute of Medicine Committee on Regulating Occupational Exposure to Tuberculosis for helpful reviews of successive drafts of this paper.

REFERENCES

1. Centers for Disease Control and Prevention. *Reported Tuberculosis in the United States.* Annual Reports. Centers for Disease Control and Prevention. Atlanta: 1999.
2. Sepkowitz KA. Tuberculosis and the health care worker: a historical perspective. *Annals of Internal Medicine* 1994; 120:71–79.
3. Bowden KM, McDiarmid MA. Occupationally acquired tuberculosis: what's known. *Journal of Occupational Medicine* 1994; 36:320–325.
4. Markowitz SB. Epidemiology of tuberculosis among health care workers. *Occupational Medicine* 1994; 9:589–608.
5. McGowan JE Jr. Nosocomial tuberculosis: new progress in control and prevention. *Clinical Infectious Diseases* 1995; 212:489–505.
6. Menzies D, Fanning A, Yuan L, Fitzgerald M. Tuberculosis among health care workers. *New England Journal of Medicine* 1995; 332:92–98.
7. Sepkowitz KA. AIDS, tuberculosis, and the health care worker. *Clinical Infectious Diseases* 1995; 20:232–242.
8. Pugliese G, Tapper ML. Tuberculosis control in health care. *Infections Control and Hospital Epidemiology* 1996; 17:819–827.
9. Blumberg HM. Tuberculosis infection control. In Reichman LB, Hershfield ES (editors). *Tuberculosis. A Comprehensive International Approach* 2nd ed. New York: Marcel Dekker, Inc., 2000; pp.609–643.
10. Daniel TM, Debanne SM. Estimation of the annual risk of tuberculous infection for white men in the United States. *Journal of Infectious Diseases* 1997; 175:1535–1537.
11. Styblo K. The relationship between the risk of tuberculous infection and the risk of developing infectious tuberculosis. *Bulletin of the International Union against Tuberculosis* 1985; 60:117–119.
12. Engel A, Roberts J. Tuberculin skin test reaction among adults 25-74 years, 1971-1972. DHEW publication no. (HRA) 77-1649. Washington, DC: U.S. Department of Health, Education, and Welfare, 1977.
13. World Health Organization. WHO report on the global tuberculosis epidemic 1998. Geneva, Switzerland: World Health Organization, 1998.
14. Rhoades ER, Alexander CP. Reactions to the tuberculin tine test in Air Force recruits. *American Review of Respiratory Diseases* 1968; 98:837–841.
15. Trump DH, Hyams KC, Cross ER, Struewing JP. Tuberculosis infection among young adults entering the US Navy in 1990. *Archives of Internal Medicine* 1993; 153:211–216.
16. Reichman LB, O'Day R. Tuberculous infection in a large urban population. *American Review of Respiratory Diseases* 1978; 117:705–712.
17. Barnard MW, Amberson JB Jr, Loew MF. Tuberculosis in adolescents. A study of 1000 school-children in New York City made under the auspices of the Bellevue-Yorkville Health Demonstration in 1930. *American Review of Tuberculosis* 1931; 23:593–641.
18. Edwards LB, Smith DT. Community-wide tuberculin testing study in Pamlico County, North Carolina. *American Review of Respiratory Diseases* 1965; 92:43–54.
19. Rosenthal SR, Afremow ML, Nikurs L, Loewinsohn E, Leppmann M, Katele E, Liveright D, Thorne M. BCG vaccination and tuberculosis in students of nursing. *American Journal of Nursing* 1963; 63:88–93.
20. Edwards LB, Acquaviva FA, Livesay VT, Cross FW, Palmer CE. An atlas of sensitivity to tuberculin, PPD-B, and histoplasmin in the United States. *American Review of Respiratory Diseases* 1969; 99(suppl.):1–132.
21. Hanzel GD, Rogers KD. Multiple-puncture and Mantoux tuberculin tests in high school students. A comparative study. *Journal of the American Medical Association* 1964; 190: 1038–1042.
22. Tuberculosis Program, National Communicable Disease Center, US DHEW PHS. Tuberculin testing in special tuberculosis projects 1966, 1967. Summary tables. Atlanta: Public Health Service, U.S. Department of Health, Education, and Welfare, 1968.

23. Vennema A, Ruggiero D. Tuberculin-sensitivity and risk of infection in New York City school children in 1980-81. *Bulletin of the International Union against Tuberculosis* 1984; 59:138–140.

24. McKenna MT, Hutton M, Cauthen G, Onorato IM. The association between occupation and tuberculosis. A population-based study. *American Journal of Respiratory and Critical Care Medicine* 1996; 154:587–593.

25. *Bulletin of the National Tuberculosis and Respiratory Disease Association.* 1969; 55:1–16.

26. Ruben FL, Norden CW, Schuster N. Analysis of a community hospital employee tuberculosis screening program 31 months after its inception. *American Review of Respiratory Diseases* 1977; 115:23–28.

27. Vogeler DM, Burke JP. Tuberculosis screening for hospital employees. A five-year experience in a large community hospital. *American Review of Respiratory Diseases* 1978; 117:227–232.

28. Berman J, Levin ML, Orr ST, Desi L. Tuberculosis risk for hospital employees: analysis of a five-year tuberculin skin testing program. *American Journal of Public Health* 1981; 71:1217–1222.

29. Aitken ML, Anderson KM, Albert RK. Is the tuberculosis screening program of hospital employees still required? *American Review of Respiratory Diseases* 1987; 136:805–807.

30. Louther J, Rivera P, Feldman J, Villa N, DeHovitz J, Sepkowitz KA. Risk of tuberculin conversion according to occupation among health care workers at a New York City hospital. *American Journal of Respiratory and Critical Care Medicine* 1997; 156:201–205.

31. Fella P, Rivera P, Hale M, Squires K, Sepkowitz K. Dramatic decrease in tuberculin skin test conversion rate among employees at a hospital in New York City. *American Journal of Infection Control* 1995; 23:352–356.

32. Maloney SA, Pearson ML, Gordon MT, Del Castillo R, Boyle JF, Jarvis WR. Efficacy of control measures in preventing nosocomial transmission of multidrug-resistant tuberculosis to patients and health care workers. *Annals of Internal Medicine* 1995; 122:90–95.

33. Blumberg HM, Watkins DL, Berschling JD, Antle A, Moore P, White N, Hunter M, Green B, Ray SM, McGowan JE. Preventing the nosocomial transmission of tuberculosis. *Annals of Internal Medicine* 1995; 122:658–663.

34. Sotir MJ, Khan A, Bock NN, Blumberg HM. Risk factors for tuberculin skin test (TST) positivity and conversion among employees at a public inner-city hospital in a high incidence area (abstract). Journal of Investigative Medicine 1997; 45:64A.

35. Blumberg HM, Sotir M, Erwin M, Bachman R, Shulman JA. Risk of house staff tuberculin skin test conversion in an area with a high incidence of tuberculosis. *Clinical Infectious Diseases* 1998; 27:826–833.

36. Sepkowitz KA, Friedman CR, Hafner A, Kwok D, Manoach S, Floris M. Martinez D, Sathianathan K, Brown E, Berger JJ, Segal-Maurer S, Kreiswirth B, Riley LW, Stoeckle MY. Tuberculosis among urban health care workers: a study using restriction fragment length polymorphism typing. *Clinical Infectious Diseases* 1995; 21:1098–1101.

37. Rattner SL, Fleischer JA, Davidson BL. Tuberculin positivity and patient contact in healthcare workers in the urban United States. *Infection Control and Hospital Epidemiology* 1996; 17:369–371.

38. Ball R, Van Wey M. Tuberculosis skin test conversion among health care workers at a military medical center. *Military Medicine* 1997; 162:338–343.

39. Boudreau AY, Baron SL, Steenland NK, Van Gilder TJ, Decker JA, Galson SK, Seitz T. Occupational risk of *Mycobacterium tuberculosis* infection in hospital workers. *American Journal of Industrial Medicine* 1997; 32:528–534.

40. Bailey TC, Fraser VJ, Spitznagel EL, Dunagan WC. Risk factors for a positive tuberculin skin test among employees of an urban, midwestern teaching hospital. *Annals of Internal Medicine* 1995; 122:580–585.

41. Fraser VJ, Kilo CM, Bailey TC, Medoff G, Dunagan WC. Screening of physicians for tuberculosis. *Infection Control and Hospital Epidemiology* 1994; 15:95–110.

42. Christie CD, Constantinou P, Marx ML, Willke MJ, Marot K, Mendez FL, Donovan J, Thole J. Low risk for tuberculosis in a regional pediatric hospital: nine-year study of community rates and the mandatory employee tuberculin skin-test program. *Infection Control and Hospital Epidemiology* 1998; 19:168–174.
43. Van Drunen N, Bonnicksen G, Pfeiffer AJ. A survey of tuberculosis control programs in seventeen Minnesota hospitals: implications for policy development. *American Journal of Infection Control* 1996; 24:235–242.
44. Managan LP, Bennett CL, Tablan N, Simonds DN, Pugilese G, Collazo E, Jarvis WR. Nosocomial tuberculosis prevention measures among two groups of US hospitals, 1992 to 1996. *Chest* 2000; 117:380–384.
45. U.S. Department of Labor. Occupational Safety and Health Administration. Occupational exposure to tuberculosis; proposed rule. *Federal Register* 1997; 62:54160–54308.
46. National Center for Health Statistics, Centers for Disease Control and Prevention, U.S. Department of Health and Human Services. *An Overview of Nursing Homes and their Current Residents*: Data from the 1995 National Nursing Home Survey. Atlanta: Centers for Disease Control and Prevention, 1997: pp.97–250.
47. Centers for Disease Control. Prevention and control of tuberculosis in facilities providing long-term care to the elderly. Recommendations of the Advisory Committee for Elimination of Tuberculosis. *Morbidity and Mortality Weekly Report* 1990; 39(RR-10):7–13.
48. Hutton MD, Cauthen GM, Bloch AB. Results of a 29-state survey of tuberculosis in nursing homes and correctional facilities. *Public Health Reports* 1993; 108:305–314.
49. Stead WW. Tuberculosis among elderly persons: an outbreak in a nursing home. *Annals of Internal Medicine* 1981; 94:606–610.
50. Munger R, Anderson K, Leahy R, Allard J, Kobayashi JM. Tuberculosis in a nursing care facility—Washington. *Morbidity and Mortality Weekly Report* 1983; 32:121–128.
51. Price LE, Rutala WA. Tuberculosis screening in the long-term care setting. *Infection Control* 1987; 8:353–356.
52. Pelletier AR, DiFerdinando GT Jr, Greenberg AJ, Sosin DM, Jones WD Jr, Bloch AB, Woodley CL. Tuberculosis in a correctional facility. *Archives of Internal Medicine* 1993; 153:2692–2695.
53. Steenland K, Levine AJ, Sieber K, Schulte P, Aziz D. Incidence of tuberculous infection among New York State prison employees. *American Journal of Public Health* 1997; 87: 2012–2014.
54. Campbell R, Sneller V-P, Khoury N, Hinton B, DeSouza L, Smith S, Howard J, Ciofalo F, Welsh AL, Krycia W, Mycroft F, Hooper K, Goldman L, Royce S, Dorfman B, Morita S, Coulter S, Rutherford GW. Probable transmission of multidrug-resistant tuberculosis in a correctional facility—California. *Morbidity and Mortality Weekly Report* 1993; 42:48–51.
55. Prendergast T, Hwang B, Alexander R, Charron T, Lopez E, Culton J, Bick J, Shalaby M, Dewsnup D, Meyer H, Horowitz E, Khoury N, Mohle-Boetani J, Royce S, Chin D, Petrillo S, Miguelino V, Desmond E, Harrison R, Cone J, Greene C, Joseph M, Waterman S. Tuberculosis outbreaks in prison housing units for HIV-infected inmates—California, 1995–1996. *Morbidity and Mortality Weekly Report* 1999; 48:79–82.
56. Koo DT, Baron RC, Rutherford GW. Transmission of *Mycobacterium tuberculosis* in a California state prison, 1991. *American Journal of Public Health* 1997; 87:279–282.
57. Bergmire-Sweat D, Barnett BJ, Harris SL, Taylor JP, Mazurek GH, Reddy V. Tuberculosis outbreak in a Texas prison, 1994. *Epidemiology and Infection* 1996; 117:485–492.
58. Jones TF, Craig AS, Valway SE, Woodley CL, Schaffner W. Transmission of tuberculosis in a jail. *Annals of Internal Medicine* 1999; 131:557–563.
59. Johnsen C. Tuberculosis contact investigation: two years of experience in New York City correctional facilities. *American Journal of Infection Control* 1993; 21:1–4.

60. Erdil M, Stahl K. Prevalence of tuberculosis skin test reactivity in preplacement applicants to the Connecticut Department of Corrections from 1991 to 1992. *Journal of Occupational Medicine* 1993; 35:1178–1179.

61. Brudney K, Dobkin J. Resurgent tuberculosis in New York City. Human immunodeficiency virus, homelessness, and the decline of tuberculosis control programs. *American Review of Respiratory Diseases* 1991; 144:745–749.

62. Frieden TR, Sterling T, Pablos-Mendez A, Kilburn JO, Cauthen GM, Dooley SW. The emergence of drug-resistant tuberculosis in New York City. *New England Journal of Medicine* 1993; 328:521–526.

63. Nardell E, McInnis B, Thomas B, Weidhaas S. Exogenous reinfection with tuberculosis in a shelter for the homeless. *New England Journal of Medicine* 1986; 315:1570–1575.

64. Nolan CM, Elarth AM, Barr H, Saeed AM, Risser DR. An outbreak of tuberculosis in a shelter for homeless men. A description of its evolution and control. *American Review of Respiratory Disease* 143(2):257–261, 1991.

65. Barnes PF, El-Hajj H, Preston-Martin S, Cave MD, Jones BE, Otaya M, Pogoda J, Eisenach KD. Transmission of tuberculosis among the urban homeless. *Journal of the American Medical Association* 1996; 275:305–307.

66. Curtis AB, Ridzon R, Novick LF, Driscoll J, Blair D, Oxtoby M, McGarry M, Hiscox B, Faulkner C, Taber H, Valway S, Onorato IM. Analysis of *Mycobacterium tuberculosis* transmission patterns in a homeless shelter outbreak. *International Journal of Tuberculosis and Lung Disease* 2000; 4:308–313.

67. Layton MC, Cantwell MF, Dorsinville GJ, Valway SE, Onorato IM, Frieden TR. Tuberculosis screening among homeless persons with AIDS living in single-room-occupancy hotels. *American Journal of Public Health* 1995; 85:1556–1559.

68. Pierce JR, Sims SL, Holman GH. Transmission of tuberculosis to hospital workers by a patient with AIDS. *Chest* 1992; 101:581–582.

69. Hoch DE, Wilcox KR Jr. Transmission of multidrug-resistant tuberculosis from an HIV-positive client in a residential substance-abuse treatment facility—Michigan. *Morbidity and Mortality Weekly Report* 1991; 40:129–131.

70. Howell JT, Scheel WJ, Pryor VL, Tavris DR, Calder RA, Wilder MH. *Mycobacterium tuberculosis* transmission in a health clinic—Florida, 1988. *Morbidity and Mortality Weekly Report* 1989; 38:256–264.

71. Zahnow K, Matts JP, Hillman D, Finley E, Brown LS Jr, Torres RA, Ernst J, El-Sadr W, Perez G, Webster C, Barber B, Gordin FM. Rates of tuberculosis infection in healthcare workers providing services to HIV-infected populations. *Infection Control and Hospital Epidemiology* 1998; 19:829–835.

72. Prezant DJ, Kelly KJ, Mineo FP, Janus D, Karwa ML, Futterman N, Nolte C. Tuberculin skin test conversion rates in New York City Emergency Medical Service health care workers. *Annals of Emergency Medicine* 1998; 32:208–213.

73. Kao AS, Ashford DA, McNeil MM, Warren NG, Good RC. Descriptive profile of tuberculin skin testing programs and laboratory-acquired tuberculous infections in public health laboratories. *Journal of Clinical Microbiology* 1997; 35:1847–1851.

74. Ussery XT, Bierman JA, Valway SE, Seitz TA, DiFerdinando GT Jr, Ostroff SM. Transmission of multidrug-resistant *Mycobacterium tuberculosis* among persons exposed in a medical examiner's office, New York. *Infection Control and Hospital Epidemiology* 1995; 16:160–165.

75. Gershon RRM, Vlahov D, Escamilla-Cejudo JA, Badawi M, McDiarmid M, Karkashian C, Grimes, M, Comstock GW. Tuberculosis risk in funeral home employees. *Journal of Occupational Environmental Medicine* 1998; 40:497–503.

76. Sterling TR, Pope DS, Bishai WR, Harrington S, Gershon RR, Chaisson RE. Transmission of *Mycobacterium tuberculosis* from a cadaver to an embalmer. *New England Journal of Medicine* 2000; 342:246–248.

77. Lauzardo M, Duncan H, Hale Y, Lee P. Transmission of *Mycobacterium tuberculosis* to a funeral director during routine embalming (abstract). *American Journal of Respiratory and Critical Care Medicine* 2000; 161:A299.

78. Price LE, Rutala WA, Samsa GP. Tuberculosis in hospital personnel. *Infection Control* 1987; 8:97–101.

79. Beck-Sagué C, Dooley SW, Hutton MD, Otten J, Breeden A, Crawford JT, Pitchenik AE, Woodley C, Cauthen G, Jarvis WR. Hospital outbreak of multidrug-resistant *Mycobacterium tuberculosis* infections. Factors in transmission to staff and HIV-infected patients. *Journal of the American Medical Association* 1992; 268:1280–1286.

80. Panlilio AL, Burwen DR. Tuberculin skin testing surveillance of health-care workers (HCWS) (abstract). *American Journal of Respiratory and Critical Care Medicine* 1996; 153 (suppl):A133.

81. Sinkowitz RL, Fridkin SK, Managan L, Wenger PN, Jarvis WR. Status of tuberculosis infection control programs at United States Hospitals, 1989 to 1992. *American Journal of Infection Control* 1996; 24:226–234.

82. Ferebee SH. Controlled chemoprophylaxis trials in tuberculosis. A general review. *Advances in Tuberculosis Research* 1970; 17:28–106.

83. Myers JA, Bearman JE, Botkins AC. Natural history of tuberculosis in the human body. IX. Prognosis among students with tuberculin reaction conversion before, during and after medical school. *Diseases of the Chest* 1966; 50:120–132.

84. Myers JA, Bearman JE, Botkins AC. Natural history of tuberculosis in the human body. IX. Prognosis among students with tuberculin reaction conversion before, during and after school of nursing. *Diseases of the Chest* 1968; 53:687–698.

85. Sepkowitz KA. Tuberculin skin testing and the health care worker: lessons of the Prophit survey. *Tuberculosis and Lung Disease* 1996; 77:81–85.

86. Barrett-Connor E. The epidemiology of tuberculosis in physicians. *Journal of the American Medical Association* 1979; 241:33–38.

87. Edwards LB, Livesay VT, Acquaviva FA, Palmer CE. Height, weight, tuberculous infection, and tuberculous disease. *Archives of Environmental Health* 1971; 22:106–112.

88. Horwitz O, Wilbek E, Erickson PA. Epidemiologic basis of tuberculosis eradication. *Bulletin of the World Health Organization* 1969; 41:95–113.

89. Medical Research Council. BCG and vole bacillus vaccines in the prevention of tuberculosis in adolescence and early adult life. *Bulletin World Health Organization* 1972; 46:371–385.

90. Comstock GW. Community research in tuberculosis. Muscogee County, Georgia. *Public Health Reports* 1964; 79:1045–1056.

91. Comstock GW, Woolpert SH, Livesay VT. Tuberculosis studies in Muscogee County, Georgia. Twenty-year evaluation of a community trial of BCG vaccination. *Public Health Reports* 1976; 91:276–280.

92. Comstock GW, Livesay VT, Woolpert SF. The prognosis of a positive tuberculin reaction in childhood and adolescence. *American Journal of Epidemiology* 1974; 99:131–138.

93. Comstock GW, Edwards PQ. The competing risks of tuberculosis and hepatitis for adult tuberculin reactors. *American Review of Respiratory Diseases* 1975; 111:573–577.

94. Selwyn PA, Hartel D, Lewis VA, Schoenbaum EE, Vermund SH, Klein RS, Walker AT, Friedland GH. A prospective study of the risk of tuberculosis among intravenous drug users with human immunodeficiency virus infection. *New England Journal of Medicine* 1989; 320:545–550.

95. Selwyn PA, Sckell BM, Alcabes P, Friedland GH, Klein RS, Schoenbaum EE. High risk of active tuberculosis in HIV-infected drug users with cutaneous anergy. *Journal of the American Medical Association* 1992; 268:504–509.

96. Di Perri G, Cruciani M, Danzi MC, Luzatti R, De Checchi G, Malena M, Pizzighella S, Mazzi R, Solbiati M, Concia E, Bassetti D. Nosocomial epidemic of active tuberculosis among HIV-infected patients. *Lancet* 1989; 2:1502–1504.

97. Daley CL, Small PM, Schecter GF, Schoolnik GK, McAdam RA, Jacobs WR Jr, Hopewell PC. An outbreak of tuberculosis with accelerated progression among persons infected with the human immunodeficiency virus. *New England Journal of Medicine* 1992; 326: 231–235.

98. Combs DL, O'Brien RJ, Geiter LJ. USPHS tuberculosis short-course chemotherapy trial 21: effectiveness, toxicity, and acceptability. The report of final results. *Annals of Internal Medicine* 1990; 112:397-406.

99. Rieder HL, Kelly GD, Bloch AB, Cauthen GM, Snider DE Jr. Tuberculosis diagnosed at death in the United States. *Chest* 1991; 100:678–681.

100. Goble M, Iseman MD, Madsen RN-C, Waite D, Ackerson L, Horsburgh CR Jr. Treatment of 171 patients with pulmonary tuberculosis resistant to isoniazid and rifampin. *New England Journal of Medicine* 1993; 328:527–532.

D

Effects of CDC Guidelines on Tuberculosis Control in Health Care Facilities

Keith F. Woeltje, M.D., Ph.D. [*]

SUMMARY

In response to nosocomial outbreaks of tuberculosis among patients and health care workers, the Centers for Disease Control and Prevention (CDC) released tuberculosis control guidelines in 1990. These were later expanded and revised in 1994. The CDC guidelines rely on a series of controls: administrative, engineering, and personal respiratory protection. Administrative controls include the prompt identification and isolation of patients who may have pulmonary tuberculosis. Engineering controls include proper ventilation for isolation rooms and other areas, possibly supplemented by ultraviolet germicidal irradiation or high-efficiency particulate air (HEPA) filtration. Personal respiratory protection consists of some form of mask or respirator worn by a health care worker to minimize the risk of inhaling infectious airborne droplet nuclei.

Implementation of control measures in outbreak settings has been shown repeatedly to stop the outbreak. Although many steps may be started at once, the bulk of the evidence suggests that the CDC controls are hierarchical, in that administrative controls are most important (if tuberculosis is not suspected, the other controls will not be initiated), followed by the engineering controls, and lastly, the type of personal respiratory equipment. In nonoutbreak settings having these measures in place almost certainly reduces the risk for health care workers and patients of nosocomial exposure to tuberculosis. However, studies trying to correlate health care worker infections with adherence to tuberculosis

[*]Assistant Professor of Medicine, Section of Infectious Diseases, Medical College of Georgia, Augusta.

controls in low- to moderate-risk situations have had mixed results. This may be due to underlying differences in the baseline purified protein derivative (PPD) conversion rates in different hospitals. In addition to the adoption of the whole guidelines, a number of studies have focused on parts of the guidelines. This is particularly true of administrative controls. It is in this area where the most variability in practice will arise, particularly in designing criteria for patient isolation, owing to the wide differences in patient populations seen at different hospitals.

Although compliance with the guidelines in the early 1990s was suboptimal, a number of studies show significant improvements in guideline compliance. However, there are many areas that still have considerable room for improvement, particularly in the education of health care workers about tuberculosis. Information on implementation of the guidelines outside of the inpatient setting of acute-care hospitals is scarce. Some evidence exists that many emergency departments are making progress.

The cost of implementation of the guidelines can be substantial, but many of these costs are one-time facility improvements. Although the ongoing costs of a tuberculosis control program can be substantial, these programs may be relatively cost-effective compared with the costs incurred in evaluating patients or healthcare workers exposed to a non-isolated tuberculosis patient.

INTRODUCTION

Summary of 1990 and 1994 CDC Guidelines

After decades of declining rates of tuberculosis in the United States, case rates leveled off and then increased in the late 1980s and early 1990s (1, 2). A number of factors led to the reversal of the previous trend: decreased public health infrastructure, the human immunodeficiency virus (HIV) epidemic, and an influx of immigrants from areas where tuberculosis is endemic (3). The problem was compounded by the fact that many physicians and other healthcare workers had very little experience with tuberculosis. They often did not suspect the diagnosis when a patient with the disease first presented and, even if suspected, often had little appreciation for the infection control issues involved. Almost inevitably, a number of nosocomial outbreaks of tuberculosis occurred, including outbreaks involving multidrug-resistant tuberculosis (MDR tuberculosis) (4, 5, 6, 7, 8, 9, 10). In December 1990, CDC published "Guidelines for Preventing the Transmission of Tuberculosis in Health-Care Settings, with Special Focus on HIV-Related Issues" (11) in response to these outbreaks. Subsequently, these guidelines were expanded and refined with the publication in October 1994 of "Guidelines for Preventing the Transmission of *Mycobacterium tuberculosis* in Health-Care Facilities, 1994" (12).

The 1994 CDC guidelines include recommendations for assignment of responsibility for tuberculosis control. A risk assessment for the facility (and potentially for individual wards and areas within the facility) is suggested. This risk assessment takes into account the number of tuberculosis patients seen at the facility, the number of tuberculosis patients in the surrounding community, and whether or not there is evidence of increased health care worker PPD skin test conversions. The extent to which other control actions are taken would then depend on the risk of the facility. For example, a baseline PPD test for new employees is recommended for essentially all facilities, but the frequency of routine serial testing would be determined by the risk assessment. The guidelines also suggest health care worker education consistent with the duties/training of the employee. Good cooperation with local health departments is also stressed. Although the bulk of the guidelines are targeted to acute-care hospitals, tuberculosis control in other settings such as dental clinics, physicians' offices, and long-term-care facilities are also briefly discussed.

The core of the 1994 CDC guidelines is a series of control measures for handling patients suspected of having tuberculosis. Three categories of controls are described: administrative, engineering, and personal respiratory protection. Administrative controls include prompt recognition of patients who may have tuberculosis with subsequent rapid isolation of these patients, efficient diagnostic evaluation, and criteria for releasing patients from isolation. Other administrative controls include practices such as keeping patients on tuberculosis isolation in their room unless medically necessary. Engineering controls involve primarily ventilation. tuberculosis isolation rooms should have negative pressure, $\geq$ six air changes per hour (ACH), and exhaust air directly to the outside (or HEPA filter the air before recirculation if this is not possible). Engineering controls also include having good general ventilation, especially in areas where patients may congregate. Ultraviolet germicidal irradiation (UVGI) may be used as an adjunct to both general ventilation and tuberculosis isolation room ventilation. Finally, the guidelines discuss personal respiratory protection for health care workers who are likely to be exposed to tuberculosis aerosols (e.g., while in a tuberculosis isolation room). The respirator should be compliant with Occupational Safety and Health Administration (OSHA) requirements, and used as part of a comprehensive respiratory protection program.

Focus of Review

The author was directed to "prepare a technical background paper reviewing the literature and data on the effects of the CDC guidelines on tuberculosis control in health care facilities." This paper is being written as background for an Institute of Medicine report on occupational exposure to tuberculosis. Although the 1994 guidelines do include employee tuberculin skin testing programs and personal respiratory equipment, this paper will not address these particular aspects because the topics will be covered in other background papers. One important exception is that employee PPD test conversion rates will be discussed as a marker for the effectiveness of different tuberculosis control plans.

Although the 1994 CDC guidelines are the most current, as summarized above, these guidelines are an extension and revision of the 1990 guidelines. Thus, this paper will review the impact of implementation of policies following both sets of guidelines. As with the guidelines, this paper will focus primarily on the inpatient, acute-care setting. This is partly out of necessity, as there is a paucity of data on implementation of the guidelines in other settings.

Methods

To find papers for review, a MedLine search using Ovid (Ovid Technologies, New York, New York) was performed. The database was searched from the most recent update available in mid-June 2000 back through 1991. Initial search terms were Tuberculosis/pc,ep,tm (Prevention & Control, Epidemiology, Transmission) AND Health facilities. The search was further limited to English-language articles. This yielded 257 references. Abstracts of these references were reviewed to choose appropriate articles. Additional Medline search strategies included Guidelines AND Tuberculosis/pc (which added 5 references not previously obtained), and (Tuberculosis OR Mycobacterium tuberculosis) AND Occupational exposure (which yielded 64 additional references, only 2 of which were useful). The author's files served as another source of articles. Finally, potentially useful references found while reading the initial papers were also reviewed. Although the guidelines are generally applicable, because the expectation of implementation is primarily in U.S. hospitals, papers regarding health-care facilities outside of the United States were not included. Not all papers reviewed were included in the final document—papers were chosen either for the strength of their data or because they contributed a unique view into the implementation of the CDC standards.

IMPACT OF FOLLOWING THE GUIDELINES

Studies of Implementation of Entire Guidelines

Studies Showing Resolution of Outbreaks

The strongest evidence for the beneficial impact of the CDC guidelines comes from institutions where control measures were implemented in response to nosocomial transmission of tuberculosis to patients and/or health care workers. Implementation of these measures then led to decreases in nosocomial cases of tuberculosis infection or disease.

Wenger and coworkers (13) reported the experience of Jackson Memorial Hospital, Miami, Florida, following an outbreak of MDR tuberculosis from 1988 to 1990 on an HIV ward (4, 14). Control measures were implemented over time, starting in March 1990. The measures implemented included the following:

March

 • Stricter enforcement of isolation policy to include isolation of any HIV-positive patient with an abnormal chest radiograph (CXR)
 • Change in criteria for stopping isolation from discontinuation after 7 days on therapy to discontinuation only after three negative smears for acid-fast bacilli (AFB) (or after reduction in AFB on three smears plus a clinical response)
 • Enforcement of policy to keep tuberculosis patients in their rooms unless medically necessary and having patients wear a surgical mask when out of their rooms
  • Sputum induction done only in isolation rooms
  • Initial therapy for tuberculosis with four drugs

April (through April 1991)

 • The 6 tuberculosis isolation rooms (of 23) without negative pressure were repaired, and the ventilation in the other rooms was made more consistent

June

 • Aerosolized pentamidine administered only in isolation room

September

 • Change from cup-type surgical mask to submicron mask for health care workers

A review of admissions of HIV-positive patients with MDR tuberculosis was performed, covering three time periods: initial period (January 1990 to May 1990), early follow-up (June 1990 to February 1991), and late follow-up (March 1991 to June 1992). There was a decrease in MDR tuberculosis patient-days over the three periods (222/100 real days initially, then 119/100, and finally 16/100). Fifteen patients with MDR tuberculosis were admitted during the initial period: 12 (80 percent) had been exposed while on the HIV ward. Eleven patients were admitted during the follow-up periods, only five of whom had been exposed on the ward, all during the initial period. No known patient exposures occurred during the follow-up periods.

Health care worker PPD test results were also reviewed over the same time periods. A total of 39 health care workers were previously PPD negative and tested (25 during the initial period, 17 during early follow-up, and 23 during the late follow-up). There was a total of 10 PPD conversions: 7/25 (28 percent) in the initial period, 3/17 (18 percent) in early follow-up, and 0/23 in late follow-up ($P < 0.01$). Of the three PPD conversions during the early follow-up period, two were linked to exposure to a patient with MDR tuberculosis who was not isolated on admission because of the fact that he was on therapy and had been AFB smear negative at the time of a recent hospital discharge. However, he subsequently proved to be smear positive. This led to an additional policy that any patient with a history of MDR tuberculosis would be isolated regardless of previous smear and treatment status.

The authors point out that it is difficult to know what components of the control measures were most important. However, the early implementation of administrative controls linked with beginning improvements in engineering controls led to a reduction in nosocomial transmission of MDR tuberculosis to other patients, as well as a reduction in PPD conversions in health care workers.

Similarly, Maloney and colleagues (15) detailed control methods implemented in June through October 1991 after an outbreak of MDR tuberculosis at Cabrini Medical Center in New York City. Control measures included improved isolation criteria (not detailed in the paper, but 90 percent of patients with MDR tuberculosis were isolated on admission, compared with isolation of 40 percent of patients preintervention) and molded surgical masks for employees (June): improved lab services (July); increase from 0/10 tuberculosis isolation rooms with negative pressure to 16/27 with negative pressure (September); and a chamber for sputum induction and pentamidine administration (October).

With the adoption of these measures the number of patients with MDR tuberculosis who had previously been admitted to Cabrini fell from 24 in the preintervention period (January 1990 through June 1991) to 6 in the postintervention period (July 1991 through August 1992). Three of the six postintervention patients also had documented non-hospital or preintervention exposures documented. In the postintervention period only 1 patient was found to have had a documented nosocomial exposure during a previous hospitalization, as opposed to 20/24 (83%) in the preintervention period.

Implementation of control measures led to no change in the overall rate of PPD conversions (~3 percent). However the rate of conversion on the HIV and medical wards fell from 16.7 percent during the preintervention period to 5.1 percent postintervention ($p = 0.02$), with no change on wards that did not usually house tuberculosis patients. The postintervention PPD rates on HIV and medicine wards became essentially the same as the rates on other wards (5.1 percent versus 4.0 percent; $p = 0.5$).

Again, the impact of the individual control measures could not be determined, but clearly, the overall impact was significant. The authors note that the overall PPD conversion rate was unchanged. They highlight the importance of determining job-specific rates.

Blumberg and colleagues (16) reported the efforts made at Grady Memorial Hospital in Atlanta. These were in response to nosocomial transmissions of drug-sensitive tuberculosis in 1991 and early 1992 (5). Control measures implemented included the following:

March 1

• Expanded isolation policy—all patients with known or suspected tuberculosis (including all patients for whom AFB smear and culture were ordered), also any patient with HIV infection (or risk for HIV infection with unknown serology) with abnormal CXR. Increased surveillance by infection control to ensure that patients for whom smears ordered were in isolation.

• Isolation stopped only after three negative AFB smears (previously stopped after 2 weeks of therapy)
   • Increased physician education
   • Window fans added to 90 rooms to provide negative pressure

June 1

• Submicron masks used for personal respiratory protection

July 1

• PPD testing done every 6 months now included nonemployee health care workers (e.g., attendings, house staff, medical students)
   • tuberculosis nurse epidemiologist hired

To determine the effectiveness of these measures the authors reviewed tuberculosis exposure episodes (from July 1, 1991, to June 30, 1994) and PPD conversions (from January 1, 1992 to June 30, 1994). Over the 3-year period there were 752 admissions (673 patients) with tuberculosis; for 461 admissions (61 percent) the patients had positive AFB smears and were considered infectious. The results for these patients are shown in Table D-1.

Employee PPD conversion rates fell steadily from 3.3 percent to 0.4 percent during the postintervention period (for trend, $p < 0.001$). For the January–June 1994 PPD conversions (23/5,153 [0.4 percent]) no clustering by work area was noted. In fact only 10 health care workers had direct patient contact on wards where tuberculosis patients were housed, 4 had patient contact on low-risk tuberculosis areas (e.g., neonatal intensive care unit [ICU]), and 9 had no patient contact, suggesting that more than half of the conversions may have been community acquired.

Tuberculosis isolation rooms were tested with smoke approximately every 3 months. The failure rate ranged from 6.1 percent to 21.7 percent (mean, 16.5 percent). One room tested with sulfur hexafluoride had 4.9 ACH. The author suggest that their data imply that the improvements in PPD conversion rates were primarily the result of improved administrative controls since changes mirrored improved isolation as a result of the new policies. They argue that since room negative pressure was demonstrated to be frequently suboptimal, engineering controls were not the major factor in the improvements. Likewise submicron masks appeared to be adequate. The new policies resulted in only one of eight patients placed on tuberculosis isolation having culture-confirmed tuberculosis.

Columbia-Presbyterian Medical Center in New York City had control measures detailed by Bangsberg and colleagues (17). They revised their tuberculosis control guidelines to be consistent with the CDC guidelines. Prior to June, 1992, medical house staff were PPD tested at baseline and were then instructed to be tested annually by their primary physicians. Starting in June 1992, PPD testing was done every 6 months on medical house staff. The overall rate of participation was 92 percent.

Revised tuberculosis control measures included stricter isolation policy (implemented in May 1992) so that patients with HIV infection or HIV infection risk factors or who were homeless and presented with pneumonia or evidence of tuberculosis were placed in tuberculosis isolation until three sputum samples were AFB negative and the patient was judged noninfectious by pulmonary and infectious disease consultants. Tuberculosis isolation rooms were installed in the emergency department (ED) in July 1992. A tuberculosis service was implemented at the end of June 1993. In July 1993 3M respirators (type not stated) were instituted.

TABLE D-1. Results of Interventions at Grady Memorial Hospital

Measure	Pre-intervention (7/91–2/92)	Post-intervention (3/92–6/94)	p
No. of tuberculosis admissions	184	568	
No. of tuberculosis admissions/ month (AFB +)	23 (12.9)	20 (12.8)	
No. of exposure episodes/month	4.4	0.6	
No. of exposure days/month	35.4	3.3	< 0.001
No. of patients not appropriately isolated/total no. of patients	35/103 (34%)	18/358 (5%)	< 0.001
No. of HIV infected patients admissions associated with exposure episodes/total no. of admissions	22/33 (67%)	7/143 (5%)	< 0.001

TUBERCULOSIS IN THE WORKPLACE

The number of patients with pulmonary tuberculosis appropriately isolated during January through June 1992 (preintervention) was only 29/71 (38 percent). This increased to 29/45 (64 percent) from January to December 1992. Subsequent isolation rates continued to improve slightly: 60/82 (72 percent) from January to June 1993 and 33/44 (75 percent) from July to December 1993 ($p < 0.01$ for trend). Results considering only HIV infected patients were similar.

PPD conversion rates among house staff were as follows: June 1992, 10 percent (5.8/100 person-years); December 1992, 3 percent (5.1/100 person-years); June 1993, 0 percent; December 1993, 1 percent (2.3/100 person-years); June 1994, 0 percent. Conversion rates were calculated per 100 person-years of exposure because of varying exposure times possible at the June 1992 testing (12–36 months, depending on the year of the resident).

Because the biggest drop occurred between December 1992 and June 1993, the authors imply that isolation policy and possibly the tuberculosis isolation rooms in the ED were most important in leading to the improvements. Clearly their expanded isolation policy resulted in much better isolation of patients with pulmonary tuberculosis over this time period.

Stroud and colleagues (18) reviewed the effects of control measures at Roosevelt during three 15-month periods: period I, January 1989 to March 1990; period II, April 1990 to June 1991; and period III, July 1991 to September 1992. Period I was essentially a preintervention period, during which there was an outbreak of nosocomial tuberculosis (7). Patients with suspected tuberculosis were admitted to private room (only 1 of 16 with negative pressure), doors were often left open, and isolation was discontinued without negative AFB smears. Surgical masks were used for respiratory protection. Most rooms, however, did exhaust to the outside.

During period II administrative controls were enforced—a lower threshold for initiating isolation was set, more aggressive evaluation for possible tuberculosis was started, and more aggressive treatment regimens were started if there was no response to initial therapy. An effort was made to keep HIV-infected patients off wards with tuberculosis patients.

In period III engineering controls were phased in. From July to December 1991, 11 rooms were fitted with UVGI. From November 1991 through January 1992 seven of these rooms were fitted with exhaust fans for ≥6 ACH and negative pressure. Isolation chambers were used for sputum induction/aerosolized pentamidine administration. Surgical masks (Technol 47080070) were used through all three study periods. With the implementation of administrative controls during periods II and III, patients with pulmonary tuberculosis were more likely to be isolated on admission (44 percent versus 0 percent during period I). The median delay before isolation initiated (2 versus 6 days) also improved.

During period I, the likelihood of an HIV-infected patient getting tuberculosis decreased with distance from source patient room (but oddly, not related to the amount of time spent on the ward). Smear negative patients were not a source of nosocomial infection in period I. Crude rates of nosocomial tuberculosis were reduced from 8.8 percent during period I to 2.6 percent during period II and to 0 percent in period III. During period II, there was no association of nosocomial tuberculosis with distance from the source patient's room.

The impact on health care worker PPD conversion rates could not be determined due to insufficient data. However, during period II plus period III, PPD conversion rates were higher on tuberculosis wards than on other wards (5/29 versus 0/15; $p = 0.15$).

The impact of implementing the CDC guidelines on employee PPD conversion rates at St. Clare's Hospital in New York was reported by Fella and colleagues (19). Beginning in 1991, all health care workers with patient contact had PPD testing every 6 months; others were tested annually. Two-step testing of new employees was implemented in February 1993. Prior to 1991, no negative-pressure isolation rooms were available at St. Clare's. The implementation of control measures and PPD conversion rates are shown in Table D-2.

In an abstract presented at the 1994 Annual Conference of the Society for Occupational and Environmental Health—Tuberculosis Control in the Workplace: Science, Implementation, and Prevention Policy, Koll and colleagues (20) summarized data from Beth Israel Medical Center (BIMC) in New York City. The hospital had large numbers of tuberculosis patients and admissions in the early 1990s. A comprehensive tuberculosis policy (based on the 1990 CDC guidelines) was implemented in mid-1992. tuberculosis isolation rooms with negative pressure, ≥6 ACH, and UVGI were

TABLE D-2. PPD Conversions and Interventions at St. Clare's Hospital

Year	Interval	No. PPD Positive/ No. tested	Rate (%)	PRP	Environmental Interventions
1991	Jan–June	30/145	20.7	Technol shield	Negative-pressure rooms
	July–Dec	11/158	7.0	Technol shield	
1992	Jan–June	7/219	3.2	Particulate respirator UVGI	
	July–Dec	14/227	6.2	Particulate respirator	
1993	Jan–June	10/249	4.0	Dust-mist-fume respirator	
	July–Dec	9/154	5.8	Dust-mist-fume respirator	

NOTE: PRP = personal respiratory protection.

made available. Automatic door closers were installed. HEPA filters were used for recirculated air. A protocol for rapid identification of patients with possible tuberculosis was instituted. Surgical masks were replaced with submicron masks. Strict adherence to tuberculosis isolation precautions was promoted with patient education and incentives. Booths were used for aerosolized pentamidine administration and sputum induction. An annual PPD program for health care workers was implemented, with testing of high-risk health care workers every six months. The impact of the policies on health care worker PPD conversion is noted in Table D-3.

The reason for such small numbers of respiratory therapist conversions was not noted in the abstract. The authors noted that the rate of compliance with PPD testing in 1991 and 1992 was <75 percent; in 1993 it was 95 percent, so the reduction may have been even greater than documented. Unfortunately, rates are not provided, but overall the data are suggestive.

Grant (21) presented the results of a review of all tuberculosis cases at Parkland Memorial Hospital, Dallas, in 1994 and 1995. A variety of enhancements to the tuberculosis control policies were made from April to December 1994, including certification of PPD placement, an algorithm for tuberculosis isolation room assignment in times of low availability, standing orders for patients with suspected tuberculosis, increased UV in waiting areas, a fit testing program, increased employee PPD frequency (depending on job category), and notification of infection control by radiology of suspicious CXRs. Previously, an increase in health care worker PPD conversions had led to improvements in engineering controls, with 64 tuberculosis isolation rooms being made available.

Over the 2 years, 253 tuberculosis patients were admitted, 85 percent of whom had pulmonary disease. In 1994, all AFB smears were processed within 24 hours. Nontuberculous mycobacteria (NTM) were found in 193/407 (47 percent) patients with a positive AFB smear. Further results are presented in Table D-4.

The authors report that the data gathered each year were released along with information about the importance of compliance with the tuberculosis control protocols. They suggest that the high rate of NTM made the diagnosis of true tuberculosis more difficult. They also suggest that

TABLE D-3. PPD Conversions in Health Care Workers at BIMC

| Year | No. of Conversions | | | |
	House Staff	Nurses	RT	All Other
1991	9	14	0	7
1992	4	9	0	7
1993	1	7	0	6

NOTE: RT = respiratory therapists.

TABLE D-4. Results of Tuberculosis Control Measures at Parkland
Memorial Hospital

Measure	Percent 1994	1995	*p*
Patient isolated on admission day	87	79	
Patient isolated by 2nd hospital day	89	83	
Patient isolated within 72 hours	91	86	
Patient never isolated	4.1	7.5	
Employee tuberculosis exposure rate	18	25	0.03
Health care worker compliance with PPD testing	49	74	
PPD conversions	2.7	3.5	

interpretation of apparent increased PPD conversion rates may be spurious because some employees not tested in 1994 may already have had positive PPD test results and would not have been counted as conversions in 1995.

This paper highlights the fact that despite implementation of a protocol and other measures, reductions in employee skin test conversions is not inevitable. Clearly, Parkland suffered from continued delayed isolation of patients and even an increase in employee exposures. This occurred despite an apparently energetic infection control program.

Very little is known about tuberculosis control in nonhospital settings. Nolan and colleagues (22) reported on the control of an outbreak in a shelter for homeless men in Seattle. During December 1986 and January 1987, seven cases of tuberculosis were diagnosed in shelter clients. This prompted mass PPD testing of all the residents of the shelter. Anyone with a positive PPD test result (≥ 5 millimeter) or symptoms suggestive of tuberculosis were offered chest radiographs. This resulted in the identification of six additional asymptomatic cases of tubreculosis. Persons with tuberculosis were excluded from the shelter, and isoniazid (INH) therapy for latent tuberculosis infection was offered to everyone with a positive PPD test result. The air-handling system (which provided minimal air changes—air was recirculated for economy of heating) was reengineered. Thirty-six UVGI lights were installed in the duct system. The intensity-time dosage was considered adequate to kill 95 percent of the *Mycobacterium tuberculosis* organisms exposed to it. These interventions led to an interruption of the outbreak. Only five residents were found to have active tuberculosis over the next 2 years. Although this shelter did not follow the CDC guidelines in the strictest sense, their control plan included implementation of administrative controls (identification of cases with subsequent isolation [i.e., removal from the shelter]) and engineering controls. Provision of therapy for latent tuberculosis infection (LTBI) was likely also an important aspect in preventing further cases of active disease in those already infected.

Studies Correlating Implementation and Outcomes

Although not as compelling as a directed study of the impact of control measures, studies correlating implementation of control measures with relevant outcomes can also provide insight into the efficacy of the CDC guidelines.

One such example is from a Society for Healthcare Epidemiology of America (SHEA)-CDC survey of 1989–1992 tuberculosis control practices reported by Fridkin and colleagues (23, 24). The survey was sent to all members of SHEA in March 1993. Members from 210 hospitals responded. Part II of the results (24) focused on the efficacy of control measures. It showed that "high-risk" employees (e.g., respiratory therapists and bronchoscopists) were more likely than other health care workers to have PPD conversion if ≥6 tuberculosis patients per year admitted, if the hospital was "large" (≥437 beds), or if MDR tuberculosis was present. The most significant impact on both high risk and other PPD conversions was whether the hospital admitted ≥6 tuberculosis patients (for non-high risk health care workers, PPD conversions of 1.2 percent in high-volume hospital versus 0.6 percent in low-volume hospitals; for high-risk health care workers, PPD conversion rates were 1.9 percent versus 0.2 percent).

The authors evaluated four criteria from the 1990 CDC guidelines: (a) placing known/suspected tuberculosis patients into single patient room (or cohorting), (b) negative-pressure ventilation, (c) air exhaust directly to outside, and (d) ≥6 ACH. Hospitals with ≥ tuberculosis patients meeting all four criteria had PPD conversion rates of 0.60 percent, whereas they were 1.89 percent for hospitals that did not ($p = 0.02$). Hospitals meeting at least criteria a to c had PPD conversion rates of 0.62 percent whereas the rate was 1.83 percent for those that did not ($p = 0.03$). The data suggested that having negative pressure or outside exhaust versus not having one or the other also reduced rates, but this did not reach statistical significance. The use of a submicron mask versus a surgical mask made no difference in conversion rates. For hospitals with less than six tuberculosis admissions per year, no difference in PPD conversion rates could be shown to be related to control measures.

A similar survey on tuberculosis control measures was sent to members of the Association for Professionals in Infection Control and Epidemiology (APIC) in March 1993, as reported by Sinkowitz and colleagues (25). It also covered practices from 1989 to 1992. Data were obtained from 1,494 hospitals. Compared with the SHEA-CDC survey, the hospitals in this APIC survey were more likely to be a community hospital and more likely to not have any tuberculosis admissions in 1992. Results of the survey are summarized in Table D-5.

Whether or not tuberculosis isolation rooms met CDC criteria was also reviewed, but the data are not summarized here.

TABLE D-5. Results of CDC-APIC Tuberculosis Control Survey

Measure	Percent			
	1989	1990	1991	1992
Hospital admitted patient with tuberculosis	46.4	49.6	53.0	56.6
PPD conversion rate (pooled average)	0.39	0.42	0.47	0.51
Respiratory protection provided				
Surgical mask	96.8	95.8	91.3	66.8
Submicron mask	2.5	3.4	6.8	19.0
Dust-mist respirator	0.3	0.5	1.1	10.9
Dust-mist-fume respirator	0	0	0.3	2.4
HEPA respirator	0	0	0.2	0.5

Slightly different than in the SHEA-CDC study, bronchoscopists at hospitals with one to five tuberculosis patients per year were more likely than other health care workers to convert their PPD test results. This was not true for hospitals with ≥6 tuberculosis patients per year. Like the CDC-SHEA survey, the type of respiratory protection in use did not correlate with PPD conversion rates. However, unlike the CDC-SHEA survey, PPD conversion rates at hospitals were not related to control measures.

A result similar to that of the APIC result was found in a review of tuberculosis control measures in the 13 hospitals of a midwestern health system, as reviewed by Woeltje and colleagues (26). This survey was performed in 1994–1995. All hospitals had a tuberculosis plan, and all had annual testing of at least selected employees as recommended by the guidelines. Six of 13 (46 percent) of the hospitals were considered very low risk, 6 (46 percent) were considered low risk, and 1 (6 percent) was considered intermediate risk.

Tuberculosis isolation rooms were available at 10/13 (77%) of hospitals; however, only 44 to 100 percent of rooms (median, 88 percent) actually had negative pressure. Dust-mist-fume respirators were used most commonly. PPD conversion rates in 1994 ranged from 0 to 1.0 percent (median, 0.3 percent). The hospital location (urban/rural), type of respiratory protection, tuberculosis risk category, number of tuberculosis isolation rooms, percentage of tuberculosis isolation rooms that were actually at negative pressure, and number of tuberculosis cases were not correlated with PPD conversion. Only the tuberculosis case rate approached significance ($p = 0.06$, but this may have been spurious, as noted in the discussion section of this paper). In the discussion the authors note that actual compliance with CDC guidelines fell short of the hospitals' written policies.

Studies Showing Stable Control

Although not as compelling as studies showing the before-and-after effects of implementing control measures, the experiences of hospitals (especially those with large numbers of tuberculosis patients) that have low nosocomial tuberculosis rates and health care worker PPD conversion rates by following the CDC guidelines provide further assurance of the effectiveness of the guidelines.

An extremely detailed search for possible cases of nosocomial transmission of tuberculosis was done at Cook County Hospital in Chicago, where French and colleagues performed DNA fingerprinting on one isolate from every patient with tuberculosis for 1 year, from April 1995 through March 1996 (27). A comprehensive record review of patients whose isolates were in a fingerprint cluster was done to determine chance of cross-transmission. Overall, 91/168 (54 percent) isolates were in 15 clusters. There were six clusters of 2 isolates, 7 clusters of 3 to 8 isolates each, one cluster of 16 isolates, and one cluster of 29 isolates. The risk factors for clustering were birth in United States, male sex, African-American ethnicity, alcohol or illicit drug abuse, and homelessness. On multivariate analysis, only male sex and birth in the United States were associated with clustering.

For 13 of 15 clusters (46 patients), no instances were identified where two patients were inpatients or outpatients at same time. For the two largest clusters, 148 instances of two patients being on hospital grounds at same time were found. For 144/148 instances, cross-transmission was thought to be unlikely because of different sensitivity patterns (32 instances) or lack of geographic overlap of patients (112 instances). Of four remaining instances, the site of possible cross-transmission was ED (3 instances), and the HIV clinic (1 instance). In one case the possible source patient had only extrapulmonary tuberculosis, so nosocomial transmission was thought to be unlikely. In another case, only 5 weeks elapsed from the time of exposure to the diagnosis of fibrotic pulmonary disease in an immunocompetent patient. Cross-transmission in this case was thought to be implausible.

Of two remaining instances, the same source patient was involved. In one instance the source patient (patient A, HIV positive, CD4 count of 423 cells per milliliter) had a CXR consistent with miliary tuberculosis. The patient was masked and placed in isolation within 1.25 hours of admission. Patient B (also HIV positive) was brought to the ED by ambulance after patient A had been placed in isolation. Patient B had a history of a positive PPD test result and so was masked and placed in an isolation room 50 yards from patient A. Eight months later patient B developed pulmonary tuberculosis. Given the prompt masking and isolation of both patients and a history of a positive PPD, nosocomial transmission to patient B was thought to be unlikely (albeit possible, since droplet nuclei can stay suspended for some time).

The last possible patient exposure occurred in the HIV clinic. Patient C (also HIV positive) was in a clinic concurrent with patient A 5 weeks before patient A was diagnosed. Patient A had complained of low-grade fevers and weight loss, but a lack of cough and pulmonary signs was specifically documented. Four months later patient C developed pulmonary tuberculosis caused by an isolate with the same fingerprint as that of the isolate from patient A. Despite a documented lack of pulmonary symptoms, nosocomial transmission was thought to be possible.

During the study period eight patients with pulmonary tuberculosis were not isolated before the diagnosis was made. Two had isolates in clusters: six did not. A total of 186 employees had follow-up testing with no PPD conversions. In fact, 28 of 70 (40 percent) health care workers with PPD conversions over the entire study period had no adult patient care responsibilities.

The authors state that their hospital follows guidelines consistent with the CDC guidelines, although details are not provided. This paper suggests that even in a hospital with a large number of tuberculosis admissions, the CDC guidelines are effective at preventing nosocomial transmission. Of the two possible cases of nosocomial transmission, no breakdown in following the guidelines occurred. This points out that unless every patient is isolated for every visit, some nosocomial transmission of tuberculosis may be unavoidable.

Jernigan and colleagues (28) reported on a retrospective questionnaire that was sent to 52 former residents who had done a total of 70 6-week (420 physician-weeks) rotations at a tuberculosis sanatorium affiliated with the University of Virginia. There were 10 unprotected exposures to tuberculosis patients during training reported by the former house staff, 2 of which occurred at the sanatorium. No PPD conversions were reported during residency. The sanatorium had tuberculosis isolation rooms with negative pressure as well as UVGI (details were not given), and only simple surgical masks were used at the facility. Since "administrative controls" are somewhat built in at a sanatorium (in that tuberculosis is presumably known in all patients prior to their arrival), this suggests that even in a potentially high-risk environment, routine engineering controls and simple personal respiratory protection are adequate.

Studies of Specific Aspects of the Guidelines

Administrative Controls

The major role of administrative controls is to ensure that patients with pulmonary tuberculosis are promptly isolated. In most settings this requires isolating many patients who prove not to have tuberculosis for every patient who actually does have tuberculosis. As pointed out in the CDC guidelines, criteria for isolation must be derived locally, taking into account the local prevalence and presentations of tuberculosis. Many different isolation strategies have been reported.

Pegues and colleagues (29) studied the impact at the Massachusetts General Hospital from 1993 through 1994 after the implementation in 1993 of a tuberculosis isolation algorithm. The algorithm includes typical signs and symptoms (chronic cough, fever, weight loss, etc.) and risk factors (HIV infection, homeless, intravenous drug abuse [IVDA], jail, immigration from a country where tuberculosis is endemic, etc.), as well as the CXR. If the patient had a normal CXR, then the patient was not placed in isolation. If the CXR was abnormal, then a risk evaluation was done. If low risk, the patient was placed in a private room until one smear was AFB negative. If the patient was at moderate risk (i.e., had risk factors or a suspicious CXR), the likely degree of infectivity was considered. If the patient was judged to be likely infectious (as determined by the presence of a cavity on CXR or cough/sputum production by history), then the patient was placed in a tuberculosis isolation room. Otherwise the patient was placed in a lesser isolation room until three sputum samples were shown to be AFB negative.

There were 31 case patients with pulmonary tuberculosis over the 2-year study period (out of 58 patients with + AFB smears). All had an abnormal CXR, and 9/31 (29 percent) had cavitary disease. Ages ranged from 7 months to 97 years.

Isolation was initiated within 24 hours of admission in 19/31 (61 percent), 17 in the ED. Of 12 patients not isolated appropriately, 7 were eventually isolated (after 2 to 31 days; median, 9 days), and 5 were never isolated during admission (range, 3 to 28 days; median, 4 days). Reasons for inappropriately not isolating the patients included misclassified risk factors for five patients (three with HIV infection); seven patients had atypical or misinterpreted (but abnormal) CXRs and were not captured by the algorithm because they had no risk factors. No data on the total number of patients isolated are presented.

The 12 patients inappropriately not isolated led to 136 patient-exposure days. Of 11 roommates and 281 employees exposed, no PPD conversions or cases of active tuberculosis were found.

In the discussion the authors note that if the five patients who should have been isolated by the algorithm had been isolated, the sensitivity would be 77 percent. Inclusion of other risk factors (such as end-stage renal disease and residence at a long-term-care facility) would have improved the sensitivity, but at the cost of much more overisolation. Unfortunately, there is no discussion as to whether the new algorithm led to improvements in isolation practices compared with the previous policies.

The results of a survey including isolation practices in 159 Veterans Affairs hospitals (100% response, but not on all questions) were reported by Roy (30). Overall, 1,063 patients/month were isolated (median, 3 per facility). In 1993, a total of 974 patients were diagnosed with pulmonary tuberculosis (median, 3 per facility). The ratio of patients isolated/patients with pulmonary tuberculosis ranged from 1 to 120 (median, 12). There was no correlation between this ratio and the number of tuberculosis patients at the facility. Unfortunately there are no data presented on health care worker PPD conversion rates. Nevertheless, the variability in the degree of overisolation is striking. The methods used to determine who should be isolated were not discussed.

Columbia University has a renowned medical informatics group, and not surprisingly, an informatics approach to tuberculosis isolation was evaluated there, as reported by Knirsch and colleagues (31).

A clinical protocol for tuberculosis isolation was implemented in 1992 (17). Tuberculosis isolation was to be initiated (and continued until three negative AFB smears were obtained) in patients with a CXR suggesting tuberculosis (e.g., cavitary lesion, or any abnormality on CXR for patients with HIV infection) plus HIV risk factors or homelessness. Overall prompt isolation of tuberculosis patients improved from 51 percent in 1992 to 75 percent in 1993.

An automated protocol of computer screening of records was developed in 1995 using the CXR as the starting point. CXR reports were already automatically parsed at Columbia, so terms suggesting tuberculosis could be checked for. If the CXR was abnormal, immunodeficiency status was checked from other records (e.g., laboratory and pharmacy records). The hospital epidemiologist was notified via a computer generated e-mail to review the record for anyone meeting the preselected criteria. In 1995–1996 the combined clinical and automated protocol correctly isolated 34/43 (79 percent) of patients with tuberculosis. The clinical system alone would have isolated 30/43 (70 percent). The automated alert system flagged the records of 22/43 patients (51 percent). The automated protocol generated 15 alerts for every culture-positive tuberculosis patient, which was thought to be a tolerable number. By its nature, the system failed to detect patients with a normal CXR and patients with an abnormal CXR but no evidence of HIV infection—these accounted for most of the 21 percent not isolated by either system.

An effort to improve the isolation protocol at Grady was reported by Bock and colleagues (32). The charts of 376 patients (12 percent of all medicine admissions) on tuberculosis isolation from October through December 1993 were reviewed shortly after admission. Of these, 53 had pulmonary tuberculosis and 51 (96 percent) had been appropriately isolated. The two patients missed should have been isolated under existing protocols. Thus, 7.4 patients were isolated for every case of tuberculosis (positive predictive value, 14 percent).

A total of 295 of these patients (42 with tuberculosis) agreed to be interviewed. The authors evaluated 15 variables available on admission.

On univariate analysis, the presence of a cavity or upper lobe infiltrate was most predictive of tuberculosis. On multivariate analysis those factors remained significant, and a history of knowing someone with tuberculosis and a self-report of a previous positive PPD test result were also predictive. A self-report of INH preventative therapy in the past was protective. When stratified by HIV infection status, for patients without HIV infection, only radiological finding were significant, whereas in patients with HIV infection the radiological findings were not predictive.

A model was made including CXR findings, history of a positive PPD test result without INH therapy, and a history of knowing someone with tuberculosis. If this model were applied to the patient data set, only 129 of 295 patients would have been placed on isolation (a 56 percent reduction), including 34 of 42 patients with tuberculosis (overisolation factor, 3.8). Of the eight patients who would not have been isolated, four were smear positive. The hypothetical policy had a sensitivity of 81 percent, and a positive predictive value of 26 percent. The authors concluded that since the policy was supposed to prevent nosocomial transmission of tuberculosis, the hypothetical policy was not acceptable because of its lower sensitivity.

The impact of a tuberculosis team on appropriate isolation was noted by Fazal and colleagues (33). In April 1993, a tuberculosis team was started at the Bronx-Lebanon Hospital, New York. At the same time an isolation algorithm was implemented, so that patients with suspected tuberculosis would promptly be placed in isolation and AFB sputum would be obtained. The team consisted of infectious disease physician, an internist, and a physician's assistant. Daily rounds were conducted, and a team member was available 24 hours/day for questions. The time to appropriate isolation of tuberculosis patients was evaluated from September 1992 through October 1993 (7 months each pre- and postteam). Results of the team approach are shown in Table D-6.

No differences in demographics or number with MDR tuberculosis were noted. The degree of "overisolation" was not discussed, but the discussion does comment that isolation rooms were more readily available postteam due to more appropriate use. Length of stay decreased due to more timely smears and improved discharge planning (weekly rounds with community tuberculosis clinic staff). Despite the improvements, failure to isolate all AFB+ patients on admission was still a problem. Their guidelines were to undergo further evaluation and refinement.

Decreasing the delays in "ruling out" tuberculosis was also the focus of a study by Harmon and Roche (34) at a Hartford, Connecticut, hospital. Initial data were gathered on 52 patients on tuberculosis isolation over a 2-month period. A total of 36/52 (69 percent) were on tuberculosis precautions on the day of admission, and 43/52 (83 percent) were on tuberculosis isolation within 24 hours of admission. Only 33 had tuberculosis

TABLE D-6. Effects of Forming a Tuberculosis Team on Patient Isolation Practices

Measure	Preteam	Postteam	p
No. of AFB+ tuberculosis patients admitted	46	39	
No. (%) of AFB+ patients isolated within 24 hours	16 (35)	23 (59)	0.03
Mean no. of days patients not isolated	19.0	3.5	0.002
Median no. of days patients not isolated	12	0	
No. (%) of patients never isolated	19 (41)	2 (5)	

ruled out with three negative smears—this took a mean 6.6 days (range, 3 to 13). Continuous quality improvement (CQI) methods were used to design a protocol to improve the process of ruling out tuberculosis. Post-intervention, 28 patients were evaluated on protocol. Fifteen (54 percent) were ruled out within 4 days, the target goal. Mean time to stopping isolation was 4.9 days (range, 3 to 19 days, $p < 0.001$). No data were presented on how many patients were actually ruled in. Because a historical comparison group was used, the reduction in evaluation may have been due to the increased attention to tuberculosis, not the protocol per se. Nevertheless, their efforts succeeded in reducing the delays associated with ruling out tuberculosis.

Some hospitals have taken a very broad policy in isolating patients to rule out tuberculosis. An increase in health care worker PPD conversion from 0.3 to 1.7 percent between January and June 1991 at the University of Louisville Hospital was attributed to a failure to follow 1990 CDC guidelines (35). This led to the mandatory isolation of all patients presenting with community-acquired pneumonia (until two AFB smears were negative, or until tuberculosis was "ruled out on clinical grounds"). This policy was started in July 1991. Uyamadu and colleagues (36) reported that from July 1991 through December 1994, 70 patients with pulmonary tuberculosis were admitted, 33 (47 percent) of whom were AFB positive. All but one (who presented with mental status changes) were isolated on admission. The health care worker PPD conversion rate fell to an average of 0.6 percent (range, 0.3 to 0.8 percent per 6-month follow-up period).

No clear discussion of how much overisolation occurred. The authors state that "25 percent of patients being isolated will not meet CDC criteria for high risk for tuberculosis." This suggests that 75 percent would meet criteria for risk and so would have had to be isolated anyway. But this still does not address how many patients without tuberculosis were isolated for every patient with tuberculosis. Still, this paper suggests that aggressive isolation will reduce employee tuberculosis infection rates, as marked by a reduction in the PPD conversion rates.

Additional model algorithms for determining the need for isolation have been reported by Trovillion and colleagues (37) from Barnes-Jewish

Hospital in St. Louis, El-Solh and colleagues (38) from Eire County Medical Center (affiliated with the State University of New York at Buffalo), and Redd and Susser (39) from the ED at Columbia in New York City. These algorithms encompass various risk factors available from history, as well as CXR results. They are all somewhat similar. The studies by El-Solh and colleagues and by Redd and Susser evaluate the potential utility of the algorithms. Data on actual implementation are lacking, however.

Engineering Controls

General/Ventilation

Most studies evaluating control methods have been in settings where multiple changes in control measures have occurred at once, so attributing results to just ventilation is difficult. Behrman and Shofer (40) reported on the ED of the University of Pennsylvania in Philadelphia. Baseline PPD results of ED staff and other hospital employees were similar. Attending physicians were not included because non-ED data were not complete. On a 1-year follow-up, health care workers in the ED had 6/50 (12 percent) conversions, versus 51/2,514 (2 percent) conversions for other health care workers.

A new ED facility with four tuberculosis isolation rooms, improved air flow throughout the ED, and Plexiglas shields and laminar air flow for registrars was opened in January of the third testing (2-year follow-up) period. With the implementation of these measures, PPD conversions were 0/64 for ED health care workers versus 36/3,000 (1.2 percent) for other health care workers. The authors noted that the numbers of tuberculosis patients seen in the ED did not decline over the study period. They also noted that their protocols (early triage, use of approved respirators) did not change during periods. The authors conclude that the drop in the PPD conversion rate was due to improved engineering controls, which were primarily changes in ventilation.

Ultraviolet Germicidal Irradiation

Since UVGI is mentioned only as a supplemental means of engineering control of tuberculosis, there are few new data on its use or effectiveness alone. Stead and colleagues (41) reported that tuberculosis isolation rooms at the University of Arkansas hospital had 15 ACH and UVGI. The use of masks was optional (the paper does not state whether actual use was common or not). There were 16 patients with tuberculosis in 1992, including a man with cavitary MDR tuberculosis disease whose case was presented as a case report at the beginning of the article. The annual PPD conversion rate was 0.7 percent overall. Only 1/137 employees exposed to the case patient converted his PPD (and he was exposed while the patient was in the ICU on a ventilator, with negative AFB smears at the time). The report of Stead and colleagues implies that it was UVGI that was responsible for low PPD conversion rate, even though they had terrific ventilation. He cites one reference (42) regarding PPD conversion, despite 11 ACH in support of this. He also cites older data (43) on UVGI being effective even if no negative-pressure ventilation is available.

The paper by Jernigan et al. (28) cited previously included an interesting statement regarding National Jewish Hospital in Denver. A "personal communication" from L. J. Burton is cited stating that only two PPD conversions had occurred at National Jewish Hospital over a 10-year period, both associated with failure of an ultraviolet light system on a ward. I could not find a publication to confirm this.

Several recent reviews by Nardell (44), Macher (45), and Riley (46) present information on older studies on the efficacy of UVGI.

PROGRESS IN ADOPTION OF THE GUIDELINES

Degree of Implementation

General

Initial studies early in the 1990s suggested poor initial implementation of the 1990 CDC guidelines. Manangan and colleagues (47) reported on a 1992 survey of 180 Texas hospitals (of 475 in the state, of which 151 [83 percent] responded). In 1991, 122/151 (81 percent) had at least 1 tuberculosis admission (up from 98/151 [65 percent] in 1989). Overall, tuberculosis isolation rooms of any sort were not available at 25/140 (18 percent). Seventy-two percent of hospitals had at least one room meeting all CDC criteria. Of the hospitals that had tuberculosis isolation rooms, the rooms had negative pressure in 108/133 (81 percent), ≥6 ACH in 97/131 (74 percent), and air directly vented to outside in 109/131 (83 percent). Only 53/121 (44 percent) hospitals routinely checked the negative pressure in the tuberculosis isolation rooms. The rooms had a private bathroom in 125/134 (93 percent) hospitals. At 94/143 (66 percent) the door was kept closed at all times. Eighty-two percent of hospitals had only surgical masks available for health care workers. Ninety-seven percent performed baseline PPD testing, but only 91 percent performed PPD testing after an exposure.

Van Drunen (48) and colleagues presented data from a Minnesota survey of 17 hospitals carried out by APIC for 1989–1991. Overall there was a wide variety of practice. A total of 13/17 (76 percent) had tuberculosis isolation rooms available. Only three hospitals performed annual PPD tests; many hospitals let employees self-read the PPD test results. All of the hospitals used surgical masks for personal respiratory protection. There were a total of 33 exposure events involving 1,031 health care workers (445 patient days). However, the rate of PPD conversion following exposure was only 0.97 percent. Although the authors indicate that their data show that practices in Minnesota hospitals were "reasonably consistent with critical elements of the 1990 CDC guidelines" full compliance was apparently uncommon.

McDiarmid and colleagues (49) reported on the results of OSHA inspections performed from May 1992 through October 1994. An OSHA database of reports (for 262/272 cases) as well as supplemental questionnaires completed by OSHA compliance officers (for 149/272 cases) were reviewed.

In May 1992 OSHA region II (New York, New Jersey, Puerto Rico, Virgin Islands) developed enforcement guidelines based on the CDC 1990 guidelines. In the fall of 1993 OSHA issued national guidelines (50). A total of 272 facilities were inspected by OSHA; of these 53 percent were in New York and New Jersey. Hospitals made up 45 percent of inspected facilities, nursing homes made up 17 percent, prisons made up 13 percent, shelters made up 5 percent, and other made up 20 percent (e.g., outpatient drug treatment centers, physician offices, Emergency Medical Services). Complaints of employees/unions prompted 71 percent of the inspections.

Overall 66/117 (56 percent) had a tuberculosis control program, and 77/97 (79 percent) screened patients/clients for tuberculosis on admission. A total of 60/117 (51 percent) had some form of tuberculosis isolation available, and 54/129 (42 percent) had negative-pressure isolation rooms. "Adequate" personal protective equipment was provided at 33/114 (29 percent) (surgical masks were provided at 21 percent of facilities, dust-mist respirators were provided at 38 percent, and no masks were provided at 14 percent). Seventy-nine percent performed at least annual PPDs. Overall hospitals had better compliance.

Only 54/101 facilities (53 percent) appropriately recorded positive PPD test results on the OSHA 2000 log. Following exposure incidents, facilities applied an average of 79 (standard deviation [SD] = 179) PPDs, finding mean of 0.75 (SD = 1.5) converters, with 0.20 (SD = 0.9) active cases of tuberculosis found among converters.

Forty-two percent of facilities received citations under the general-duty clause; 39 percent were cited for noncompliance with respiratory protection standard; 20 percent were cited for noncompliance with the recording and reporting standard. OSHA also requires room placarding—10 percent of facilities were cited in violation of this.

The authors note a high degree of noncompliance during the study period; however, since most inspections were instigated by complaints, the selection of facilities may have been biased toward those with poorer compliance. Also, the time distribution of surveys was not noted. Thus, low compliance may also reflect a lag time in planning and implementing a comprehensive program, especially if many surveys were at the early end of the survey period.

Although these initial studies suggested poor initial implementation of the guidelines, with time implementation overall seems to have improved. Part I of the 1993 SHEA-CDC survey reported by Fridkin et al. (23) covered the status of tuberculosis control practices from 1989 to 1992. The results were as follows. Members from 210 (out of 359 possible) hospitals responded to the survey.

Tuberculosis isolation rooms meeting all CDC criteria were available at 113/181 (62 percent) hospitals. A total of 205/205 (100 percent) placed suspected tuberculosis patients in private rooms, 138/181 (76 percent) had negative pressure, 140/181 (77 percent) had air exhaust directly to the outside, and 158/189 (84 percent) reported ≥6 ACH. UVGI was used in 14/196 (7 percent). Employee PPD testing at 199 reporting hospitals was done annually at 127 (64 percent), every 6 months at 10 (5 percent), every 2 years at 13 (7 percent), and at varied times depending on risk at 48 (24 percent). Personal respiratory protection provided varied of the time period, as shown in Table D-7.

The authors note that there was still room for improvement in having appropriate tuberculosis isolation rooms available, but noted that the high cost of construction would likely make this a slow process. They also noted a trend toward the adoption of more compliant personal respiratory protection consistent with the 1990 CDC guidelines.

The results of a survey of U.S. hospitals by the Hospital Infections Program (HIP) of CDC were reported by Manangan and colleagues (51). A sample of US hospitals from the American Hospital Association database was surveyed in 1992. The response rate was 763/1076 (71 percent). In 1996, hospitals that had had ≥6 tuberculosis admissions in 1991 were resurveyed.

The 1992 survey showed that from 1989 to 1991 there was an increase in the proportion of hospitals admitting patients with tuberculosis and in

TABLE D-7. Personal Respiratory Protection Trends from 1993 CDC-SHEA Survey

Respiratory Protection	Percent			
	1989	1990	1991	1992
Surgical mask	95	94	92	57
Submicron mask	4	5	5	20
Dust-mist respirator	1	1	3	13
Dust-mist-fume respirator	0	0	0	10
HEPA respirator	0	0	0	0

the numbers of tuberculosis patients admitted. Only 536/755 (71 percent) had tuberculosis isolation rooms meeting 1990 CDC criteria. A total of 648/727 (89 percent) had no appropriate tuberculosis isolation rooms in the ED. In 334/545 (61 percent), the air flow of tuberculosis isolation rooms was not routinely checked; of 211 hospitals that did routinely check air flow, 81 (38 percent) checked it annually, but only 28 (13 percent; 5 percent of total) checked it at least monthly. In 339/775 (44 percent) hospitals, doors to tuberculosis isolation rooms were left open at least some of the time. Patients were allowed out of isolation for other than medical reasons (e.g., to go to a lounge) in 451/734 (61 percent) hospitals by policy and in 517/734 (70 percent) in practice. Nosocomial transmission of tuberculosis to health care workers was reported by 96/716 (13 percent) hospitals, and 14/728 (2 percent) reported transmission to patients. For the 1996 survey, 136 hospitals resurveyed—103 (76 percent) responded. Comparisons of the answers in hospitals that responded in both 1992 and 1996 are shown in Table D-8.

The survey showed improvement in isolation rooms and maintenance. In 1992 few hospitals had implemented the 1990 guidelines, but the authors suggest that by 1996 "most had made progress in implementing recommendation in the 1994 CDC tuberculosis guidelines." There was even a suggestion of reductions in nosocomial transmission of tuberculosis.

TABLE D-8. Comparison of 1992 and 1996 Responses to HIP (CDC) Survey

Measure	1992	1996
Tuberculosis isolation rooms meet CDC guidelines	59/92 (64)	99/103 (96)
Routine check for negative pressure in tuberculosis isolation rooms	72/85 (49)	96/99 (97)
At least monthly check	5/35 (14)	76/90 (84)
Mask use		
Surgical mask	101/101 (100)	1/103 (1)
Particulate respirator	8/101 (8)	40/103 (39)
Dust-mist-fume respirator		4/103 (4)
HEPA respirator		36/103 (35)
N95 respirator		85/103 (83)
PPD testing program		
Covered Personnel		
Nurses	103/103 (100)	103/103 (100)
RT	102/103 (100)	103/103 (100)
House staff	55/81 (69)	65/73 (89)
Attendings	43/86 (50)	65/94 (69)
Perform PPD after exposure	98/101 (97)	102/103 (99)
Maintain yearly reports	64/98 (65)	93/98 (95)

NOTE: Data represent number in that category/total number (percent).

Manangan and colleagues (52) also reported on results from New Jersey hospitals. In April 1992, a questionnaire was sent to all 96 New Jersey hospitals; 53 (55 percent) responded. In December 1996, a repeat survey was sent to the original 53 respondents, with 49 (92 percent) returning the survey (hospital mergers effectively changed the numbers to 51 and 47). The results are shown in Table D-9.

The health care worker PPD conversion rate peaked in 1991 and then fell (1989, 0.81 percent; 1991, 1.15 percent; 1996, 0.44 percent) and the total number of PPD tests done increased. However, in 1996 only 27/47 (57 percent) of hospitals could report the number of employees who had had a PPD test.

Like the national survey, the results from New Jersey showed increased compliance with tuberculosis precautions. The decline in the PPD conversion rate suggests, however, that there was also a drop in the number of tuberculosis patients admitted over the time period in the survey.

Likewise, a recently published survey of Maryland acute-care hospitals in 1997 was compared with a similar survey in 1992 and shows significant improvements in guideline compliance (53). The results are shown in Table D-10. However, only 41/56 (73 percent) hospitals responded, so the results may be overly optimistic.

Tuberculosis isolation procedures in 22 New York City hospitals from 1992 through 1994 were observed by Stricof and colleagues (54). Results are presented in Table D-11, shown as the percentage of room observations.

TABLE D-9. Results of New Jersey Hospital Survey

Measure	1992	1996
No. tuberculosis isolation rooms meeting CDC criteria	21/51 (41)	2/47 (4)
Had copy of 1994 CDC guidelines	n/a	47/47 (100)
Surgical mask used for PPE	28/51 (55)	
N95 mask for PPE		45/47 (96)
Hospitals with nosocomial tuberculosis	2	0

NOTE: Data represent number in the category/total number (percent). n/a = not available
PPE = personal protective equipment

TABLE D-10. Results of Maryland Hospital Survey

Measure	Percent		
	1992	1997	p
Tuberculosis isolation rooms meeting CDC criteria		100	
Tuberculosis rooms routinely checked	50	90	<0.01
EDs with tuberculosis isolation rooms available	50	90	<0.01
Compliant respirator used	24	100	<0.01
Protocol for identifying high-risk patient		49	
At least annual PPD test for health care workers	50	98	<0.01

TABLE D-11. Tuberculosis Isolation Practices in New York City
Hospitals, 1992–1994

Measure	Percent			p
	1992	1993	1994	
Tuberculosis patients in shared rooms	12.8	10.5	0	
No private toilet in room	19.7	6.7	5.3	
Room with negative pressure	51.3	70.5	80.3	<0.001
Room with HEPA filtration	1.7	20.0	27.6	
Room with no negative pressure/HEPA/UVGI	32.5	14.3	6.6	
Room door left open	5.1	3.8	5.3	
Window in room open	19.7	12.4	9.2	
Tuberculosis patient isolated on admission	75		84	0.02
Patient not isolated until + AFB reported	15	10	7	0.009
Dust-mist respirator	28		76	<0.001
AFB done 7 days/week	40		95	
Tuberculosis case reported to health department	80		100	

The discussion notes that improvements in case follow-up led to a decreased length of stay, so that fewer patients were in the hospital at any given time. Overall, there was significant improvement in compliance with CDC guidelines, although glitches (e.g., open doors and windows) persisted.

Unfortunately, as noted previously, survey results may give an incomplete picture. Sutton and colleagues (55) reported the results of a questionnaire and direct observation at three California hospitals (two county, one private-community) in an area where tuberculosis is highly endemic. This was done over 1 year (1994–1995, [exact dates not given]).

All of the hospitals had written tuberculosis plans consistent with CDC guidelines, but none of the hospitals performed routine assessment of their tuberculosis control practices. There were 13–17 tuberculosis isolation rooms available, including at least 1 each in the ICU and ED, at each hospital. Negative pressure was documented in 18/25 (72 percent) tested rooms, and 19/22 (86 percent) tested rooms had ≥6 ACH (6/16 [38 percent] had ≥12 ACH, even though they were not new rooms). However, only 1/27 (4 percent) rooms tested met recommended airflow pattern, and 20/24 (83 percent) had poor-fair air mixing (>10 seconds for puff of smoke to disperse, equivalent to ≥2 breaths for health care workers). The latter measurements are rarely reported in other studies.

One hospital provided HEPA masks with a fit testing program, one used dust-mist (DM) masks without a fit testing program, and one used DM masks but had HEPA masks with fit testing available (but the paper notes that in practice these were not used).

Practices noted on direct observations included lack of regular checks of negative pressure; windows that could be opened (with potential changes in airflow) in 44 percent of rooms; no engineering controls in a chest clinic that saw tuberculosis patients; and unmasked tuberculosis patients leaving room to smoke, use a phone, watch television, use a bathroom (the number of tuberculosis isolation rooms without bathrooms was not stated).

Thus, measures that would have been on a typical survey tool would have shown good results. However, the practices were sometimes poor. In addition, parameters that are rarely checked (e.g., airflow patterns and air mixing) may not be optimal according to the guidelines, even if other criteria for a tuberculosis isolation room are met. The actual significance of this is unknown.

Tuberculosis control practices at facilities for children were the focus of an APIC-CDC survey of children's hospitals and hospitals with pediatric units with >30 beds (56, 57). The survey covered 1990 to 1994. Overall, 195/284 (69 percent) hospitals responded (including 63/83 [76 percent] of freestanding children's hospitals). Part I of the survey (56) reviewed isolation policies. There was an increase in total tuberculosis cases tuberculosis and resistant tuberculosis reported over the survey period.

Control practices implemented by the hospitals included the following:

- 175/178 (98 percent) isolated patients with cavitary disease
- 176/179 (98 percent) isolated patients with AFB+ smears
- 120/175 (69 percent) isolated patients with miliary tuberculosis
- 138/175 (79 percent) isolated patients with AFB + gastric aspirates
- 9/179 (5 percent) allowed patient to leave room for nonmedical reason
- 96/139 (69 percent) restricted parents/adult visitors to isolation room
- 57/135 (42 percent) denied visiting privileges of parents until a tuberculosis evaluation done
- 40 percent of hospitals inappropriately required patients to wear dust-mist-fume (DMF) or HEPA masks when out of room

A total of 14 "clusters" of ≥ 2 PPD conversions among health care workers were reported from 11/191 (6 percent) hospitals, with one child PPD conversion reported.

Part II of the survey (57) reviewed the physical facilities available for tuberculosis control at the hospitals. Results included the following:

- 166/194 (86 percent) had facilities to care for a child with tuberculosis
- 78/190 (41 percent) had a pediatric-specific tuberculosis policy
- 83/187 (44 percent) stated that 1994 OSHA compliance memorandum caused change in policy
- 158/171 (92 percent) had isolation room with ≥ 6 ACH
- 153/170 (90 percent) vented air directly to outside

- 153/170 (90 percent) had negative pressure
- 158/177 (89 percent) used private rooms for isolation
- 23/170 (14 percent) used UV in room, 4/170 (2 percent) used UV on exhaust
- 32/167 (19 percent) used portable HEPA in rooms
- 73/174 (42 percent) had isolation rooms in outpatient areas
- All had an employee PPD program
- 182/186 (98 percent) performed at least annual PPD testing for health care workers
- 182/184 (99 percent) used the Mantoux test
- 114/167(68 percent) used two-step testing of new employees

From 1991 to 1994 surgical mask use dropped from ~86 percent for procedures/isolation room use to <33 percent. The use of DM and DMF masks increased, as did HEPA mask use (from 3 hospitals in 1991 to 62 hospitals in 1994). Overall compliance was thought to be good.

Rapid Specimen Processing

Rapid processing of smears for AFB and cultures is part of the CDC guidelines. This is to allow the prompt diagnosis of tuberculosis and also to allow patients without tuberculosis to have isolation discontinued in a timely fashion. Tokars and colleagues (58) reported on a survey of labs by the HIP and the Division of Tuberculosis Elimination at CDC. A total of 1,076 hospitals with ≥100 beds were surveyed in 1992 with a 70 percent response. Twenty percent of the responding labs were resurveyed in 1995. The results for hospitals included in both surveys are shown in Table D-12.

The discussion notes an overall improvement in following recommended procedures, with a concomitant decrease in reporting times. The authors suggest that if tuberculosis case rates continue to decline, consolidation of tuberculosis testing to a smaller number of labs may be desirable, especially since there is still considerable room for improvement in meeting recommended techniques.

TABLE D-12. Improvements in Laboratory Testing for Tuberculosis

Recommended Test	1992	1995
Fluorochrome stain for microscopy for AFB	44%	73%
Radiometric methods for primary culture	27%	37%
Rapid method for M. tuberculosis identification	59%	88%
Radiometric method for sensitivity testing	55%	75%
Median time for reporting smear for AFB	2 days	1 day
Median time to M. tuberculosis identification	40 days	21 days
Median time to susceptibility report	45 days	35 days

Education

LoBue and Catanzaro (59) studied health care worker compliance with tuberculosis control policies at the University of California at San Diego. This hospital implemented tuberculosis control policies consistent with the 1990 CDC guidelines in 1992 (60). Direct observations of health care worker behavior was made over a 14-week period (the year is not given). There were 115 sessions of 60 to 120 min for 52 patients on isolation, with a total of 541 health care worker observations made

Overall, 64 violations were observed—36 failures to maintain isolation (e.g., leaving door open) and 28 failures to use masks properly. Residents/fellows had 0.34 violations/observation, medical students had 0.28 violations/observation, prison guards had 0.5 violations/observation, and housekeepers had 0.38 violations/observation. Respiratory therapists had 5 violations in 3 observations (1.67 violations/observation), but these data were not included in analysis because there were less than five observations. Aides/transport and nurses did very well (0.02 and 0.08 violations/observation, respectively); they also had the most observations.

Physicians in training (medical students, residents, and fellows) committed 45 percent of violations (contributing 17 percent of observations). Of 29 violations, 8 were judged to be "technical" and of no clinical significance, in that an order to discontinue isolation was made prior to or shortly after observation (but a sign was still on the door, so it was counted as a violation).

Overall compliance was judged to be OK, but the authors suggest that additional education was needed, especially among physicians in training. As in other papers, this study points out that having a policy consistent with the CDC guidelines is not the same as following the policy.

Lack of health care worker knowledge at the University of Massachusetts was the focus of a study by Lai and colleagues (61). A test was administered in August 1993 to 200 health care worker with patient contact. Ninety-five (48 percent) reported having some tuberculosis education within the previous 2 years.

Overall, 195 (98 percent) knew that tuberculosis could be spread by coughing/sneezing. However, 55 (28 percent) thought that it could be spread by shaking hands. A total of 175 (88 percent) knew that masks should be used when entering the room of a tuberculosis patient. However, 70 (35 percent) would also use gowns. The study showed a surprisingly high lack of knowledge of how tuberculosis is transmitted.

IMPLEMENTATION IN NON-INPATIENT SETTINGS

Studies of tuberculosis control outside of the acute-care hospital inpatient setting are uncommon. Many of the articles retrieved by literature search are simply reviews of tuberculosis and tuberculosis control with some suggestions at implementing control measures in whatever setting rather than studies of actual practices or outcomes.

Emergency Departments

Moran and colleagues (62) reported the results of a 1993 CDC survey of tuberculosis control practices in the ED. Written policies for managing patients with suspected tuberculosis in the triage and waiting areas were available at 159/282 (56.4 percent) hospitals. A total of 214/280 (76.4 percent) had written policies for the ED proper. The decision to isolate patients was usually made in triage (235/286 [82.2 percent] hospitals). Written criteria for this decision were available in 105/286 (44.7 percent) hospitals. Patients suspected of having tuberculosis were given a mask in 228/246 (91.9 percent) of institutions. A total of 5/247 (1.7 percent) had tuberculosis isolation rooms in the triage/waiting area, while 56/286 (19.6 percent) had tuberculosis isolation room in the ED proper. UVGI was used in 15/277 (5.4 percent) triage/waiting areas and in 21/264 (8 percent) EDs proper. Air was recirculated in 211/262 (81 percent) of triage areas and 205/258 (79 percent) of EDs proper.

An employee PPD program was in place at 283/286 (99 percent). A total of 186 (65.7 percent) were tested annually, 58 (20.5 percent) were tested every six months, and 18 (6.4 percent) were tested only at hire. For 1991, 34/211 (16.1 percent) had >1 PPD conversion; for 1992 this changed to 63/234 (26.9%). The overall rate of PPD conversion in 1991 was 78/7,348 (1.1 percent) whereas it was 141/8,698 (1.6 percent) in 1992.

This study showed that in the early 1990s, compliance with suggested control measures for EDs was suboptimal, along the lines of general compliance discussed above.

Dental Clinics

Murphy and Younai (63) report on a study done at the New York University College of Dentistry. This school runs an extremely busy clinic with 288,000 patient visits/contacts per year in New York City. From 1991 it had gradual implementation of annual PPD testing for faculty, staff, and students. For the 1993–1994 testing period, there was a 20.9 percent conversion rate in employees (56 percent of these conversions were in employees with no patient contact) and a 15 percent conversion rate in students. To evaluate for possible tuberculosis exposures in the clinic, the authors conducted a retrospective review of patients referred out for a medical condition from August 1994 through July 1995. A total of 96/1,259 (0.4 percent) of the referrals were potentially related to tuberculosis—a review of those who returned to dental care and had records available showed no cases of patients with active tuberculosis at time of their dental visit. These chart review data were also reported separately in greater detail (64).

The authors conducted a survey of 54 dental schools and received 24 (44 percent) responses. A total of 14/24 (58 percent) had no PPD data available, and 5 (21 percent) had no data available but were planning to start testing. Of five (21 percent) with data, only three shared their results. At one dental clinic on the West Coast, the PPD conversion rate was approximately 1 percent. At another West Coast school, the conversion rate for faculty was 1.6 percent, for students it was 2 percent, and for staff it was 1.8 percent. At the third school, in the Midwest, the only positive PPD results were in foreign-born students.

A 1-year study, completed in July 1995, of student conversions during the 3rd year (the first clinical year) revealed a 10.6 percent conversion rate. It was unclear if students had received two-stage testing for their initial tests.

The control plan for the facility involved a risk analysis, after which the facility was designated very low risk (i.e., tuberculosis in the community but not the facility). The paper speculates that a lot of the skin test conversion may have been community acquired. Administrative controls included obtaining a detailed history from every new patient and an abbreviated history on patient return to screen for tuberculosis; patients with suspicious findings were sent to a designated clinic for more detailed evaluation. HEPA masks were made available and were to be used for high-risk patients. Engineering controls are not required at that risk level, and none were specifically planned.

Although no cases of tuberculosis were found by their chart review, given the high prevalence of tuberculosis in New York City during that time period and given the high rates of PPD conversions in students and faculty, a higher-level risk assessment would seem more appropriate. An argument could be made for implementing more aggressive control measures, especially engineering controls in common areas, and perhaps better personal protective equipment for the staff.

COSTS OF IMPLEMENTING GUIDELINES

Entire Guidelines

Kellerman and colleagues (65) calculated the costs from 1989 to 1994 of implementing the CDC guidelines at three New York City hospitals (Roosevelt, Cabrini, St. Clare's) and a Miami hospital (Jackson) that had had nosocomial outbreaks. Also included was one low-risk hospital in Nebraska (Regional West) for comparison. The hospitals provided estimates of nursing time for placing and reading PPD tests, supply costs, and costs of follow-up of those with positive PPD test results. The absolute costs of an employee PPD program ranged from $330 to $58,380 per year. The cost per health care worker tested ranged from $3.53 to $12.94. Additional personnel costs for administering a tuberculosis control program ranged from $10,000 (0.25 full-time equivalents [FTE]) to $137,400 (2 FTE). Capital costs for environmental controls ranged from $54,000 to $554,900. Maintenance costs (including increased utility costs due to increased ventilation) were estimated at $4,000 to $25,000 per year.

Kellerman and colleagues (66) also evaluated the costs of tuberculosis control in children's hospitals in 1994–1995. The Baby and Children's Hospital–New York Presbyterian Medical Center (BCH-NYPMC) Children's Hospital and Health Center–San Diego (CHHC-SD), and the pediatric ward at the University of California at San Diego (UCSD) were surveyed. Costs per health care worker for PPD testing ranged from $6.91 to $12.49, with total costs of the program running $2,470 to $26,577 per year. Construction costs for that year ranged from $12,800 to $24,500. Total respirator costs for a year were $1,360 at BCH-NYPMC (with fit testing by manufacturer), $1,680 at CHHC-SD (fit testing was available but was not used), and $480 at UCSD (no fit testing).

While the "data" aspects of the implementation of control measures at Roosevelt in New York City were reviewed by Stroud et al. (18), Williams et al. (67) provided a discussion of the "soft" aspects of the control program. A primary barrier early on was a lack of tuberculosis knowledge by health care workers, which required providing significant education efforts. Because much of the tuberculosis at Roosevelt came through the ED, the medical director there played a key role in educating that department. This led to more timely isolation in the ED.

They noted that a key priority was enlisting the collaboration of the admitting department so that patients could be moved out of the ED in a timely fashion. They developed a system of bed triage based on estimated risk so that tuberculosis isolation rooms would be used appropriately in times of shortage.

Getting health care workers to implement controls was hampered by the perception that prevention of tuberculosis outbreaks was solely the responsibility of infection control, which had "failed" since an outbreak had occurred. Also, the increased numbers of patients on isolation increased the *perception* that more tuberculosis patients were being admitted, increasing employee fear and anger. However, the concerns of health care workers did spark increased compliance with routine PPD testing.

The authors noted that one key difficulty was keeping patients in their rooms. They tried offering incentives (e.g., free television, free incoming phone calls, special food choices) as suggested in the CDC guidelines, but noted that the actual impact was small. Although this paper does not address any dollar costs in implementing control measures, it provides an excellent review of the social costs of an outbreak and associated controls.

Isolation/Administrative Controls

A significant fraction of the ongoing cost of a tuberculosis program may be in evaluating patients who do not have tuberculosis but who meet criteria to be evaluated. Scott and colleagues (68) evaluated the experience at the University of Iowa Hospital and Clinics. All patients with a positive sputum culture for tuberculosis between January 1, 1987, and September 24, 1992, were considered a case. Forty-four patients were identified, and charts were available for review for 43. Control patients were chosen randomly from patients who had had sputum submitted for AFB but who had negative cultures. Since bronchoscopy specimens were routinely sent for AFB smear and culture regardless of clinical suspicion of tuberculosis, patients who had specimens only from bronchoalveolar lavage were excluded. Of 92 potential controls for every case, 43 random controls chosen matched by location (inpatient/outpatient) and service.

Of the case patients, 39 (91 percent) were smear positive; 25 (58 percent) were positive on the first smear. Only one test for AFB was sent from 48 percent of the control subjects. Of 24 inpatients with pulmonary tuberculosis, only 10 (42 percent) were isolated upon admission. A total of 37/43 (86 percent) case patients had a CXR consistent with tuberculosis, as did 7/43 (16 percent) controls. If same rate held for all patients, ~670 patients would have had abnormal CXRs. The six other case patients had abnormal CXRs, but not "typical" for tuberculosis. From July 1, 1991, through June 30, 1992, there were 12 "exposure" workups for an AFB+ smear, with 363 contacts. Only 4 of the 12 had tuberculosis; the others had infection with non-tuberculous mycobacteria (NTM).

Scott and colleagues (68) calculated the cost of diagnosing a case of tuberculosis: $18.30 was spent for an AFB smear and culture. Control patients had an average of 2 sputum specimens sent, while case patients had an average of 3.2 specimens sent. With 92 control patients for every tuberculosis patient, this led to a cost of $3,426 per case of tuberculosis diagnosed. The authors also estimated that 15 minutes/person of nurse epidemiologist time was spent tracing and contacting health care workers exposed to a case of tuberculosis, with an additional $6.00 to $11.00 per employee for PPD testing.

The authors state that a policy of isolating everyone for whom an AFB smear was sent would be unreasonable, causing a 92-fold overuse of isolation rooms. However, this is within the range reported in the Veterans Affairs hospital study by Roy et al. (30). Although not discussed, if only the estimated 670 patients with "typical" CXRs were isolated, the over-isolation ratio would be ~18:1, which does not seem unreasonable.

It would seem that the ordering of testing of sputum for AFB at Iowa at that time period was excessive, especially given that almost half of the control patients had only one sputum specimen sent. Despite this apparent interest in diagnosing tuberculosis, only 42 percent of tuberculosis patients were isolated on admission. One wonders if physicians are lulled into complacency about tuberculosis since so many of the positive AFB smears proved to be NTM. This increase in NTM compared with tuberculosis has been reported elsewhere (21, 69) as well.

Although the authors did not calculate this, using their estimate of 30 contacts per case, the 14 nonisolated tuberculosis patients would have exposed 420 health care workers at a cost of 105 nurse epidemiologist hours ($2,100 at the $20/hour they estimated), plus an additional $2,520 to $4,620 for PPD testing.

Kerr and Savage (70) calculated the potential cost of exposure to a single nonisolated patient in a postanesthesia care unit (PACU). Based on traffic in the PACU and typical recovery times, they estimated that a patient with tuberculosis would expose 24 other patients, 10 PACU staff, 38 operating room staff, and 9 ancillary staff (total 81). Cost and time estimates were from Brown et al. (70) and Scott et al. (67). Their results follow:

Cost per contact identification		$17.00
PPD testing cost		$8.21
Total contact tracing/testing	$25.21 * 81 =	$2,042.01
Legal/risk management		$550.00
Infectious disease consult		$200.00
Total initial costs		$2,792.01
Follow-up 65 with negative initial		
PPD test	$8.21 * 65 =	$533.65
Follow-up for 16 PPD conversions		
Physician visit, smear, CXR	$88.30 * 16 =	$1,412.80
Follow-up for 3 with active disease		
Hospital costs	$12,369.00 * 3 =	$37,107.00
Physician visits	$1,785.00 * 3 =	$5,355.00
Follow-up for 13 with latent tuberculosis		
6 months of INH @ $7.20/month		$562.38
Monthly nurse visits @ $20.00/month		$1,560.00
Follow-up physician exam @ $45.00		$585.00
Follow-up CXR @ $25.00		$325.00
Grand Total		$57,477.84

Although one can take exception to some of the estimates, the values chosen for baseline PPD test positivity, PPD conversion, and development of active disease are all within reasonable ranges. The conversion rates were cited from Griffith and colleagues (72). The rate of developing active tuberculosis seems high (albeit possible), and the need for inpatient therapy seems unlikely. For outpatient therapy of tuberculosis, Brown et al. (71) list $2,300/case for drug-susceptible tuberculosis (health department data). Nevertheless it is clear that one tuberculosis exposure can be quite expensive if one figures in all the costs involved and not just contact tracing and a single round of PPD testing.

A study submitted for publication by Topal and colleagues (73) and associates at Yale University reviewed their experience with isolation protocols. Because their case finding included all patients for whom a sample for testing for AFB was sent, even if only from a bronchoscopy specimen, it is difficult to compare their results with those of others.

Their initial protocol required tuberculosis isolation if a patient had cough for ≥2 weeks AND infiltrate on CXR AND a risk factor (tuberculosis exposure/history of tuberculosis or positive PPD/HIV infection/homelessness/IV drug use/alcohol use OR [fever + weight loss + night sweats]). Patients were evaluated from October 1996 through June 1997. In the initial group, 48/141 (34 percent) of isolated patients (19 percent of total patients for whom cultures for AFB testing were sent) did not meet isolation criteria and were considered over-isolated. Twenty-one of these were HIV-infected patients. At least one patient who was over-isolated by their criteria had tuberculosis. This patient had a cough and an abnormal CXR, but no clinical symptoms or risk factors on their list. He was from India and had been isolated anyway. A total of 13/115 patients for whom AFB tests were ordered and who were not placed on isolation actually met the criteria, and should have been isolated. One such patient with tuberculosis exposed 200 health care workers (no PPD conversions were found on follow-up).

The protocol was revised to allow for clinical concern in HIV-infected patients. The revised protocol also included foreign birth in an area with high prevalence of tuberculosis as a risk factor. A postintervention study was done from January through June 1998, after educating health care workers about the new guidelines. Only 12.6 percent of the group were over-isolated, and only 2 (1.5 percent) patients were under-isolated. Thus, their educational intervention was successful, and apparently, with the new criteria, no patient with tuberculosis was not isolated. Overall, the new criteria had increased sensitivity (80 versus 100 percent) with a loss of specificity (50 to 40 percent).

Although it is not clear from the data in the results, the authors state in the discussion that their over-isolation ratio was 25:1 in the post-intervention period. Their cost estimate for smears for AFB and culture was $50.00 (it is implied that this is for three sputum samples). Thus, laboratory costs for a 25:1 over-isolation are $1,250 spent for every case of tuberculosis diagnosed. They also estimate respirator costs at $5.00 to $6.50 per day ($0.50/mask with 10–13 used/day), and with a mean duration in tuberculosis isolation of 4.2 days, respirator cost would be about $700 for 25 patients. This leads to a total laboratory and isolation cost of under $2,000 for every patient actually diagnosed with tuberculosis (the authors actually calculate a cost of approximately $3,000 per case, but their calculation assumes that every patient isolated stays on isolation for the duration of their stay, about 10 days). If one patient exposed 400 health care workers (as had happened at Yale in 1993), labor costs alone were estimated at $11,000. Thus, even if there were no PPD converters, they suggest that their 25:1 over-isolation ratio may be cost-effective.

Education

Trovillion and colleagues (37) reported on the costs of implementing an educational program. A tuberculosis protocol was introduced at Barnes-Jewish Hospital in St. Louis in the summer of 1995. An estimated 3,000 employees with patient contact (35 percent of total) needed training. Because this was beyond the means of the infection control practitioners, 146 volunteer trainers were instructed and provided with training materials. These trainers then provided training sessions at their respective locations.

Only 924 employees (31 percent) received training within 6 weeks as was requested. By the end of 5 months, 1,909 (64 percent) of targeted employees had been trained. The sessions tended to last ~20 minutes because of time constraints, not the 40 minutes envisioned during the training of the trainers.

The estimated costs were infection control program development time (40 hours) ($1,386) + training packets ($812) + employee time away from workplace to provide/attend training ($23,855), for a total of $26,053. Excluding the cost for the employees to attend, which would be incurred by any training method, this format was thought to be a cost-effective way of providing efficient training. No hard evidence of the effectiveness of the training was obtained, but the discussion mentions that staff seemed to be more knowledgeable.

REFERENCES

1. American Thoracic Society. Control of tuberculosis in the United States. *American Review of Respiratory Diseases* 1992;146:1623–1633.
2. Centers for Disease Control and Prevention. Tuberculosis morbidity–United States, 1997. *Morbidity and Mortality Weekly Report* 1998;47:253–257.
3. Brudney K, Dobkin J. Resurgent tuberculosis in New York City. Human immunodeficiency virus, homelessness, and the decline of tuberculosis control programs. *American Review of Respiratory Diseases* 1991;144:745–749.

4. Fischl MA, Uttamchandani RB, Daikos GL, Poblete RB, Moreno JN, Reyes, et al. An outbreak of tuberculosis caused by multiple-drug-resistant tubercle bacilli among patients with HIV infection. *Annals of Internal Medicine* 1992;117:177–183.

5. Zaza S, Blumberg HM, Beck-Sague C, Haas WH, Woodley CL, Pineda M, et al. Nosocomial transmission of Mycobacterium tuberculosis: role of health care workers in outbreak propagation. *Journal of Infectious Diseases* 1995;172:1542–1549.

6. Pearson ML, Jereb JA, Frieden TR, Crawford JT, Davis BJ, Dooley SW, et al. Nosocomial transmission of multidrug-resistant Mycobacterium tuberculosis. A risk to patients and health care workers [see comments]. *Annals of Internal Medicine* 1992;117:191–196.

7. Edlin BR, Tokars JI, Grieco MH, Crawford JT, Williams J, Sordillo EM, et al. An outbreak of multidrug-resistant tuberculosis among hospitalized patients with the acquired immunodeficiency syndrome. *New England Journal of Medicine* 1992;326:1514–1521.

8. Dooley SW, Villarino ME, Lawrence M, Salinas L, Amil S, Rullan JV, et al. Nosocomial transmission of tuberculosis in a hospital unit for HIV-infected patients. *Journal of the American Medical Association* 1992;267:2632–2634.

9. Ikeda RM, Birkhead GS, DiFerdinando GTJ, Bornstein DL, Dooley SW, Kubica GP, et al. Nosocomial tuberculosis: an outbreak of a strain resistant to seven drugs. *Infection Control and Hospital Epidemiology* 1995;16:152–159.

10. Jarvis WR. Nosocomial transmission of multidrug-resistant Mycobacterium tuberculosis. *American Journal of Infection Control* 1995;23:146–151.

11. Dooley SWJ, Castro KG, Hutton MD, Mullan RJ, Polder JA, Snider DE, Jr. Guidelines for preventing the transmission of tuberculosis in health-care settings, with special focus on HIV-related issues. *Morbidity and Mortality Weekly Report* 1990;39:1–29.

12. Centers for Disease Control and Prevention. Guidelines for Preventing the Transmission of *Mycobacterium tuberculosis* in Health-care Facilities, 1994. *Morbidity and Mortality Weekly Report* 1994;43:1–132.

13. Wenger PN, Otten J, Breeden A, Orfas D, Beck-Sague CM, Jarvis WR. Control of nosocomial transmission of multidrug-resistant Mycobacterium tuberculosis among health-care workers and HIV-infected patients. *Lancet* 1995;345:235–240.

14. Beck-Sague C, Dooley SW, Hutton MD, Otten J, Breeden A, Crawford JT, et al. Hospital outbreak of multidrug-resistant Mycobacterium tuberculosis infections. Factors in transmission to staff and HIV-infected patients. *Journal of the American Medical Association* 1992;268:1280–1286.

15. Maloney SA, Pearson ML, Gordon MT, Del Castillo R, Boyle JF, Jarvis WR. Efficacy of control measures in preventing nosocomial transmission of multidrug-resistant tuberculosis to patients and health care workers. *Annals of Internal Medicine* 1995;122:90–95.

16. Blumberg HM, Watkins DL, Berschling JD, Antle A, Moore P, White N, et al. Preventing the nosocomial transmission of tuberculosis. *Annals of Internal Medicine* 1995;122:658–663.

17. Bangsberg DR, Crowley K, Moss A, Dobkin JF, McGregor C, Neu HC. Reduction in tuberculin skin-test conversions among medical house staff associated with improved tuberculosis infection control practices. *Infection Control and Hospital Epidemiology* 1997;18:566–570.

18. Stroud LA, Tokars JI, Grieco MH, Crawford JT, Culver DH, Edlin BR, et al. Evaluation of infection control measures in preventing the nosocomial transmission of multidrug-resistant Mycobacterium tuberculosis in a New York City hospital. *Infection Control and Hospital Epidemiology* 1995;16:141–147.

19. Fella P, Rivera P, Hale M, Squires K, Sepkowitz K. Dramatic decreases in tuberculin skin test conversion rate among employees at a hospital in New York City. *American Journal of Infection Control* 1995;23:352–356.

20. Koll B, Raucher B, Nadig R, McKinley FW, Asnino C, Vernon E, Sommerville D. Effectiveness of a tuberculosis control plan in reducing PPD skin test conversions among health care workers. In: Anonymous. tuberculosis control in the workplace: science, implementation, and prevention policy. 1994 Annual Conference of the Society for Occupational and Environmental Health. December 1-3, 1994, Rockville, Maryland. Abstracts. *Infection Control and Hospital Epidemiology* 1994;15:764–775.

21. Grant PS. Evaluation of infection control parameters according to the 1994 Centers for Disease Control and Prevention Tuberculosis guidelines: a 2-year experience. *America Journal of Infection Control* 1998;26:224–231.

22. Nolan CM, Elarth AM, Barr H, Saeed AM, Risser DR. An outbreak of tuberculosis in a shelter for homeless men. A description of its evolution and control. *American Review of Respiratory Diseases* 1991;143:257–261.

23. Fridkin SK, Manangan L, Bolyard E, Jarvis WR. SHEA-CDC TB survey, Part I: Status of TB infection control programs at member hospitals, 1989–1992. Society for Healthcare Epidemiology of America. *Infection Control and Hospital Epidemiology* 1995;16:129–134.

24. Fridkin SK, Manangan L, Bolyard E, Jarvis WR. SHEA-CDC TB survey, Part II: Efficacy of TB infection control programs at member hospitals, 1992. Society for Healthcare Epidemiology of America. *Infection Control and Hospital Epidemiology* 1995;16:135–140.

25. Sinkowitz RL, Fridkin SK, Manangan L, Wenger PN, Jarvis WR. Status of tuberculosis infection control programs at United States hospitals, 1989 to 1992. APIC. Association for Professionals in Infection Control and Epidemiology. *American Journal of Infection Control* 1996;24:226–234.

26. Woeltje KF, L'Ecuyer PB, Seiler S, Fraser VJ. Varied approaches to tuberculosis control in a multihospital system. *Infection Control and Hospital Epidemiology* 1997;18:548–553.

27. French AL, Welbel SF, Dietrich SE, Mosher LB, Breall PS, Paul WS, et al. Use of DNA fingerprinting to assess tuberculosis infection control. *Annals of Internal Medicine* 1998; 129:856–861.

28. Jernigan JA, Adal KA, Anglim AM, Byers KE, Farr BM. Mycobacterium tuberculosis transmission rates in a sanatorium: implications for new preventive guidelines. *American Journal of Infection Control* 1994;22:329–333.

29. Pegues CF, Johnson DC, Pegues DA, Spencer M, Hopkins CC. Implementation and evaluation of an algorithm for isolation of patients with suspected pulmonary tuberculosis. *Infection Control and Hospital Epidemiology* 1996;17:412–418.

30. Roy MC, Fredrickson M, Good NL, Hunter SA, Nettleman MD. Correlation between frequency of tuberculosis and compliance with control strategies. *Infection Control and Hospital Epidemiology* 1997;18:28–31.

31. Knirsch CA, Jain NL, Pablos-Mendez A, Friedman C, Hripcsak G. Respiratory isolation of tuberculosis patients using clinical guidelines and an automated clinical decision support system. *Infection Control and Hospital Epidemiology* 1998;19:94–100.

32. Bock NN, McGowan JEJ, Ahn J, Tapia J, Blumberg HM. Clinical predictors of tuberculosis as a guide for a respiratory isolation policy. *American Journal of Respiratory and Critical Care Medicine* 1996;154:1468–1472.

33. Fazal BA, Telzak EE, Blum S, Pollard CL, Bar M, Ernst JA, et al. Impact of a coordinated tuberculosis team in an inner-city hospital in New York City. *Infection Control and Hospital Epidemiology* 1995;16:340–343.

34. Harmon JC, Roche JM. Development of a research-based protocol to rule out tuberculosis by means of continuous quality improvement techniques. *American Journal of Infection Control* 1995;23:329–336.

35. Ramirez JA, Anderson P, Herp S, Raff MJ. Increased rate of tuberculin skin test conversion among workers at a university hospital. *Infection Control and Hospital Epidemiology* 1992;13:579–581.

36. Uyamadu N, Ahkee S, Carrico R, Tolentino A, Wojda B, Ramirez J. Reduction in tuberculin skin-test conversion rate after improved adherence to tuberculosis isolation. *Infection Control and Hospital Epidemiology* 1997;18:575–579.

37. Trovillion E, Murphy D, Mayfield J, Dorris J, Traynor P, Fraser V. Costs of implementing a tuberculosis control plan: a complete education module that uses a train-the-trainer concept. *American Journal of Infection Control* 1998;26:258–262.

38. El-Solh A, Mylotte J, Sherif S, Serghani J, Grant BJ. Validity of a decision tree for predicting active pulmonary tuberculosis [published erratum appears in *Am J Respir Crit Care Med* 1997 Dec;156(6):2028]. *American Journal of Respiratory and Critical Care Medicine* 155:1711–1716.

39. Redd JT, Susser E. Controlling tuberculosis in an urban emergency department: a rapid decision instrument for patient isolation. *American Journal of Public Health* 1997;87: 1543–1547.

40. Behrman AJ, Shofer FS. Tuberculosis exposure and control in an urban emergency department. *Annals of Emergency Medicine* 1998;31:370–375.

41. Stead WW, Yeung C, Hartnett C. Probable role of ultraviolet irradiation in preventing transmission of tuberculosis: a case study. *Infection Control and Hospital Epidemiology* 1996;17:11–13.

42. Kantor HS, Poblete R, Pusateri SL. Nosocomial transmission of tuberculosis from unsuspected disease. *American Journal of Medicine* 1988;84:833–838.

43. Stead WW. Clearing the air: the theory and application of ultraviolet air disinfection [letter]. *American Review of Respiratory Diseases* 1989;140:1832.

44. Nardell EA. Interrupting transmission from patients with unsuspected tuberculosis: a unique role for upper-room ultraviolet air disinfection. *American Journal of Infection Control* 1995;23:156–164.

45. Macher JM. The use of germicidal lamps to control tuberculosis in healthcare facilities [review]. *Infection Control and Hospital Epidemiology* 1993;14:723–729.

46. Riley RL. Ultraviolet air disinfection: rationale for whole building irradiation. *Infection Control and Hospital Epidemiology* 1994;15:324–325.

47. Manangan LP, Perrotta DM, Banerjee SN, Hack D, Simonds D, Jarvis WR. Status of tuberculosis infection control programs at Texas hospitals, 1989 through 1991. *American Journal of Infection Control* 1997;25:229–235.

48. Van Drunen N, Bonnicksen G, Pfeiffer AJ. A survey of tuberculosis control programs in seventeen Minnesota hospitals: implications for policy development. *American Journal of Infection Control* 1996;24:235–242.

49. McDiarmid M, Gamponia MJ, Ryan MAK, Hirshon JM, Gillen NA, Cox M. Tuberculosis in the workplace: OSHA's compliance experience. *Infection Control and Hospital Epidemiology* 1996;17:159–164.

50. Decker MD. OSHA enforcement policy for occupational exposure to tuberculosis. *Infection Control and Hospital Epidemiology* 1993;14:689–693.

51. Manangan LP, Simonds DN, Pugliese G, Kroc K, Banerjee SN, Rudnick JR, et al. Are US hospitals making progress in implementing guidelines for prevention of Mycobacterium tuberculosis transmission? *Archives of Internal Medicine* 1998;158:1440–1444.

52. Manangan LP, Collazo ER, Tokars J, Paul S, Jarvis WR. Trends in compliance with the guidelines for preventing the transmission of Mycobacterium tuberculosis among New Jersey hospitals, 1989 to 1996. *Infection Control and Hospital Epidemiology* 1999;20:337–340.

53. Fuss EP, Isreal E, Baruch N, Roghmann M-C. Improved tuberculosis infection control practices in Maryland acute care hospitals. *American Journal of Infection Control* 2000; 28(2):133–137.

54. Stricof RL, DiFerdinando GTJ, Osten WM, Novick LF. Tuberculosis control in New York City hospitals. *American Journal of Infection Control* 1998;26:270–276.

55. Sutton PM, Nicas M, Reinisch F, Harrison RJ. Evaluating the control of tuberculosis among healthcare workers: adherence to CDC guidelines of three urban hospitals in California [see comments]. *Infection Control and Hospital Epidemiology* 1998;19:487–493.

56. Kellerman SE, Simonds D, Banerjee S, Towsley J, Stover BH, Jarvis W. APIC and CDC survey of Mycobacterium tuberculosis isolation and control practices in hospitals caring for children. Part 1: Patient and family isolation policies and procedures. Association for Professionals in Infection Control and Epidemiology, Inc. *American Journal of Infection Control* 1998;26:478–482.

57. Kellerman SE, Simonds D, Banerjee S, Towsley J, Stover BH, Jarvis W. APIC and CDC survey of Mycobacterium tuberculosis isolation and control practices in hospitals caring for children. Part 2: Environmental and administrative controls. Association for Professionals in Infection Control and Epidemiology, Inc. *American Journal of Infection Control* 1998;26:483–487.

58. Tokars JI, Rudnick JR, Kroc K, Manangan L, Pugliese G, Huebner RE, et al. U.S. hospital mycobacteriology laboratories: status and comparison with state public health department laboratories. *Journal of Clinical Microbiology* 1996;34:680–685.

59. LoBue P, Catanzaro A. Healthcare worker compliance with nosocomial tuberculosis control policies. *Infection Control and Hospital Epidemiology* 1999;20:623–624.

60. LoBue PA, Catanzaro A. Effectiveness of a nosocomial tuberculosis control program at an urban teaching hospital. *Chest* 1998;113:1184–1189.

61. Lai KK, Fontecchio SA, Kelley AL, Melvin ZS. Knowledge of the transmission of tuberculosis and infection control measures for tuberculosis among healthcare workers. *Infection Control and Hospital Epidemiology* 1996;17:168–170.

62. Moran GJ, Fuchs MA, Jarvis WR, Talan DA. Tuberculosis infection-control practices in United States emergency departments. *Annals of Emergency Medicine* 1995;26:283–289.

63. Murphy DC, Younai FS. Obstacles encountered in application of the Centers for Disease Control and Prevention guidelines for control of tuberculosis in a large dental center. *American Journal of Infection Control* 1997;25:275–282.

64. Murphy DC, Younai FS. Risk of tuberculosis transmission in dentistry. Results of a retrospective chart review. *AAOHN Journal* 1997;45:377–385.

65. Kellerman S, Tokars JI, Jarvis WR. The cost of selected tuberculosis control measures at hospitals with a history of Mycobacterium tuberculosis outbreaks. *Infection Control and Hospital Epidemiology* 1997;18:542–547.

66. Kellerman S, Saiman L, Soto-Irizarry M, San Gabriel P, Larsen CA, Besser, et al. Costs associated with tuberculosis control programs at hospitals caring for children. *Pediatric Infectious Disease Journal* 1999;18:604–608.

67. Williams J, Schneider N, Gilligan ME. Implementing a tuberculosis control program. *American Journal of Infection Control* 1995;23:152–155.

68. Scott B, Schmid M, Nettleman MD. Early identification and isolation of inpatients at high risk for tuberculosis. *Archives of Internal Medicine* 1994;154:326–330.

69. Cox JN, Brenner ER, Bryan CS. Changing patterns of mycobacterial disease at a teaching community hospital. *Infection Control and Hospital Epidemiology* 1994;15:513–515.

70. Kerr CM, Savage GT. Managing exposure to tuberculosis in the PACU: CDC guidelines and cost analysis. *Journal of Perianesthesia Nursing* 1996;11:143–146.

71. Brown RE, Miller B, Taylor WR, Palmer C, Bosco L, Nicola RM, et al. Health-care expenditures for tuberculosis in the United States. *Archives of Internal Medicine* 1995;155:1595–1600.

72. Griffith DE, Hardeman JL, Zhang Y, Wallace RJ, Mazurek GH. Tuberculosis outbreak among healthcare workers in a community hospital. *American Journal of Respiratory and Critical Care Medicine* 1995;152:808–811.

73. Topal JE, Reagan-Cirincione P, Weinstein JA, Dembry LM, Hierholzer WJ Jr. Optimizing the use of airborne precautions for patients with suspected pulmonary tuberculosis in an intermediate risk healthcare facility. Submitted for publication. 2000.

E

OSHA in a Health Care Context

Scott Burris, J.D., and Jamie Crabtree, B.A. *

This appendix summarizes requirements of the Occupational Safety and Health Act for the development, enforcement, and adjudication of new safety and health standards, with particular emphasis on the current proposal to regulate occupational exposure to tuberculosis.

Occupational safety and health, like other core public health concerns, was historically a matter of state, rather than federal, oversight. States directly attempted to promote occupational safety and health by passage of industrial safety legislation and indirectly by passage of worker's compensation schemes. Although commentators disagree about the overall effectiveness of state safety measures (Chelius, 1977; McLaury, 1981), by the late 1960s, support had grown for a uniform national workplace safety regime. Citing statistics placing the cost of workplace injuries at more than $8 billion annually (Senate Report No. 1282, 1970), the U.S. Congress passed the Occupational Safety and Health Act of 1970 (the Act).

THE OCCUPATIONAL SAFETY AND HEALTH
ACT IN FORM AND FUNCTION

The Act covers private employers in the 50 states and all U.S. territories and guarantees workers a workplace safe from the threat of workplace accidents and exposure to toxic substances (Occupational Safety

---

*Scott Burris, J.D., Professor of Law, Temple University Beasley School of Law, Philadelphia, Pennsylvania. Jamie Crabtree, J.D. Candidate Temple University Beasley School of Law.

and Health Act of 1970). The Act imposes upon covered employers a "general duty" to provide a safe workplace to employees and created the Occupational Safety and Health Administration (OSHA) to adopt and enforce rules. For clarity and ease of enforcement, the Act also authorized OSHA to create specific standards for particular industries or risks. Several other agencies were created to conduct research, try enforcement cases, or otherwise contribute to the workplace safety system. Individuals and organizations in the private sector also play a considerable role in shaping OSHA's standards and priorities.

Political Bodies Responsible for Administering OSHA

The administration of the Act is comprised of four basic functions: *research* on workplace risks and risk reduction; the development of specific safety standards (called *rulemaking*); *enforcement* of the rules through education and technical assistance, as well as investigation and punishment of violations; and *adjudication and judicial review* of standards and enforcement measures. In all these functions, OSHA and other federal agencies must comply with both the substantive and procedural requirements of the Act and other related federal rules, which prescribe what rules agencies like OSHA may make and how it must go about making them.

Research

Several entities conduct research or provide information to OSHA (Figure E-1). The National Institute for Occupational Safety and Health (NIOSH) is the principal government agency charged with conducting research regarding workplace hazards. NIOSH is part of the Centers for Disease Control and Prevention (CDC), within the Department for Health and Human Services. Unlike OSHA, NIOSH has no regulatory or enforce-

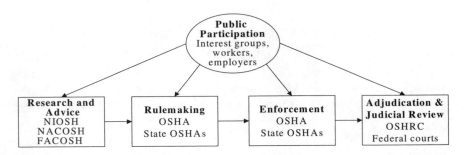

FIGURE E-1. OSHA processes and personae.

ment authority. It does have the authority to enter workplaces and question employees as part of its research activities. NIOSH may examine medical records or conduct medical examinations upon consenting employees, and may involve employees in data collection with the employees' consent. NIOSH and OSHA have entered into cooperative agreements under which NIOSH advises OSHA on the development of new standards, and assists in ensuring employer compliance by offering training and education (Rothstein, 1998).

The National Advisory Committee on Occupational Safety and Health (NACOSH) advises the U.S. Department of Labor and the U.S. Department of Health and Human Services on the feasibility of and alternatives to new standards. Its 12 members include representatives of labor, management, the public, and occupational safety professionals. The Federal Advisory Council on Occupational Safety and Health (FACOSH) advises the Secretary of Labor on occupational safety and health among federal agencies. The Secretary may create additional advisory committees to aid OSHA in the promulgation of new standards. These committees may be permanent committees to advise the Secretary on safety and health in a single industry or temporary committees created to advise the Secretary on issuing a single standard (Rothstein, 1998).

Rulemaking

The Act creates a duty for each covered employer to provide "to each of his employees employment and places of employment which are free from recognized hazards that are causing or are likely to cause death or serious physical harm to his employees" (Occupational Safety and Health Act of 1970). This is known as the general-duty clause of the Act. The Act authorizes OSHA to interpret and enforce this general rule and also to issue more specific standards for particular industries or hazards. The decision to issue a specific standard initiates a process known in administrative law as rulemaking. Rulemaking is subject to substantive and procedural rules that are discussed in detail later in this appendix.

OSHA is part of the U.S. Department of Labor and is headed by the Assistant Secretary of Labor for OSHA. Staff in Washington, D.C., make policy and develop new standards in accordance with the research results and advice of NIOSH, the various advisory boards, and the many other public and private individuals and organizations with an interest in worker health and safety. Public participation is required by the statute and formalized in U.S. Department of Labor regulations providing for "written petitions" submitted to the Secretary by "any interested person" suggesting a new standard. These petitions must include the rule proposed, a statement of reasons for the new standard, and a statement of its intended effect (29 C.F.R. 1911.3).

The Act also allows states to operate their own occupational safety and health regulatory systems. States that exercise this option are called "state plan jurisdictions" and have taken regulatory authority back from OSHA by creating and submitting for approval to the Secretary of Labor their own regulatory plan for occupational safety and health. A more detailed discussion of state plan jurisdictions and the requirements for approval by the Secretary is included below.

Enforcement

Enforcement of the Act is an OSHA function. In states that have their own occupational safety and health systems, state agencies also carry out enforcement activities. Enforcement activities include

- analyzing the compliance reports that employers are required to submit on a regular basis,
- conducting inspections on the agency's own initiative or in response to incidents or complaints,
- citing employers for violations, and
- providing training and technical support.

OSHA's enforcement is conducted by Area Directors placed throughout the country who are responsible for providing explanations to any questions received from affected parties in the area for which the Director is responsible, responding to complaints made by employees covered by OSHA protection, scheduling and conducting the periodic inspections required by the Act, determining when employers should be cited for violations, and assigning any fines as the result of a violation. Under the authority of the Area Directors are Compliance Safety and Health Officers, or Compliance Officers, whose responsibility it is to inspect individual work sites, counsel employers regarding compliance concerns, as well as submit reports to the area directors regarding these investigations. These reports provide Area Directors with a means to assess employer compliance for purposes of issuing citations and violations (Rothstein, 1998).

The Act requires some employers to maintain records regarding the injury and illness rates of the individual facility, which must be available on site for review during inspections. These reports help OSHA decide what industries or sites should be targeted for inspections and assess how well the Act and state plans are being implemented. Standards designed to address toxic substances also include exposure control plans. These plans identify the workers who are in danger of exposure to toxic substances in order to ensure proper training and medical surveillance.

OSHA's Compliance Officers conduct two types of inspections: periodic "programmed inspections" scheduled by OSHA Area Directors and inspections made in response to complaints, deaths, or other indicators of an imminent danger. The thoroughness of the inspection can vary depending upon the illness and injury rate for the particular employer. However, at the end of an inspection the Compliance Officer counsels the employer and employee representatives accompanying the inspection on how to improve the safety and health plan in their workplace. The Compliance Officer submits a report regarding the inspection to the Area Director, who determines if there are violations. Once a determination has been made after an inspection that a standard is being violated, a citation is sent to the employer with a detailed description of the violation and a date by which the condition should be corrected. This notice will also include the amount of the proposed penalty. If the employer fails to contest the citation within 15 days, the citation becomes a final order of the Occupational Safety and Health Review Commission (OSHRC) (see adjudication section below) and the penalty a fine which is owed. If contested, the Commission will hold a hearing to determine the level of violation and fine.

The sanctions for violating the Act are a function of the seriousness of the risk created and the perceived motives and past behavior of the employer. The more serious the risk and the more it was known to and disregarded by the employer, the more serious the violation and the higher the penalty. A *de minimus* violation occurs when the employer is technically not in compliance with a standard but the violation has no direct effect on safety and health. This violation is different from all other OSHA violations in that it carries no penalty and is not contestable under OSHA's adjudication process. OSHA issues a *nonserious violation* when the noncompliant condition has an effect on safety and health, but it is not likely to result in death or serious physical harm. *Serious violations* are issued for conditions likely to result in death or serious physical harm. *A repeated violation* arises when the same employer has been cited at least once before, and a final order was issued for a substantially similar violation. OSHA may issue a *willful violation* when the employer has blatantly violated the Act demonstrating indifference to complying with its standards (Rothstein, 1998; Occupational Safety and Health Act of 1970).

Violation Categories and Fines	
De minimus notice	$0
Nonserious	$0–$7,000
Serious	$1–$7,000
Repeated	$0–$70,000
Willful	$5,000–$70,000
Failure to abate	$0–$7,000/day
Failure to post	$0–$7,000/day

A violation must be corrected within a specified time, and failure to correct can itself be a violation. The *failure to abate violation* carries one of the most severe penalties, with fines ranging from $1,000 to $7,000 per day. In order to impose this violation OSHA must show that the original citation was upheld in the adjudicatory process (see below), a reinspection uncovered violation of the exact same condition, and the condition continues to present a hazard (Rothstein, 1998; Occupational Safety and Health Act of 1970). *Failure to post* is a record-keeping violation arising out of the enforcement process. An employer must post notice to his employees of violations as well as year-end summaries of injury and illness (Occupational Safety and Health Act of 1970). In addition to these civil penalties, the Act does provide for criminal penalties in cases where employer neglect is extreme and results in the death of an employee (Occupational Safety and Health Act of 1970).

The employer's demonstrated good faith, history of compliance with the Act, and the size of the employer's financial resources may all influence the penalty (Occupational Safety and Health Act of 1970). Good faith can be judged by examining the employer's overall safety plan, not just the particular standard for which it was cited. The employer's track record with OSHA may help to a large degree if it shows a history of a willingness to comply. OSHA considers the size of the business and may impose lesser penalties on smaller businesses in order not to unduly hamper the employer's ability to stay in business. The gravity of the harm the noncompliant condition creates is a large factor taken into consideration since the overall aim of the statute is to improve safety and health of employees (Rothstein, 1998).

OSHA has the resources to inspect only a fraction of workplaces (Rabinowitz and Shapiro, 2000). The success of the Act's scheme therefore requires a high degree of voluntary compliance by employers. The deterrent effect of fines and unannounced inspections makes some contribution, but the agency also uses positive methods of training and technical assistance to facilitate employer compliance with standards. Some research suggests that the cooperative approach to regulation under OSHA such as facilitation of worker involvement in safety programs actually has a greater deterrent effect on workplace hazards than do coercive measures such as fines (Rabinowitz and Shapiro, 1997; Gray and Scholz, 1997)

Although the Act also imposes upon *employees* a duty to comply with OSHA's rules, regulations, and standards, OSHA may not levy fines or otherwise punish employees for failure to comply. The sections of the Act addressing enforcement proceedings only refer to employers, and the legislative history confirms congressional intent to hold employers ultimately liable for compliance (*Atlantic & Gulf Stevedores, Inc.,* v. *Occupational Safety & Health Review Commission,* 1976). In practice, employers enforce employee compliance through their own disciplinary practices (Rothstein, 1998).

Adjudication and Judicial Review

The agency responsible for administering the Act's adjudicatory process is OSHRC. OSHRC is an independent agency within the executive branch exercising quasijudicial powers. It consists of three members appointed by the President. The OSHRC members appoint Administrative Law Judges, who are stationed throughout the country in OSHA's regional offices. These judges hear challenges to enforcement penalties issued to employers, including challenges to the factual basis of the alleged violation and challenges to the validity of the standard being enforced. They weigh evidence, listen to testimony and issue a ruling on the challenges that come before them. Decisions of the judges can be appealed to the three commission members. Upon making a determination regarding the validity of the judge's decision, OSHRC issues a final ruling that may be appealed in federal court (Rothstein, 1998).

Federal courts hear two kinds of cases under the Act: appeals from final decisions of OSHRC and "preenforcement" challenges to new standards when they are issued. Although the validity of the standard can be attacked in both types of action, in practice new OSHA standards are invariably challenged in federal court upon issuance. These preenforcement challenges must be filed within 59 days of the publication of the final rule in the *Federal Register*, and employers must obey the rule during the months and years of litigation.

There are three levels of federal courts. Normally litigation in the federal system is initiated in the District Courts that are responsible for conducting trials. However, appeals from the final order of OSHRC or from OSHA's decision to issue a new standard go directly to the Circuit Courts of Appeals (Occupational Safety and Health Act of 1970). Decisions of the Courts of Appeals can be appealed to the Supreme Court, which has the discretion to hear the case or leave the lower court decision unreviewed.

In appellate courts, what is known as *the standard of review* governs the scope of the court's inquiry into the decision being appealed. More than one standard of review may apply; for example, courts usually review findings of fact differently than conclusions of law in the same case. The standards applied in the review of OSHA and OSHRC were set by Congress in the Act. When reviewing OSHA's standard promulgation and OSHRC's factual findings, courts are limited to determining whether or not the decision at issue was "supported by substantial evidence on the record considered as a whole" (Occupational Safety and Health Act of 1970). Substantial evidence is "such relevant evidence as a reasonable mind might accept as adequate to support a conclusion" (*American Textile Manufacturers Institute, Inc.* v. *Donovan*, 1981). OSHRC's decision to impose a penalty will be reversed only if the reviewing court decides it was "arbitrary and capricious" or an "abuse of discretion" — i.e., an unreasonable exercise of the agency's power that evinces clear disregard of its statutory role (Rothstein, 1998; *Brennan* v. *OSHRC*, 1973). There has been some variation over time and across the judicial circuits in the stringency of review, which has led to some strategic "forum-shopping" by challengers to OSHA rules (Cherrington, 1994).

State Plan Jurisdictions

Upon passage of the Act, all state safety and health regulations covered by OSHA were preempted by OSHA standards. However, the Act included a provision for allowing states to take jurisdiction back from OSHA by creating a state plan to regulate occupational safety and health (Occupational Safety and Health Act of 1970). The most significant difference between state plan and OSHA jurisdictions is the scope of workplace coverage. State plans are required by the Act to cover the employees of the state and its political subdivisions in addition to private workplaces (Occupational Safety and Health Act of 1970). Two state plan jurisdictions, Connecticut and New York, only cover public employees, leaving occupational safety and health of private workplaces in the hands of OSHA (Rothstein, 1998).

Beyond the required additional coverage, states may choose to cover parties not covered by the Act, such as volunteers. Other than this, state plan jurisdictions and OSHA jurisdictions operate in much the same way. State plans must designate a state agency responsible for the plan's enforcement. The plan must include a means to adopt new safety and health standards, and these standards must be at least as stringent as those adopted by OSHA. The means of abating the hazardous condition being regulated does not have to be identical to the means outlined in OSHA's standard, but the protective effect of the state standard must be equal or greater to the protective effect of the OSHA standard (Occupational Safety and Health Act of 1970). The plan to regulate Occupational Exposure to Tuberculosis calls for state plan jurisdictions to adopt the new rule or one at least as effective within 6 months of the rule's final approval by OSHA (Occupational Exposure to Tuberculosis, 1997).

The enforcement of standards in state plan jurisdictions does not differ substantially from that in OSHA jurisdictions (Occupational Safety and Health Act of 1970). Unannounced inspections must be included, and employers may ultimately pay a fine for violating safety and health standards. State plan jurisdictions may also have a steeper fine structure than OSHA's. In order to monitor the effectiveness of the state plan, state plan jurisdictions must require employers to continue to provide OSHA with required information as though no plan were in place. OSHA may also inspect workplaces in state plan jurisdictions to monitor the effectiveness of the state's efforts at regulating workplace safety and health.

State Plan States

Alaska	New York*
Arizona	North Carolina
California	Oregon
Connecticut*	Puerto Rico
Hawaii	South Carolina
Iowa	Tennessee
Kentucky	Utah
Maryland	Vermont
Michigan	Virginia
Minnesota	Virgin Islands
Nevada	Washington
New Mexico	Wyoming

*Covers only employees of the state and its political subdivisions.

RULEMAKING

The starting point for understanding the Act's requirements is the general-duty clause: "Each employer shall furnish to each of his employees employment and a place of employment which are free from recognized hazards that are causing or are likely to cause death or serious physical harm to his employees" (Occupational Safety and Health Act of 1970). It represents a catchall means for OSHA to enforce basic safety in the workplace on matters concerning which OSHA has not promulgated a specific standard. Currently, OSHA enforcement of tuberculosis prevention is based in part on the authority of the general-duty clause (Occupational Exposure to Tuberculosis, 1997).

When OSHA concludes that a workplace hazard is best addressed by a specific standard, it initiates the rulemaking process to promulgate a standard. The standards that OSHA adopts require a specific plan to abate workplace risks through use of protective equipment, environmental controls, workplace practices, or a combination of these measures. Standards may be designed to prevent a particular hazard or protect against a type of hazard existing throughout many industries. For example, parts of OSHA's current regulation of TB risk come under existing general industry standards that require employers "to provide respiratory protection equipment" (29 C.F.R. 1910.34) and use "accident prevention tags to warn of biological hazards" (29 C.F.R. 1910.145 (f)). The proposed rule to regulate occupational exposure to tuberculosis is hazard specific. Where a hazard is covered by more than one OSHA standard, the employer must adhere to the standard most specifically designed to address the hazard (29 C.F.R. 1910.12; Rothstein, 1998).

On October 8, 1993, in response to the citizen petition requesting a permanent tuberculosis standard and an Emergency Temporary Standard,[1] OSHA issued enforcement guidelines to protect workers exposed to tuberculosis based on the general-duty clause and the existing respiratory hazard and biohazard warning standards. OSHA initiated rulemaking proceedings for a specific standard to prevent occupational exposure to tuberculosis (Occupational Exposure to Tuberculosis, 1997).

Like all executive branch agencies, OSHA is limited in its power by the legislation creating it and by legal doctrines generally applicable to administrative agencies. These limitations constrain the process by which OSHA adopts a new standard, the content of the new standard, and even what it may undertake to regulate in the first instance. We turn now to an examination of these limitations. Whether or not OSHA successfully promulgates a new standard within these parameters is ultimately a question for reviewing courts, and the prospect of review has a strong influence on OSHA's rulemaking work.

THE PROCEDURAL REQUIREMENTS

Under U.S. law, there are procedural requirements that all agencies engaged in rulemaking must observe (Administrative Procedure Act, 1994). These rules specify that an agency proposing to issue a regulation must give the public notice of its proposed action. Once this notice is provided, the agency must allow the public an opportunity to review and comment upon the proposed regulation. The agency may also be required to hold hearings to obtain further public input and to answer questions. Once the agency has completed obtaining all of the public input, it must consider and respond to the comments when it formulates the final regulations. Over time the implementation of certain executive orders and other acts of Congress have added more procedural steps for agencies making regulations.

Procedural requirements of the statute provide that a new OSHA standard shall be adopted according to the following procedure:

- A notice of proposed rulemaking is placed in the *Federal Register*.
- Interested parties have 30 days following publication of the notice to submit written data or comments. This is known as the comment period, and may be extended or reopened at the discretion of the agency.

---

[1]Emergency temporary standards may be issued by OSHA to protect workers from "grave danger" and are effective for only 6 months; however, this power is only used in extraordinary circumstances as it allows OSHA to exert its authority without observing the procedural requirements detailed in this section.

- An interested party may file *an objection* to the rulemaking (i.e., to the making of any rule, as opposed to a comment on the proposed rule) during the comment period. The filing of an objection requires the agency to hold hearings.
- In order to hold hearings OSHA must publish notice of the objections filed along with the dates, times, and places for the hearings in the *Federal Register* within 30 days of the close of the comment period.
- Within 60 days of completion of the last hearing or the last day for submission of comments if no hearings were required, the Secretary may issue a decision regarding the approval or disapproval of the new standard. The Secretary has the discretion to exceed this period.

When promulgating new standards OSHA must also comply with requirements imposed by other congressional acts and executive orders in the name of regulatory reform (McGarity, 1996). These include environmental impact statements, unfunded mandates analysis, and regulatory flexibility analysis. All agencies are required under the National Environmental Policy Act of 1969 to prepare Environmental Impact Statements when taking an action that will have an effect on the quality of the environment. Even if a new standard will have no effect on the quality of the environment, OSHA still must conduct the analysis and provide the basic notice that its action will have no environmental effect prior to instituting the new rule (Occupational Exposure to Tuberculosis, 1997). OSHA must provide notice that it undertook an analysis calculating the most cost-effective means of accomplishing its regulatory objective in order to fully comply with the Unfunded Mandates Reform Act of 1995. This is required when any executive agency action imposes costs in excess of $100 million per year on the private sector (Unfunded Mandates Reform Act of 1995). Finally, OSHA must assess the nonregulatory alternatives to achieving the same benefit of the regulation, perform a limited cost-effectiveness analysis, and conduct a costs minimization analysis for small business in order to comply with the Regulatory Flexibility Act and Executive Order 12866, which governs regulatory planning and review in the executive branch. This Executive Order requires administrative agencies to engage in regulatory flexibility analysis to determine among other things if the costs of the regulation are justified by its benefits. The cost-benefit and costs minimization analyses are discussed below in the section on substantive rulemaking requirements, as they have some impact on understanding how OSHA is tabulating the effect of its proposed standard and how OSHA developed some portions of the content of its standard. OSHA did not find that there were nonregulatory alternatives to accomplishing the same goal as the proposed standard (Occupational Exposure to Tuberculosis, 1997).

THE SUBSTANTIVE REQUIREMENTS FOR RULEMAKING

OSHA's proposed standard to regulate occupational exposure to tuberculosis arises under its authority to control exposure to toxic substances. The Act requires OSHA, when it addresses a toxic substance, to

> set the standard which most adequately assures, to the extent feasible, on the basis of the best available evidence, that no employee will suffer material impairment of health or functional capacity even if such employee has regular exposure to the hazard dealt with by such standard for the period of his working life (Occupational Safety and Health Act of 1970).

We will examine judicial interpretation of this statutory provision in the following section.

As interpreted by the courts, the phrase *"the standard which most adequately assures"* sets two important characteristics of OSHA standards. First, since the phrase does not specifically enumerate the means by which OSHA standards should protect employee safety and health, the Act authorizes OSHA to impose workplace practices, environmental controls, or protective equipment—or any combination of the three—to abate occupational exposure to toxic substances. Second, the language has been read to specify the standard OSHA should use to decide among possible measures: it must select the measure or package of measures that achieves the most protective standard. Courts generally leave this decision to OSHA and are highly deferential to OSHA's findings (*American Iron and Steel Institute* v. *OSHA*, 1999).

When deciding between the various methods to abate occupational exposure to airborne toxins, OSHA regulates to reduce the source of exposure to the substance. It considers this to be the best means to protect worker safety and health (See 29 C.F.R. § 1910.134 (a)(1); Rothstein, 1998). As a result, OSHA favors the use of engineering controls to reduce occupational exposure to airborne toxins when possible. Thus, OSHA's standard to regulate occupational exposure to tuberculosis focuses on moving those who are suspected or confirmed to have tuberculosis into acid-fast bacillus (AFB) isolation rooms as soon as possible, but provides for use of respiratory masks until the transfer takes place (Occupational Exposure to Tuberculosis, 1997).

The phrase *"to the extent feasible"* requires OSHA to conduct an economic and technological feasibility analysis of its proposed standards. Economic feasibility means that the proposed standard is economically "capable of being done" (*American Textile Manufacturers Institute, Inc.* v. *Donovan*, 1981). Case law treats this is an examination of whether or not a proposed OSHA standard will impair "the long term profitability and competitiveness of the industry" being regulated (Rothstein, 1998). The focus is on ensuring that compliance with the new standard will not cause widespread business failures in the long term. When considering alternatives, OSHA may not adopt a standard it considers to be less than the most protective safety and health standard, unless it is the only standard whose costs the industry can absorb or pass along. However, OSHA may choose the least costly of two equally protective measures (Latin, 1983). The requirement to regulate to the safest possible level precludes a true cost-benefit analysis (*American Textile Manufacturers Institute, Inc.* v. *Donovan*, 1981).

Technological feasibility as required of proposed OSHA standards involves determining that the technology exists or "may reasonably be brought into existence" to comply with a new standard. This requirement's most litigated point of interpretation regards the degree to which OSHA's authority permits it to "force" industries to adopt new technology. Essentially, OSHA cannot force industries to engage in research to achieve safer workplaces, but OSHA may impose the adoption of new or existing technologies provided it is economically feasible (Latin, 1983). The technological feasibility analysis for OSHA's proposed tuberculosis standard involves the examination of the existence and costs of requiring the use of AFB isolation rooms and biological safety cabinets in facilities where the standard requires these engineering controls. OSHA noted the existence of this equipment in its report on the proposed rule and commented that they were already in widespread use (Occupational Exposure to Tuberculosis, 1997).

To satisfy provisions of Executive Order 12866 as well as its own economic and technological feasibility analyses, OSHA may tailor its standards to the industries it affects taking into consideration size, expertise, and resources of the businesses involved. OSHA may only do this "to the extent permitted by law" under the Executive Order. The determination to change the requirements for compliance from one industry to the next must bear some reasonable relationship to the decreased risk presented in that industry and its ability to comply in light of the economic means of the industry and the skill of its workers to effectively implement the use of engineering controls (Occupational Exposure to Tuberculosis, 1997).

OSHA's decision to adopt a new standard and the means chosen to abate the regulated risks must be made on "*the best available evidence.*" While OSHA must be diligent in its efforts to collect data and must draw reasonable conclusions from that data, it is not constrained to regulate only when it finds to a "scientific certainty" that the adverse effects of a toxic substance can be remedied by the standard it proposes. Nor does OSHA have to prove to a scientific certainty that the substance it proposes to regulate will ever even cause a disease (Truong, 2000). The Supreme Court noted in *Industrial Union Department, AFL-CIO* v. *American Petroleum Institute* (the Benzene case) that this provision of the statute allowed OSHA to promulgate protective standards before a disease begins to occur in the workforce. OSHA is permitted to err on the side of overprotection (*Industrial Union Department, AFL-CIO v. American Petroleum Institute*, 1980). There is no question that exposure to aerosolized *Mycobacterium tuberculosis* causes the disease tuberculosis. OSHA's determination that it has set the highest standard of protection that is economically and technologically feasible will, however, likely be tested against this "best available evidence" standard.

The goal of proposed standards must be to ameliorate the risk of "*a material health impairment*." While the statute fails to define this term and no cases exist defining "material health impairment," it is suggested that this term can fairly "be given its common workers' compensation definition of 'loss of a physical function'" (Rothstein, 1998), but OSHA regulates impairments that may not be compensable under worker's compensation. In a number of standards, including the bloodborne pathogen and lead standards, OSHA has encompassed infections or other pre-symptomatic events antecedent to serious illness as "material impairments." The proposed rule on tuberculosis reflects this view. In the proposal, OSHA discusses the risk of death and serious disease, but regards even infection alone as a material impairment (Occupational Exposure to Tuberculosis, 1997). Courts will generally defer to OSHA's decision to define an adverse health condition a *material impairment* (*AFL-CIO v. OSHA*, 1992).

In addition to these explicit statutory requirements, OSHA must show that a new standard is designed to eliminate a "*significant risk*." The significant risk requirement comes from the Benzene case, one of the first major Supreme Court interpretations of the Act. Several Justices—though not a majority of the Court—expressed the opinion that the Act did not empower OSHA to regulate every possible occupational health risk, but only those that were "significant." These Justices suggested that the determination of significance should normally be left within OSHA's discretion, but offered, by way of illustration, the suggestion that a 1 in 1,000 risk of death was clearly significant, and that a 1 in a billion risk clearly was not (*Industrial Union Department., AFL-CIO v. American Petroleum Institute*, 1980). These Justices were not writing for a majority of the Court, and were not attempting to set the threshold for regulation at exactly the 1/1,000 level. Nevertheless, if only because it provides OSHA with a concrete figure, subsequent regulations and the case law have hewn close to the 1 in 1,000 benchmark, and courts have made it clear that "OSHA has a responsibility to quantify or explain, at least to some reasonable degree, the risk posed by each toxic substance regulated" (*AFL-CIO v. OSHA*, 1992).

The subsequent case law on significant risk does not offer a coherent, simple explanation of what level of risk is considered significant, largely because the cases have dealt with such a diverse group of scientific questions and legal arguments. Given the Benzene case requirement it seems clear that "OSHA cannot impose onerous requirements on an industry that does not pose substantial hazards to workers" (*American Dental Association* v. *Martin*, 1993), but no cases since the Benzene case have squarely faced the question of how low a risk can be and still be substantial. Instead, the cases have dealt with two basic kinds of problems: the quality of OSHA's risk evidence, and the reliability of its statistical analysis of that evidence. The ultimate question for reviewing courts is whether OSHA's findings of "significant risk" are supported by substantial evidence. The standard of review colors court decisions regarding both of these problems.

Texas Independent Ginners v. *Marshall* is an example of a case turning on the quality of OSHA's evidence. OSHA had found that American cotton gin workers were at a "significant risk" of developing byssinosis due to cotton dust exposure. OSHA had relied on studies of foreign cotton ginners and American cotton manufacturing employees other than ginners to establish that the prevalence of "acute respiratory problems" among American ginners was likely to lead to byssinosis. There was no dispute that U.S. manufacturing and foreign gin workers experienced more prolonged and higher concentrations of exposure to cotton dust than did American ginners. Since OSHA had failed to offer an explanation for how these differences in working conditions would affect the ultimate occurrence of byssinosis among U.S. ginners, the reviewing court held that the studies would not suffice to constitute substantial evidence of "significant risk."

Most of the "significant risk" cases deal with OSHA's choices among statistical methods or scientific data. For example, in *ASARCO* v. *OSHA*, members of the smelting industry challenged OSHA's standard governing exposure to airborne arsenic because it relied on studies treating duration as the key factor in determining the risks of exposure. The industry, backed by its own studies, claimed that it was the level of dosage that determined the level of risk. The court rejected the challenge, reasoning that a dispute in the scientific record did not justify overruling OSHA where OSHA articulated clear reasons for choosing its study over the one in question: "where an agency presents scientifically respectable evidence which the petitioner can continually dispute with rival, and we will assume, equally respectable evidence, the court must not second guess the particular way the agency chooses to weigh conflicting evidence or resolve the dispute" (*ASARCO* v. *OSHA*, 1984).

So long as OSHA presents reasonable explanations for accepting one version of scientific analysis over another a court will not engage in an evaluation of OSHA's decision. However, if OSHA fails to explain why it chooses one method of risk calculation over another, then the court may remand the standard for OSHA to provide these explanations (*UAW* v. *Pendergrass*, 1989). Throughout OSHA's tuberculosis risk assessment OSHA provides reasons for rejecting scientific studies critical of its analysis for this very reason (Occupational Exposure to Tuberculosis, 1997). If OSHA ultimately promulgates a final tuberculosis standard, the record must reflect that OSHA considered these studies and rejected them with reasonable explanations.

OSHA has apparently adhered to the 1/1,000 level of risk as its benchmark for "significant risk" since the Benzene case decision (*UAW* v. *Pendergrass*, 1989). It is not clear, however, that OSHA is legally required to hold to this practice. It has certainly departed from the strict terms of the Benzene case standard in some cases by regulating a 1/1,000 risk of material impairment rather than death. This is what it has proposed to do in the tuberculosis rule.

DETERMINING WHOM OSHA PROTECTS AND CONTROLS

Two aspects of the Act have a considerable influence on OSHA's regulatory impact on the health care system. The first question is how the Act defines who are the "employees" and "employers" subject to OSHA's protection and control under the Act. The other is how the Act assigns responsibility for ensuring compliance with OSHA standards in workplace settings where there are multiple employers.

Statutory Definitions of Employees and Employers

The statute defines an employee as "an employee of an employer who is employed in a business of his employer which affects commerce" (Occupational Safety and Health Act of 1970). An employer is "a person engaged in a business affecting commerce who has employees, but does not include the United States or any State or political subdivision of a State" (Occupational Safety and Health Act of 1970). "State" includes the District of Columbia and U.S. territories.

The commerce clause in the Constitution authorizes Congress to regulate matters related to the interstate economy. As a result, the constitutionality of the Act or any particular regulatory measure requires a finding that covered employers have an effect on commerce that can be felt outside the state in which the employer is located. Since OSHA must establish in its enforcement proceedings that it has jurisdiction over the cited employer, it must make an initial showing that the employer is engaged in a business "affecting commerce." This is rarely a problem and easily done. OSHA commonly establishes this by showing that in the course of doing business the employer makes use of goods produced out of state. For example, in any given health care facility this will include everything from the use of computer software to cotton swabs (Rothstein, 1998).

Employees of State and Local Governments

People who are employed by states or political subdivisions of a state are not protected by OSHA standards unless the state participates as a state plan jurisdiction. It is not always easy to determine, however, whether an employer is public or private. The Secretary of Labor's regulations delineate a two-prong test for determining whether or not an entity qualifies for the political subdivision exemption from OSHA regulation: "1) whether the entity is created directly by the state so as to constitute a department or administrative arm of government, or 2) whether the entity is administered by individuals who are controlled by public officials and responsible to such officials or to the general public" (29 C.F.R. 1975.5 (b)). Courts also examine to what degree the employees of an institution are treated as state employees, considering, for example, whether the benefits package offered to employees is the same as that offered to state employees, or whether employees are subject to the same merit and promotion system as state employees. To the degree that state university hospitals and other state-run health care providers may have engaged in quasiprivatization over the past few years, these distinctions may be helpful. These issues may also arise in state facilities where the state has outsourced some of its functions to employers who are private entities.

Volunteers

Volunteers are not protected by OSHA, because its statutory mandate is to protect employees. However, OSHA indicates that the employer's assertion that a person is a volunteer and the mere absence of monetary compensation for services are not the determinative factors. OSHA has cited employers who were compensating workers in kind. OSHRC has upheld these violations (*Secretary of Labor* v. *Arlie R. Hawk General Contractor*, 1976). Finding that a volunteer is actually an employee compensated in kind turns on proof of an exchange of value that is significant enough to give rise to an employer/employee relationship. Altruistic volunteers in health care and other service settings would probably never be treated as employees, but an employer cannot avoid the requirements of OSHA by finding alternative, nonmonetary ways of paying for services (such as room and board or discounted fees).

Students

While physicians completing residency requirements would clearly fall within OSHA's protective reach since they are being compensated for their services, it is unlikely that medical students completing clinical requirements without compensation are covered by OSHA regulation.

Federal Employees

The Act requires federal agencies to develop safety standards consistent with those adopted by OSHA, maintain occupational safety and health records, and make reports to the Secretary of Labor regarding the program. The Act gave OSHA no enforcement powers as against other federal agencies, but enforcement rules were set up by presidential order as early as the Nixon administration. The current scheme for federal compliance was set out in a 1980 Executive Order of President Carter, which requires federal agencies

- to comply with OSHA standards unless the Secretary of Labor approves an alternative safety plan;
- to comply with the general-duty clause of the Act by ridding federal workplaces of all recognized hazards that cause or are likely to cause death;
- to comply with antidiscrimination requirements of the Act by allowing employees to report safety problems without fear of retaliatory action;
- to establish within each agency an occupational safety and health committee consisting of an equal number of management and nonmanagement employees to monitor the agency's safety and health performance; and
- to allow unannounced inspections by the Secretary of Labor under certain conditions (Executive Order 12196, 1980).

Employees of Veterans Administration hospitals are protected by this section.

ASSIGNING RESPONSIBILITY IN THE MULTIEMPLOYER WORKPLACE

Often there are many employers within one workplace, raising questions about which employer is responsible for complying with OSHA regulations (*American Dental Association* v. *Martin*, 1993). This situation is common in but not unique to health care, and indeed first became an issue for OSHA in the construction industry. With time, a rule emerged that limits the responsibility of an employer who does not control the physical makeup of the work site. The subcontractor-employer must make reasonable efforts to ensure that the places where its employees work is safe: it must inspect the work site, report problems to the employer who has control of the site, provide necessary safety equipment to abate the hazardous condition to the extent possible, or in extreme cases remove its employees from the site. Additionally, the subcontractor maintains responsibility for OSHA compliance that does not require control of the work site, such as initial safety training and in some instances supply of safety equipment. In short the rule mitigates against the harshness of imposing sanctions on employers who may be unable to alleviate unsafe working conditions, but it does not relieve an employer of all responsibility assigned by OSHA (Anonymous, 1976). It is also possible to assign responsibilities for compliance by contract (Occupational Exposure to Tuberculosis, 1997).

OSHA's proposed tuberculosis standard explains how responsibility would be assigned in covered multiemployer work sites and the home health care industry (Occupational Exposure to Tuberculosis, 1997). OSHA suggests that the responsibilities for compliance with respect to temporary workers supplied to workplaces covered by the rule be specified by contract. Employers providing temporary workers would be expected ordinarily to ensure that these employees receive all necessary general training required by the statute, and the "host" employer should provide any site-specific training necessary. The "provider" employer would be responsible for postexposure medical evaluation, with the host employer maintaining responsibility for ensuring compliance with the engineering and environmental controls required by the standard. Provider employers would be exempt from recordkeeping requirements related to engineering controls. Home health care workers are covered by the proposed standard as well. Employers in this industry are not responsible for the conditions of the homes served, but are to be required to provide training and ensure that their employees have respiratory masks (Occupational Exposure to Tuberculosis, 1997).

Doctors who work for corporations that have obtained use-right agreements with a covered hospital are protected under the same multiemployer work site rules as outlined above. If a doctor has his own practice for which he has created a legal entity by filing articles of incorporation, he would qualify as a protected employee of that practice since OSHA regulations have been held applicable to management as well as subordinate employees (Rothstein, 1998). If a doctor practices medicine without having created a legal entity such as a corporation to serve as the business for which he works, then he may not be under OSHA's protective reach while practicing in a hospital. In this instance OSHA would likely consider the doctor to be an independent contractor and not an employee (Rothstein, 1998).

ALTERING OSHA RULES

OSHA may respond to changes in hazards or workplace practices by amending or rescinding a standard. In doing so, OSHA must adhere to the same procedural and substantive requirements that apply to the issuance of a new standard, and the agency's action can be challenged in court (Occupational Safety and Health Act of 1970). If new information indicated that a threat to employee health and safety were grave and extraordinary in nature, the Secretary could issue an Emergency Temporary Standard effective upon publication in the *Federal Register* (Occupational Safety and Health Act of 1970). If, however, the new information indicates that a standard is no longer "necessary or appropriate" due to an overestimation or subsequent elimination of the risk it was designed to reduce, there is no similar statutory vehicle for immediate recission. Of course, OSHA could also informally stop enforcing a rule that was no longer necessary to protect worker health, at least while it was moving formally to change or rescind the standard.

OSHA might also use new information in setting the level of violation or fine in its enforcement scheme (Occupational Exposure to Tuberculosis, 1997). For example, if CDC develops new infection control guidelines that are equal to or more protective than the OSHA standard governing control of tuberculosis, OSHA could take the position that employers following the new guidelines would only be subject to citations for de minimus violations. This violation carries no penalty or stigma.

Congress may also directly disapprove a standard prior to or after its effective date (Government Organization and Employees Act, 2000). Section 801 is part of the regulatory oversight that requires the filing of reports by administrative agencies to assess a standard's societal impact such as the Unfunded Mandates Reform Act reports. Within 60 days of the filing of these reports, Congress may by joint resolution directly invalidate an OSHA standard. The President may also, in turn, mandate that the agency standard take effect if it is necessary to eliminate one of four categories of threats including "imminent" danger to public health and safety (Government Organization and Employees Act, 2000). Congressional oversight may soon increase if new proposals requiring that all administrative agency rules be subject to congressional approval are successful.

CONCLUSION: OSHA, PUBLIC HEALTH, AND CONTAGIOUS DISEASE

Effectively regulating risk presents difficult challenges to government agencies like OSHA (Kuran and Sunstein, 1999). Regulating the risk of exposure to communicable disease through OSHA has raised several serious issues. Commentators have suggested that the added costs of OSHA compliance may hurt patients by pushing poorer consumers out of the health care market (*American Dental Association* v. *Martin*, 1993) or by exposing patients and clients with tuberculosis to discrimination by institutions with an incentive to avoid costly compliance measures (Berg, 1997). It has also been claimed that OSHA simply moves too slowly to keep up with a changing risk like tuberculosis (Berg, 1997). Few if any of these assertions are backed by data, but there is no question that the effort to regulate TB has added a new page to the history of OSHA's struggles to deal with the scientific and regulatory complexity of regulating workplace risk.

REFERENCES

Administrative Procedure Act 5 U.S. C.§§551-59 West, 1994.

AFL-CIO v. *OSHA*, 965 F.2d 962 (11th Cir. 1992).

American Dental Ass'n v. *Martin*, 984 F.2d 823 (7th Cir. 1993).

American Iron and Steel Institute v. *OSHA*, 182 F.3d 1261 (11th Cir. 1999).

American Textile Manufacturers Institute, Inc. v. *Donovan*, 452 U.S. 490 (1981).

Anonymous: Recent Case: Administrative Law—Occupational Safety and Health Act—On Multiemployer Jobsite, When Employees of Any Employer Are Affected by Noncompliance with a Safety Standard, Employer in Control of Work Area Violates Act; Employer Not in Control of Work Area Does Not Violate Act, Even if his own Employees are Affected. Harvard Law Review 89:793–800, 1976.

ASARCO, Inc. v. *OSHA*, 746 F.2d 483 (9th Cir. 1984).

Atlantic & Gulf Stevedores, Inc., v. *Occupational Safety & Health Review Commission*, 534 F.2d 541 (3d Cir. 1976).

Berg, Paula E.: When the Hazard is Human: Irrationality, Inequity, and Unintended Consequences of the Regulation of Contagion. Washington University Law Quarterly 75:1367–1429, 1997.

Brennan v. *OSHRC*, 487 F.2d 438 (8th Cir. 1973).

Chelius, James Robert: The Occupational Safety and Health Problem in Workplace Safety and Health: The Role of Workers Compensation. American Enterprise Institute for Public Policy Research, Washington, D.C., 1977.

Cherrington, David R.: The Race to the Courthouse: Conflicting Views Toward the Judicial Review of OSHA Standards. Brigham Young University Law Review, 95–128, 1994.

Executive. Order No.12196, 45 Fed. Reg. 12,769 (1980).

Executive Order No. 12866, 58 Fed. Reg. 51,735 (1993).

Farmworker Justice Fund, Inc. v. *Brock*, 811 F.2d 613 (D.C. Cir. 1987)

Government Organization and Employees Act 5 U.S.C.A. §801 (West 2000).

Gray, Wayne B. and Scholz, John T.: Can Government Facilitate Cooperation?: An Informational Model of OSHA Enforcement. American Journal of Political Science 41:693–717, 1997.

Industrial Union Department, AFL-CIO v. *American Petroleum Institute*, 448 U.S. 607 (1980).

Kuran, T. and Sunstein, C.: Availability Cascades and Risk Regulation. Stanford Law Review 51:683–768, 1999.

Latin, Howard A.: The Feasibility of Occupational Health Standards: An Essay on Legal Decisionmaking Under Uncertainty. Northwestern University Law Review 78: 583–631, 1983.

McGarity, Thomas O.: The Expanded Debate over the Future of the Regulatory State. University of Chicago Law Review 63:1463–1489, 1996.

McLaury, Judson: The Job Safety Law of 1970: Its Passage was Perilous in Mintz, Benjamin, 1984. OSHA History, Law, and Policy, The Bureau of National Affairs, Inc., 1981.

National Environmental Policy Act of 1969, 42 U.S.C.A. § 4332 *et seq.* (West 1994).

Northwest Airlines, Inc., 8 OSHC 1982, 1980 OSHD ¶24,751 (1980)

Occupational Exposure to Tuberculosis, 62 Fed. Reg. 54,160-01 (1997) (to be codified at 29 C.F.R. pt. 1910).

Occupational Safety and Health Act of 1970, 29 U.S.C.A. § 651 et seq. (West 1999).

292 TUBERCULOSIS IN THE WORKPLACE

Rabinowitz, Randy S. and Shapiro, Sidney A.: Punishment Versus Cooperation in Regulatory Enforcement: A Case Study of OSHA Administrative Law Review 49:713–762, 1997.
Rabinowitz, Randy S. and Shapiro, Sidney A.: Voluntary Regulatory Compliance in Theory and Practice: The Case of OSHA. Administrative Law Review 52:97–155, 2000.
Rothstein, Mark: Occupational Safety and Health Law, 4th ed.. West Publishing Co., St. Paul, Minn., 1998.
Secretary of Labor v. *Arlie R. Hawk General Contractor*, 1976 WL 5974 (O.S.H.R.C.) S. Rep. No. 1282 at 2-4 (1970).
Texas Independent Ginners Association v. *Marshall*, 630 F.2d 389 (5th Cir. 1980).
Truong, Hiep: Daubert and Judicial Review: How Does an Administrative Agency Distinguish Valid Science from Junk Science? Akron Law Review 33:365–390, 2000.
UAW v. *Pendergrass*, 878 F.2d 389 (D.C. Cir. 1989).
Unfunded Mandates Reform Act of 1995, 2 U.S.C.A. §1532 (West 1997).

F

Respiratory Protection and Control of Tuberculosis in Health Care and Other Facilities

Philip Harber, Scott Barnhart, Douglas Hornick, and Robert Spear *

In 1994 guidelines, the Centers for Disease Control and Prevention (CDC) recommended a hierarchy of infection control measures for tuberculosis (CDC, 1994). The hierarchy consists of administrative controls, followed by engineering controls and then personal respiratory protection. This paper examines the last step in the hierarchy: the use of personal respiratory protection devices to shield health care workers when they enter areas (e.g., a tuberculosis isolation room) where the air may contain *Mycobacterium tuberculosis* aerosol.

The respiratory protection provisions of the 1997 proposed rule from the Occupational Safety and Health Administration (OSHA) (62 FR 201 [October 17, 1997]) are generally similar to the CDC guidelines. One exception—and the major area of controversy—involves the requirement for annual fit testing of individuals who use or may use personal respirators.

The next sections of this paper describe the basic components of a respiratory protection program, the types of respiratory protection devices used to prevent transmission of tuberculosis; and methods for fit testing the devices. The remainder of the paper then considers evidence about the effectiveness of respiratory protections in reducing the occupational risk of tuberculosis.

*Philip Harber is Professor at the Department of Family Medicine, University of California Los Angeles. Scott Barnhart is Medical Director, Harborview Medical Center, Seattle Washington. Douglas Hornick is Associate Professor at the Division of Pulmonary Diseases and Critical Care Medicine, University of Iowa, Iowa City. Robert Spear is Professor of Environmental Health Sciences at the University of California at Berkeley.

COMPONENTS OF A RESPIRATORY PROTECTION PROGRAM

A respiratory protection program has several components, of which the respirator (mask) device is only one (Vesley, 1995; Schaefer, 1997). Other elements include

- Assessment of individual worker's exposure to a hazard
- Selection of appropriate respirator for that exposure
- Proper maintenance and storage of reusable respirators
- Employee education and training
- Medical certification of worker's ability to wear respirator safely
- Periodic audit of the respirator program
- Designation of individual responsible for program

In addition to explaining the rationale for respirator use and the proper way to use a respirator, the education and medical evaluation components of a respirator program should explain potential adverse effects of respirator use, such as interference with voice, breathing discomfort, and stress.

A respiratory protection program involves several steps in a sequential process (Harber et al., 1999). These steps, designed for other industries but generally applicable to tuberculosis control programs, include the following:

- Identifying work sites with potential for significant exposure to an airborne hazard
- Identifying specific workers at risk and any characteristics that might make them especially at risk from the hazardous agent
- Determining the magnitude of the risk by work site and worker tasks
- Identifying a respirator that will prevent inhalation of the hazardous agent in the airstream
- Assessing adequacy of respirator fit (i.e., proportion of airflow actually going through the filter medium rather than between the respirator seal and the wearer's face)
- Ensuring that exposed workers actually use the respirator and use it correctly

The last element is crucial. A perfect respirator is of little value unless the proper worker uses it at the proper time. While this is intuitively obvious, not all analyses have considered this broad perspective. A quantitative analysis showed that there is an asymptotic effect of noncompliance with program elements (Harber et al., 1999). That is, a high protection factor of the device itself cannot compensate for programmatic failure or individual worker behavior deficits.

TYPES OF RESPIRATORY PROTECTION DEVICES

Respirators (respiratory personal protective devices) are widely used for protection against inhaled toxins. The two major categories of respirators are air-purifying devices and atmosphere-supplying devices. Air-purifying respirators function by partially "cleaning" the inhaled the air (filtering out hazardous agents), whereas atmosphere-supplying respirators provide an independent source of air. The 1994 CDC guidelines established performance criteria for respirators employed to prevent transmission of *M. tuberculosis*.

Currently, the National Institute for Occupational Safety and Health (NIOSH) lists four types of personal respirators for use as protection against tuberculosis. The devices are listed below in appropriate order of common use, convenience, and cost.

- N95 and other disposable particulate respirators: These respirators are relatively simple, disposable devices and are now widely used for protection against occupational tuberculosis. Although they look like surgical masks, these devices are fundamentally different in construction and function.
- Powered air-purifying respirators (PAPR): The powered air-purifying respirator provides a greater degree of protection than the N95 respirator. It consists of a tight-fitting face mask or a loose-fitting hood or helmet that is attached by a hose to a battery-operated fan that blows filtered air into the mask.
- Replaceable particulate filter respirators: External air-filtering cartridges are attached externally to the mask device itself. These devices are widely used in chemical industry and other settings and come with either half-masks or full facepiece masks.
- Postive-pressure supplied-air respirators: These respirators use compressed air delivered to a half or full facepiece mask through a hose from a fixed source.

Other types of devices have been used in the past. Dust-mist (DM) and dust-mist-fume (DMF) respirators have been widely used in industry and were used for tuberculosis protection during hospital outbreaks in the late 1980s and early 1990s. High-efficiency particulate air respirators (HEPA) are effective at removing smaller particles than the DM and DMF devices and began to supplant the DM and DMF respirators for tuberculosis protection before being largely replaced by N95 devices and, infrequently, PAPRs.

The mask type for a respirator is constructed to meet the specific application needs. For tuberculosis control and a number of other uses, the mask itself generally contains the filtration medium. This contrasts with devices commonly used for many chemical exposures, in which the mask is responsible for directing airflow, but the adsorbent or filter medium is in a cartridge or canister attached to the mask.

N95 and particulate filter respirators require that the individual generate (by breathing) the negative pressure necessary to force air in through the filtration medium. PAPRs use a pump to push ambient air through the filtration medium and supply it to the mask. In addition to obviating the need for the user to perform the ventilatory effort to overcome the resistance of the filtration medium, the PAPR supplies air within the mask at positive pressure relative to the ambient atmosphere. Thus, if the facial seal is not perfect, air will tend to flow from within the mask to the outside because of the pressure gradient. In contrast, most negative-pressure respirators require inhalation effort by users to create negative pressure within the mask. For these devices, if a leak exists at the facial sealing surface, the mask will draw in ambient untreated air. Hence, PAPRs typically provide a higher degree of protection than the typical negative-pressure masks. The former are, however, cumbersome, costly to maintain, and somewhat difficult to use.

Some respirators are intended as single-use devices, designed to be discarded after one use. Others may be considered reusable, meaning that they may be employed more than once, but are not meant to be permanent and durable devices. Many of the respirators marketed for tuberculosis control fall in this category. Finally, respirators may be designed as long-lasting, multiuser pieces of equipment.

Respirators also differ in the degree to which they resemble the typical surgical mask, which is more familiar to patients and possibly less anxiety inducing than some other types of devices. Some respirators are designed so that the user exhales through the filtering medium, whereas others have special exhalation valves. Such valves may make exhalation more comfortable, but they allow patients to be exposed to unfiltered air from the wearer, so such devices are not to be used during surgery.

Masks may be constructed of a soft, flexible material or of a more rigid elastomeric material. More rigid materials generally provide a better (i.e., tighter) fit but may be more uncomfortable. Different masks cover different amounts of the face. A quarter mask covers the mouth and nose and seals between the lower lip and the chin, whereas a half mask seals underneath the chin. A full-face mask extends from below the chin to above the forehead. In general, larger masks seal more effectively than the smaller types, but they are more expensive and cumbersome.

In the United States, respirator designs must be certified by NIOSH. The certification process includes examination of the design, laboratory testing of devices supplied by the manufacturer, audit of the production process, and occasional testing of off-the-shelf devices (Hodous and Coffey, 1994).

In the early 1990s, during the resurgence of tuberculosis in United States, NIOSH classified air-purifying respirators for removing particles (appropriate for tuberculosis protection) as dust-mist, dust-mist-fume, or HEPA (high-efficiency particulate air). A large gap in the efficiency of the particulate filtration process differentiated the first two types of devices and the HEPA type. Only the HEPA type, which was much more expensive, met the performance criteria for tuberculosis protection described by CDC in the 1993 draft and 1994 final guidelines. In 1995, NIOSH certified a new class of devices known as the N95 type. This relatively inexpensive type of respirator is designed to be at least 95 percent efficient at removing particulates, which meets the CDC performance criteria.

METHODS FOR FIT TESTING OF RESPIRATORY PROTECTION DEVICES

Fit testing is the process of determining the extent to which the facial seal of the respirator prevents inward leakage of unfiltered air. It may be applied at several different points:

- To test the newly designed respirator
- To evaluate an individual worker prior to placement in a job with potential mycobacterial exposure
- To evaluate an employee whenever a new respirator type is provided
- To evaluate fit on a regularly scheduled basis (e.g., annually)

Respiratory protection programs for tuberculosis are currently exempt from the 1998 OSHA respiratory protection standard, which requires annual fit testing. Pending publication of the occupational tuberculosis standard, they are subject, instead, to special regulations that do not mandate annual testing. The 1997 proposed OSHA rule on tuberculosis would require annual fit testing.

Methods of Determining Adequacy of Fit

Respirator fit describes the degree to which the device effectively limits the air leakage around the filtration media or, in some cases, between the user's face and the sealing surface of the respirator. Traditionally, protection is described in terms of the Protection Factor (PF). This is the ratio of the material outside the mask to its concentration inside the mask. It is affected by two factors: first, the degree to which the medium cleanses air moving through it, and second, the degree of leakage at the facial sealing surface of the user. Protection factor is typically measured using a marker chemical agent.

Determination of the Protection Factor is based upon measurements using surrogate marker materials. For example, sodium chloride aerosol is commonly employed for certification of respirator design types. In industrial settings where a specific chemical agent is employed, one may measure its concentration inside and outside of the mask to develop a meaningful protection factor measurement. Or, if the agent is particularly dangerous, a marker material with similar characteristics may be employed. For tuberculosis, however, this is infeasible since measurement of tuberculosis agents in air is difficult. Therefore, protective efficacy is generally estimated based upon the respirator characteristics for chemical, rather than biologic, agents.[1]

Categories of Fit Test

There are two types of fit tests—quantitative and qualitative. In addition, workers should be trained to check the seal on their respirator at each use. The cost and applicability of these differ significantly.

In a *quantitative fit test*, the concentration of a marker material inside and outside the mask is determined empirically. Quantitative fit testing is more accurate but requires trained personnel and relatively complex equipment.

In a *qualitative fit test*, a pass/fail approach is used. An individual dons the mask, and a test material is placed in the surrounding ambient air; then, the user reports whether it passes through the respirator. For example, saccharin aerosols are detectable by their sweet taste if the respirator does not effectively remove them (e.g., because of leakage at the face seal surface). Although NIOSH recommends against it, irritant smoke is also occasionally used in a qualitative fit testing procedure.

In a user seal check (commonly called a *fit check*) *procedure*, the user performs a simple maneuver to determine if the seal is adequate in an approximate, qualitative fashion. For example, the user may obstruct the inlet ports and attempt to inhale; passage of air implies that there is significant leakage at the facial sealing surface. This type of assessment is performed by the individual each time he or she dons a mask.

During quantitative or qualitative fit tests, testers also evaluate potential physical characteristics or changes such as weight gain or loss that might affect respirator fit. Quantitative testing is difficult for certain mask

---

[1]There are several formats for expressing Protection Factor. The Assigned Protection Factor is assigned based upon the mask type design. Although it may have been based upon empiric data, it is not measured specifically for the individual user. Conversely, the Protection Factor for a particular respirator and user may be determined under laboratory testing circumstances. However, efficacy of protection (PFs) under ideal laboratory circumstances does not represent "real-life" utilization. Therefore, the Workplace Protection Factor (WPF) describes the actual Protection Factor under field-use conditions. As might be expected, there are significant disparities between the Assigned Protection Factor, the laboratory-measured Protection Factor, and the actual Workplace Protection Factor.

types. It requires a probe inside the mask to measure the concentration of the marker material. This is generally not feasible with single-use/disposable respirators. Fennelly (1997) noted that there have been very few actual quantitative fit tests with the disposable types of respirators now in common use. Until recently, probe devices were not available to perform quantitative assessment of the actual filtration efficiency of these masks when used by humans. (See Coffey et al., 1999.)

Quantitative fit testing requires technical prowess, which ideally would be supplied by a trained industrial hygienist. Although there are 7000 hospitals, there are only 5,000 industrial hygienists in United States. Therefore, if widespread use of quantitative fit testing were required for hospitals and other facilities, other alternatives might be needed.

Qualitative fit testing, which relies upon subjective responses of the user to substances such as saccharin, is less expensive and less technically demanding. It is therefore attractive to employers. Qualitative fit tests have limitations. Saccharin is avoided in many settings because of its reputation as a carcinogen, and some hospitals have stopped using irritant smoke because this may provoke asthma (Fennelly, 1997). Bitrex, an extremely bitter compound sometimes used to deter children from eating poisonous household products, may offer a good alternative.

Except during nonhuman laboratory testing in research settings, fit testing cannot be performed with the actual exposure agent of concern (mycobacteria). Nevertheless, laboratory studies have demonstrated that surrogate agents are adequate (Qian et al., 1998).

Issues in Fit Testing

The discussion above has mentioned several concerns about the role and burden of fit testing in the context of programs to prevent tranmission of *M. tuberculosis* in health care and other settings. These include the effectiveness and feasibility of quantitative versus qualitative fit testing, the selection of particular agents for use in qualitative testing, and the trade-offs between protection and worker comfort and willingness to use the masks consistently and correctly.

Traditional occupational medicine/industrial hygiene practices require that the fit testing be repeated whenever a new respirator type is chosen. This presupposes that differences among masks are so great that successful fit with one does not predict adequacy of another of the same class. Implementation of this requirement may create unique problems for tuberculosis prevention in hospitals. Workers may be employed in several different settings, and purchasing agents often change availability of particular brands based upon availability/cost. Because the at-risk population is amorphous, such a fit testing requirement might be particularly difficult to implement and enforce reliably.

EVIDENCE OF EFFECTIVENESS OF RESPIRATORY PROTECTION: FACILITY STUDIES AND SURVEYS

Unfortunately, no research has tested individually the effects of respiratory protection on health care workers' risk of acquiring tuberculosis infection or disease. Some studies do, however, include relevant findings about the mix of measures implemented following hospital outbreaks of tuberculosis in the late 1980s and early 1990s.

Three reports describe hospital responses to well-recognized outbreaks of tuberculosis (two of which involved multidrug-resistant disease) (Wenger et al., 1995; Maloney et al., 1995; Blumberg et al., 1995). In each of the hospitals, the outbreak was ended effectively using variable levels of the tuberculosis control hierarchy. Most important, nosocomial tuberculosis transmission from patient to health care worker was interrupted. Although the hospitals continued to care for substantial numbers of patients with tuberculosis, health care worker exposure incidents and tuberculosis skin test conversions dropped substantially.

Table F-1 summarizes the control measures implemented. Each institution implemented extensive administrative controls, in particular, protocols to promptly identify, isolate, evaluate, and, as appropriate, treat people with signs and symptoms of tuberculosis. Each institution also implemented variable engineering controls, usually some kind of negative-pressure isolation room. Each institution supplied workers with some kind of respiratory protection device.

It is important to note that hospital responses—including the provision of respirators to workers—predated the 1994 CDC guidelines, which specified performance criteria for respiratory protection devices. They also predated NIOSH's 1995 certification of the N95 respirator, which met the new CDC criteria but was less expensive than previously certified devices. In any case, the respiratory protection measures implemented in these institutions were less stringent than those set forth in the 1994 CDC guidelines, the 1997 proposed OSHA rule on occupational tuberculosis, or the 1998 OSHA

TABLE F-1. Measures Used to Control Outbreaks of Nosocomial Tuberculosis Transmission in Three Hospitals

	Control Measure(s) Used		
Hospital	Administrative Measures	Engineering Measures	Respiratory Protection Device
Jackson Memorial, Miami	Extensive	Extensive	Submicron
Cabrini, New York	Extensive	Exhaust fans[a]	Molded surgical
Grady Memorial, Atlanta	Extensive	Exhaust fans[a]	Submicron

[a]Exhaust fans were placed in windows to produce negative pressure in isolation rooms.
SOURCE: Adapted from McGowan (1995).

respiratory protection standard for other hazards. Again, the outbreak studies suggest that the administrative controls adopted by hospitals played the major role in ending the outbreaks and that the kinds of respiratory protections they implemented added little.

It is also illustrative to examine two reports from nonoutbreak hospitals that had relatively high admission rates for patients with active tuberculosis and had adopted tuberculosis control measures to reduce their potential for outbreaks. As summarized below, these reports also suggest a limited role for respiratory protections. Again, all control measures were adopted prior to the 1994 CDC guidelines and the NIOSH certification of N95 respirators.

In May 1992 Columbia-Presbyterian Hospital in New York City revised its infection control program to be consistent with the 1990 CDC guidelines (Bangsberg et al., 1997). The facility had not experienced an outbreak of tuberculosis, but administrators were concerned about the potential for an outbreak based on reports from other city institutions. Columbia first (May 1992) instituted extensive administrative controls that emphasized stricter respiratory isolation policies; shortly thereafter (July 1992), it installed two tuberculosis isolation rooms in the emergency department. In July 1993, the hospital began to require that medical house staff don a 3M disposable respirator to enter respiratory isolation rooms; they provided surgical masks prior to that. House staff were fit tested and instructed in the use of the new devices. The tuberculin skin test conversions among house staff dropped from 10 percent preimplementation to 0 percent to 2 percent for time intervals after implementation of the administrative controls and engineering controls but *before* the provision of new respirators. The authors felt that administrative controls were the main reason for the improvements observed.

St. Clare's Hospital in New York City implemented the 1990 CDC guidelines in 1991 (Fella et al., 1995). This hospital focused first on administrative controls (especially, early recognition and isolation of patients with active tuberculosis) and then on engineering controls (including installation of 44 negative-pressure isolation rooms in a 2-year period and installation of ultraviolet [UV] germicidal irradiation lights in patient rooms and general use-areas). The institutions made a series of changes in the respiratory protection devices provided employees (switching in January 1992 from the Technol shield to a particulate respirator, then in January 1993 to a dust-mist-fume respirator with fit testing beginning in June 1993, and, finally to HEPA respirators in 1994 after the study period ended). From 1991 to 1993, the tuberculin skin test conversion rate among health care staff fell from 20.7 percent in the first 6-month testing interval to a range of 3.2 to 6.2 percent over subsequent 6-month intervals. Changes in conversion rates were not associated with changes in personal respiratory protection.

Another report on the experience of a Chicago hospital suggests that personal respirators do not compensate for inadequate engineering controls. Kenyon and colleagues (1997) reported an outbreak of multidrug-resistant tuberculosis in a facility that had provided and fit-tested workers with high-efficiency particulate respirators but that had no isolation rooms that met CDC criteria. Delays in recognizing and treating infectious patients also contributed to the outbreak. Three of the 11 previously skin test negative workers who converted their tuberculin skin test (including one ward secretary with no patient care responsibilities) had no contact with the source case patients. The authors conclude that a respiratory protection program alone cannot protect all workers. In the absence of appropriate isolation rooms, air that escapes from rooms housing infectious patients can infect those outside the room.

Also pertinent is a survey of 52 former house staff who served in the tuberculosis facility associated with the University of Virginia between 1979 and 1987 (Jernigan et al., 1994). The 52 individuals had experienced a total of 70 6-week rotations in the facility, which had negative-pressure isolation rooms and ultraviolet germicidal radiation. A simple surgical mask (no fit-testing program) was the only form of respiratory protection used. Those surveyed reported no skin test conversions associated with the rotation.

In another survey, the Society for Healthcare Epidemiology (SHEA) surveyed member hospitals for tuberculosis control practices from 1989 to 1992 and evaluated responses from 210 hospitals (Fridkin et al., 1995a,b). Four control practices described in the 1990 CDC guidelines were evaluated: (1) placing known or suspected tuberculosis patients into a single room (or a room shared by two such patients); (2) negative-pressure ventilation of the isolation room, (3) at least 6 or greater air changes per hour in isolation rooms; and (4) air exhaust directly to the outside. For the subgroup of hospitals that admitted at least six or more tuberculosis patients per year and met all four criteria, the tuberculin skin test conversion rate among health care workers was significantly less for those hospitals compared to those for others (0.6 versus 1.89 percent; $p = 0.02$). Conversion rates were not associated with type of respiratory protection. The survey did not cover fit testing.

In all of the reports cited above, the implementation of tuberculosis control measures was associated with low levels of tuberculosis transmission among health care workers in hospitals where tuberculosis was prevalent. These data, although imperfect and limited, support CDC's emphasis on administrative controls and suggest the lesser contribution of a respiratory protection program in the hierarchy of tuberculosis infection control. Admittedly, the data lack sufficient power to support firm conclusions. Such conclusions would require well designed, prospective controlled studies to investigate specifically the independent contribution of a respiratory protection intervention. Until such data are available (and it is far from clear that the necessary studies will be undertaken), the appropriate level of respiratory protection will likely continue to be an area of debate.

MODELING STUDIES
PROJECTING EFFECTS OF RESPIRATORY PROTECTIONS

It is not a surprise to find that observational studies of the effects of implementing tuberculosis controls in health care setting have not clearly demonstrated the independent effect of the respiratory protection components of these programs. In large part, this is due to the simultaneous implementation of several control improvements with the consequent inability to contrast outcomes where individual elements of the control program are present versus when they are absent. In addition, the studies typically involve relatively small numbers of workers who convert their tuberculin skin tests following periodic (usually yearly) testing. If respirators have a small but positive effect, such studies (and epidemiologic studies generally) will lack the statistical power to detect the effects.

Much of the literature on respirator efficacy is based on theoretical and empirical data which demonstrates that respirators can reduce the exposure to airborne contaminants by factors ranging from 2.4 to greater than 200 (Barnhart et al., 1997). Two papers have modeled the potential for respirators to reduce risk for tuberculin skin test conversion based on data from a series of elegant experiments by Riley and colleagues (Riley et al., 1959, 1962). First, Riley and colleagues noted the rate at which nurses converted their skin tests in tuberculosis wards and calculated on the basis of their expected minute ventilation the estimated concentration of infectious particles in the air of these wards. Then based on these estimates they performed an experiment using guinea pigs as a bioassay and calculated the average airborne production of infectious particles generated by patients with infectious tuberculosis. These data based on direct monitoring of tuberculosis infection from airborne droplet nuclei provide, perhaps, the strongest data on risks to workers exposed to patients with infectious tuberculosis.

In two complementary papers Barnhart and colleagues (1997) and Fennelly and Nardell (1998) model the potential benefits of respiratory protection. Both papers rely on published estimates of the ability of respirators to reduce exposure to airborne particles. Inherent in this reliance is an assumption that tuberculosis particles or droplet nuclei will be filtered out by the medium just as other hazardous particles such as silica, asbestos, or plutonium are. While it is well recognized that fit factors under static conditions vary considerably from those under work conditions, the general principle of respirators reducing exposure is well accepted (Houdous and Coffey, 1994).

Barnhart and colleagues, using the data of Riley and colleagues (1959) on concentration of infectious particles, estimated that under average conditions of exposure it would take 2,650 person-hours to convert a tuberculin skin test in an unprotected worker. Risk of tuberculin skin test conversion was estimated to be reduced by the following proportions by using a respirator: surgical mask, 2.4-fold; disposable dust, fume, mist (analogous to N95), 17.5-fold; elastomeric HEPA cartridge respirator, 45-fold; and PAPR, 238-fold. Use of a dust-fume-mist respirator is estimated to increase the time to tuberculin skin test conversion from 2,650 to greater than 44,000 hours. Similar benefits were seen for increasing ventilation and use of ultraviolet germicidal irradiation. Using the data of Riley and colleagues, for a lifetime exposure to infectious patients of 250 hours, the risk of a tuberculin skin test conversion for an unprotected worker was estimated to be 9 percent. For these reasons, use of a respirator under conditions of exposure or risk was felt to be prudent. In this paper, benefit and risk are closely linked. In the absence of risk, of course, no benefit can be expected.

Fennelly and Nardell (1998) also used the data of Riley and colleagues and very similar protection factors for respirators. They tested the hypothesis "that personal respiratory protection is relatively more efficacious in decreasing the risk of infection with *Mycobacterium tuberculosis* for exposures more highly concentrated aerosols or at low room ventilation rates, and conversely that respirators are relatively less efficacious as the concentration of the infectious aerosol decreases or as room rates increase. (Fennelly and Nardell, 1998, p. 754) Their estimates showed the risk of infection decreasing exponentially with increasing room ventilation or increasing personal respiratory protection. As concentrations of the infectious particles decrease, the relative efficacy of respirators decreases. They conclude that the risk of occupational tuberculosis probably can be lowered considerably by using relatively simple respirators, but in settings of higher risk (e.g., cough-inducing procedures) more sophisticated respirators may be needed.

EVIDENCE OF EFFECTS OF WORKER TRAINING AND FIT TESTING

Among health care infection control experts, the effectiveness of respirators is less controversial than the well-established view in the occupational health world that real-world effectiveness requires that respirator use be part of a broader respiratory protection program with quite specific elements. The OSHA 1998 respiratory protection standard (29 CFR 1910.134) makes these elements explicit. They include medical evaluation of employees required to use respirators (which may be limited to a brief questionnaire), both initial and annual fit testing; employee training regarding the respiratory hazards that they face, and training in the proper use of the respirators themselves.

While respirators that fit (i.e., have an acceptably low rate of leakage around the face seal) provide greater protection than those that do not, methods to ensure good fit are imperfect and still evolving, particularly for the N95 respirators. Laboratory studies by Coffey and colleagues (1999) showed that using N95 respirators reduced exposure to aerosolized particulates and that fit testing the respirators produced substantial reductions in exposure. However, when the most rigorous criterion for fit testing was used (the 1 percent pass/fail criterion recommended by American National Standards Institute and required by OSHA), a substantial majority of tested individuals failed the fit test for 17 of the 21 devices tested, that is, most people could not be successfully fitted. The required 1 percent pass/fail criterion is thought to be needed to achieve no more than 10 percent respirator face-seal leakage during normal use in the workplace. Currently, the main certified alternative to the N95 respirator would be the PAPR, which is much more cumbersome and expensive to buy and maintain. It also can interfere with communication and cannot be used when a sterile field is needed as in surgery.

Coffey and colleagues suggested that the major source of variability is the N95 respirator design itself rather than the user-respirator interface. Several of the most inadequate devices accounted for most of the variability among test results. Interpersonal variability was lower if one excluded the worst device. The study of Chen et al. (1994) found analogous results. They demonstrated that there was considerable variability, but a single mask accounted for much of this. Excluding this one, the residual variability in leakage among the others was relatively low.[2]

At least one less extensive study has suggested that education may be as effective as fit testing in improving workers performance in adjusting their respirators correctly (Hannum et al., 1996). In that study, a hospital recruited workers to participate in one of three respirator training programs and to be tested afterward on their ability to correctly adjust the respirator's fit and seal. They concluded that training was important but that it did not matter much whether the training included direct fit testing or a classroom demonstration of proper fit checking prior to each use of a respirator. (The devices in use were HEPA respirators rather than the N95 respirators now commonly used.)

---

[2]Rather than emphasizing individual fit testing, fit testing at the premarketing stage to eliminate poor design might be more cost effective. The governmental design-certifying agency (NIOSH) could shift to manufacturers much of the burden of assuring that masks are designed to fit most users properly.

In a letter to the editor of the *New England Journal of Medicine*, Brown and colleagues (1994) discussed the value of fit testing for HEPA respirators. They report that 12 subjects passed an initial fit test but 4 of 12 failed when the test was repeated following actual use of their respirators. Deformation of the respirator was cited as the likely explanation. Thus, this short report suggests that passing a fit test may not assure adequate protection under actual use conditions. A reduction in protection may occur because of degradation of the mask, physical changes in the individual, or the need for reinforcement of proper technique.

CONCLUSION

Respiratory protection, particularly requirements for routine annual fit testing, is one of the most contentious elements of the 1997 proposed OSHA regulation on occupational tuberculosis. The challenge for policy makers is to craft reasonable, cost-effective policies in this area that (1) are based on the best available science (recognizing that much uncertainty still exists) and (2) match respiratory protection requirements to the degree of tuberculosis risk facing workers and institutions. Overall, the risk of occupational tuberculosis has been declining for health care, correctional, and other workers in recent years with adoption of community and workplace tuberculosis control measures. For example, since 1992, tuberculosis case rates have declined nationwide by 35 percent.

In some cases, research and product development efforts may help policymakers devise feasible risk-sensitive policies. For example, CDC/ NIOSH has taken steps in this direction by testing and certifying N95 respirators, which are less costly than the HEPA respirators that they have largely replaced but still meet the criteria set forth by CDC in 1994. The agency has also tested different types of N95 respirators to identify deficient models, which may suggest the need for more attention to the manufacturing and premarketing stage (before a respirator reaches a user).

Given that a major concern involves the burden of respiratory protection requirements for low-risk institutions and individuals, CDC/NIOSH should consider further research on (1) methods for risk categorization or stratification (based on probability of infection) of individuals and institutions caring for tuberculosis patients and (2) levels of respiratory protection that are appropriate (i.e., will reasonably reduce risk) for institutions or individuals with different levels of risk. Such research would provide policymakers and managers with better guidance on those situations that warrant minimal versus higher levels of respiratory protection.

REFERENCES

Bangsberg HM, et al. Reduction in tuberculin skin-test conversions among medical house staff associated with improved tuberculosis infection control practices. *Infection Control and Hospital Epidemiology*. 18:556–570, 1997.

Barnhart S, et al. Tuberculosis in health care settings and the estimated benefits of engineering controls and respiratory protection. *Journal of Occupational and Environmental Medicine*. 39(9):849–854, 1997.

Blumberg HM, Watkins DL, et al. Preventing the nosocomial transmission of tuberculosis. *Annals of Internal Medicine*. 12:658–663, 1995.

Brown V, et al. HEPA respirators and tuberculosis in hospital workers [letter; comment]. *New England Journal of Medicine*. 331(24):1659; discussion 1659–1660, 1994.

CDC (Centers for Disease and Control and Prevention). Guidelines for preventing the transmission of Mycobacterium tuberculosis in health-care facilities, 1994. *Morbidity and Mortality Weekly Report*. 43(RR-13):1–132, 1994 http://www.cdc.gov/epo/mmwr-/preview/mmwrhtml/00035909.htm.

Chen SK, et al. Evaluation of single-use masks and respirators for protection of health care workers against mycobacterial aerosols. *American Journal of Infection Control*. 22(2): 65–74, 1994.

Coffey CC, Campbell DL, Zhuang Z. Simulated Workplace Performance of N95 Respirators. *American Industrial Hygiene Association Journal*. 60:618–624, 1999.

Fella P, et al. Dramatic decreases in tuberculin skin test conversion rate among employees at a hospital in NYC. *American Journal of Infection Control*. 23:352–356, 1995.

Fennelly KP. Personal respiratory protection against Mycobacterium tuberculosis. *Clinics in Chest Medicine*. 18(1):1–17, 1997.

Fennelly KP, Nardell EA. The relative efficacy of respirators and room ventilation in preventing occupational tuberculosis. *Infection Control and Hospital Epidemiology*. 19(10):754–759, 1998.

Fridkin SK, Manangan L, et al. SHEA-CDC TB survey, Part I: Status of TB infection control programs at member hospitals, 1989–1992. *Infection Control and Hospital Epidemiology*. 16:129–134, 1995a.

Fridkin SK, Manangan L, et al. SHEA-CDC TB survey, Part II: Efficacy of TB infection control programs at member hospitals, 1992. *Infection Control and Hospital Epidemiology*. 16:135–140, 1995b.

Hannum D, Cycan K, Jones L, Stewart M, Morris S, Markowitz SM, Wong ES. The effect of respirator training on the ability of healthcare workers to pass a qualitative fit test. *Infection Control and Hospital Epidemiology*. 17(10):636–640, 1996.

Harber P, Merz B, Chi K. Decision model for optimizing respirator protection. *Journal of Occupational Medicine*. 41(5):356–365, 1999.

Hodous TK, CC Coffey. The role of respiratory protective devices in the control of tuberculosis. *Occupational Medicine*. 9(4):631–657, 1994.

Jernigan JA, Adal KA, et al. *Mycobacterium tuberculosis* transmission rates in a sanatorium: implications for new preventive guidelines. *American Journal of Infection Control*. 22:329–333, 1994.

Kenyon TA, et al. A nosocomial outbreak of multidrug-resistant tuberculosis. *Annals of Internal Medicine*. 127(1):32–36, 1997.

Maloney SA, Pearson ML, et al. Efficacy of control measures in preventing nosocomial transmission of MDRTB. *Annals of Internal Medicine*. 122:90–95, 1995.

McGowan JE. Nosocomial tuberculosis: new progress in control and prevention. *Clinical and Infectious Diseases*. 21:489–505, 1995.

Qian Y, et al. Performance of N95 respirators: filtration efficiency for airborne microbial and inert particles. *American Industrial Hygiene Association Journal*. 59(2):128–132, 1998.

Riley R, Mills C, O'Grady F, et al. Infectiousness of air from a tuberculosis ward, ultraviolet irradiation of infected air, comparative infectiousness of different patients. *American Review of Tuberculosis and Pulmonary Diseases.* 84:511–525, 1962.

Riley RL, Mills CC, Nyka W, et al. Aerial dissemination of pulmonary tuberculosis: two-year study of contagion in a tuberculosis ward. *American Journal of Hygiene.* 70: 185–196, 1959.

Schaefer JA. Respiratory protection in the health care setting. *Occupational Medicine.* 12(4): 641–654, 1997.

Sultan L, Nyka W, Mills C, O'Grady F, Wells W, Riley R. Tuberculosis disseminators, a study of the variability of aerial infectivity of tuberculosis patients. *American Review of Tuberculosis and Pulmonary Diseases.* 82:358–369, 1960.

Vesley DL. Respiratory protection devices. *American Journal of Infection Control.* 23(2):165–168, 1995.

Wenger PN, Otten J, et al. Control of nosocomial transmission of MDRTB among healthcare workers and HIV-infected patients. *Lancet.* 345:235–240, 1995.

G

Recommendations of the Institute of Medicine Committee on Eliminating Tuberculosis in the United States[1]

Recommendation 3.1   To permanently interrupt the transmission of tuberculosis and prevent the emergence of multidrug-resistant tuberculosis, the committee recommends that

• All states have health regulations that mandate completion of therapy (treatment to cure) for all patients with active tuberculosis.
• All treatment be administered in the context of patient-centered programs that are based on individual patient characteristics. Such programs must be the standard of care for patients with tuberculosis in all settings.

Recommendation 3.2   To ensure the most efficient application of existing resources, the committee recommends that

• New program standards be developed and used by CDC [Centers for Disease Control and Prevention] and state and local health departments to evaluate program performance.
• Standardized, flexible case management systems be developed to provide the information needed for the evaluation measurements. These systems should be integrated with existing case management systems and other automated public health data systems whenever possible.

---

[1]Institute of Medicine. *Ending Neglect: The Elimination of Tuberculosis in the United States* Geiter L, ed. Washington DC: National Academy Press, 2000, pp. 6–12.

Recommendation 3.3   To make further progress toward the elimination of tuberculosis in regions of the country experiencing low rates of disease, the committee recommends that

• Tuberculosis elimination activities be regionalized through a combination of federal and multistate initiatives to provide better access to and more efficient utilization of clinical, epidemiological, and other technical services.

• Protocols and action plans be developed jointly by CDC and the states for use by state and local health departments to enable planning for the availability of adequate resources.

• State and local health departments develop case management plans to ensure a uniform high quality of care for patients with tuberculosis and tuberculosis infection in their jurisdictions.

Recommendation 3.4   To maintain quality in tuberculosis care and control services in an era of increased use of managed care systems and privatization of services, the committee recommends that

• When it is determined that tuberculosis diagnosis and treatment services can be provided more efficiently outside of the public health department, the delivery of such services be governed by well-designed contracts that specify performance measures and responsibilities.

• Federal categorical funding for tuberculosis control be retained. Funding at the local level should provide sufficient dedicated resources for tuberculosis control but should be structured to provide maximum flexibility and efficiency.

• Both public and private health insurance programs be billed for tuberculosis diagnostic and treatment services whenever possible, but tuberculosis services should never be denied due to a patient's inability to make a co-payment.

Recommendation 3.5   To promote a well-trained medical (in a broad sense) workforce and educated public, the committee recommends that

• The Strategic Plan for Tuberculosis Training and Education, which contains the blueprint that addresses the training and educational needs for tuberculosis control, be fully funded.

• Programs for the education of patients with tuberculosis be developed and funded.

• Funding be provided for government, academic, and nongovernmental agencies to work in collaboration with international partners to develop training and educational materials.

Recommendation 4.1   To limit the spread of tuberculosis from infectious patients to their contacts, the committee recommends that more effective methodologies for the identification of persons with recently acquired tuberculosis infection, especially persons exposed to patients with new cases of tuberculosis, be developed and efforts be increased to evaluate appropriately and treat latent infection in all persons who meet the criteria for treatment for such infections.

Recommendation 4.2 To prevent the development of tuberculosis among individuals with latent tuberculosis infection, the committee recommends that

• Tuberculin skin testing be required as part of the medical evaluation for immigrant visa applicants from countries with high rates of tuberculosis, a Class B4 immigration waiver designation be created for persons with normal chest radiographs and positive tuberculin skin tests, and all tuberculin-positive Class B immigrants be required to undergo an evaluation for tuberculosis and, when indicated, complete an approved course of treatment for latent infection before receiving a permanent residency card ("green card"). Implementation should be in a stepwise fashion, and pilot programs should evaluate strategies and assess costs.

• Tuberculin testing be required of all inmates of correctional facilities and completion of an approved course of treatment, when indicated, be required, with referral to the appropriate public health agency for all inmates released before completion of treatment.

• Programs of targeted tuberculin skin testing and treatment of latent infection be increased for high-incidence groups, such as HIV-infected individuals, undocumented immigrants, homeless individuals, and intravenous drug abusers, as determined by local epidemiological circumstances.

Recommendation 5.1 To advance the development of tuberculosis vaccines, the committee recommends that the plans outlined in the Blueprint for Tuberculosis Vaccine Development, published by NIH [National Institutes of Health] in 1998, be fully implemented.

Recommendation 5.2 To advance the development of diagnostic tests and new drugs for both latent infection and active disease, action plans should be developed and implemented. CDC should then exploit its expertise in population-based research to evaluate and define the role of promising products.

Recommendation 5.3 To promote better understanding of patient and provider nonadherence with tuberculosis treatment recommendations and guidelines, a plan for a behavioral and social science research agenda should be developed and implemented.

Recommendation 5.4   To encourage private-sector product development, the global market for tuberculosis diagnostic tests, drugs, and vaccines should be better characterized and access to these markets for these new products should be facilitated.

Recommendation 5.5   To define the applicability of any new tools to the international arena and facilitate their development, the U.S. Agency for International Development (AID), NIH, and CDC should build upon international relationships and expertise to conduct research.

Recommendation 6.1   To decrease the number of foreign-born individuals with tuberculosis in the United States, to minimize the spread and impact of multidrug-resistant tuberculosis, and to improve global health, the committee recommends that

• The United States expand and strengthen its role in global tuberculosis control efforts, contributing to these efforts in a substantial manner through bilateral and multilateral international efforts.
• The United States contribute to global tuberculosis control efforts through targeted use of financial, technical, and human resources and research, all guided by a carefully considered strategic plan.
• The United States work in close coordination with other government and international agencies. In particular, the United States should continue its active role in and support of the Stop TB Initiative.
• AID, CDC, and NIH should jointly develop and publish strategic plans to guide U.S. involvement in global tuberculosis control efforts.

Recommendation 7.1   To build public support and sustain public interest and commitment to the elimination of tuberculosis, the committee recommends that CDC significantly increase resources for activities to secure and sustain public understanding and support for tuberculosis elimination efforts at the national, state, and local levels, including programs to increase knowledge among targeted groups of the general public.

Recommendation 7.2   To increase the effectiveness of mobilization efforts the committee recommends that the National Coalition for the Elimination of Tuberculosis continue to provide leadership and oversight and that CDC continue to work in collaboration with the coalition to secure the support and participation of nontraditional public health partners, ensure the development of state and local coalitions, and evaluate public understanding and support for tuberculosis elimination efforts with the assistance of public opinion research experts.

Recommendation 7.3 To assess the impacts of these recommendations and to measure progress toward accomplishing the elimination of tuberculosis, the committee recommends that, 3 years after the publication of this report and periodically thereafter, the Office of the Secretary of Health and Human Services conduct an evaluation of the actions taken in response to the recommendations in this report.

H

Committee Biographies

WALTER HIERHOLZER, M.D. (*Chair*), is Professor Emeritus of Internal Medicine, Infectious Diseases, and Epidemiology at the Yale University School of Medicine. He was also Director of the Department of Hospital Epidemiology and Co-director of the Department of Quality Improvement Support Services at Yale New Haven Hospital until his retirement from that institution in January 2000. From 1976 to 1985, he was the Director of the Program of Hospital Epidemiology at the University of Iowa Hospitals and Clinics, where he founded and was responsible for the Iowa Statewide Epidemiology Education and Consultation Program serving over 100 hospitals. He is the former Chair of the Centers for Disease Control and Prevention Hospital Infection Control Practices Advisory Committee, former Chair of the American Hospital Association Technical Panel on Infections within Hospitals, Past President of the Society of Healthcare Epidemiologists for America, and a member of the Joint Commission on Accreditation of Health Care Organizations Infection Control Indicators Task Force and the (Computer) Information Management Task Force.

SCOTT BARNHART, M.D., is Medical Director, Harborview Medical Center, and Associate Dean, University of Washington School of Medicine. He is past director of the University's Occupational and Environmental Medicine Program and is certified in pulmonology and occupational medicine. Dr. Barnhart has 18 years of experience in the area of clinical pulmonary and occupational medicine. He has conducted research on the structure, function, and financing of occupational health systems in the United States and Southeast Asia. His publications include work in the areas of risk assessment for intra-institutional spread of tuberculosis, benefits of engineering controls and respiratory protection, and clearance of worker populations for use of respirators.

HENRY M. BLUMBERG, M.D., is Associate Professor, Division of Infectious Diseases, Department of Medicine, at Emory University School of Medicine in Atlanta. He also serves as Hospital Epidemiologist at Grady Memorial Hospital, which is a major teaching affiliate of Emory. Dr. Blumberg has been on the Emory faculty and at Grady Hospital for the past 8 years. He is board certified in internal medicine and infectious diseases by the American Board of Internal Medicine. He is a recipient of a National Institutes of Health Tuberculosis Academic Award (1993–2001) and has played a central role in tuberculosis-related education at Emory University. He has published widely on the efficacy of tuberculosis infection control measures implemented at Grady Memorial Hospital, a 1,000-bed inner-city hospital which has cared for about 200 new tuberculosis patients per year over the past decade. He has also served as principal investigator for a Robert Wood Johnson Foundation Tuberculosis Demonstration Project in Atlanta, the Atlanta TB Prevention Coalition, which involves collaboration among a variety of major groups including public health, academic, private, and community-based organizations involved in tuberculosis education, management, and control in Atlanta.

SCOTT BURRIS, J.D., is on the faculty of Temple University School of Law, Philadelphia, where he has been since 1991. Formerly an attorney at the American Civil Liberties Union of Pennsylvania, he has also served as law clerk to Judge (now Chief Judge) Dolores Sloviter of the Third Circuit United States Court of Appeals. He is a graduate of the Yale Law School. Professor Burris is the editor of *AIDS Law Today: A New Guide for the Public* (1993), and the author or co-author of articles on the law and public health including *The Law and the Public's Health: A Study of Infectious Disease Law in the United States*, 99 Columbia L. Rev. 59 (1999). He serves on numerous advisory committees on matters relating to the intersection of public health and law.

ROBYN GERSHON, Dr.P.H., is Assistant Professor at the Joseph L. Mailman School of Public Health, Columbia University, in the Division of Sociomedical Sciences. She recently served as Associate Scientist in the Department of Environmental Health Sciences at The Johns Hopkins University School of Hygiene and Public Health. She has a doctorate in public health from Johns Hopkins University. She has conducted several research studies involving tuberculosis risk in both hospital-based and non-hospital-based health care workers, including funeral directors, emergency service employees, and most recently, correctional health care workers. She has special expertise in the area of tuberculin skin testing as well as in risk reduction methodologies, including a wide range of control measures (e.g., engineering, administrative, and work practice controls). Dr. Gershon is also a clinical microbiologist, with a master's in medical microbiology.

DOUGLAS HORNICK, M.D., is Associate Professor, Division of Pulmonary, Critical Care, and Occupational Medicine, Department of Internal Medicine, University of Iowa. He is board certified in internal medicine, with subspecialty board certification in both pulmonary and critical care medicine. His clinical and research interests focus on lung infections. He is director of the tuberculosis Chest Clinic as well as the adult Cystic Fibrosis Service at the University of Iowa. He serves as an advisor to the State Department of Health for tuberculosis-related issues and is the author of several review articles, web pages, and textbook chapters on tuberculosis. He has also served on the international consensus committee on nosocomial pneumonia, and the Microbiology, Tuberculosis and Pulmonary Infection Program committee for the American Thoracic Society.

PAMELA KELLNER, R.N., M.P.H., is the Director of the Program Development Unit for the New York City Department of Health Tuberculosis Control Program. She has also served as Deputy Director for Outreach Services, planning and providing administrative oversight for regulatory affairs, directly observed therapy, homeless services, and screening activities related to tuberculosis outbreaks and exposure incidents within large groups and special populations. She has worked as an employee health services administrator and has directed an on-site mental health program in a large urban homeless shelter.

JAMES MELIUS, M.D., Dr.P.H., is Director of the New York State Laborers' Health and Safety Trust Fund and Director of Research for the Laborers' Health and Safety Fund of North America. His work focuses on the development and promotion of health and safety programs in the construction industry. He is currently Chair of the Board of Scientific Counselors for the Agency for Toxic Substances and Disease Registries, a member of the Board of Scientific Counselors for the National Institute for Occupational Safety and Health, and a past member of the Advisory Committee for the Elimination of Tuberculosis for the Centers of Disease Control and Prevention. He worked for the National Institute for Occupational Safety and Health from 1980 to 1987, where he directed its main workplace consultation program. From 1987 to 1994, he worked for the New York State Department of Health where he directed environmental and occupational health programs including the development of a network of occupational health clinics.

STEPHEN G. PAUKER, M.D., is Vice Chairman for Clinical Affairs, Department of Medicine, and Associate Physician-in-Chief, New England Medical Center, and Sara Murray Jordan Professor of Medicine, Tufts University. Dr. Pauker is a member of the Institute of Medicine (IOM). Prior committee memberships have included IOM's Guidelines on Thyroid Cancer Screening, and the Committee to Evaluate the Artificial Heart Program of the National Heart, Lung, and Blood Institute, as well as Workshops on the National Institutes of Health Consensus Development Process and the Use of Drugs in the Elderly, both within IOM. His publications and research have focused on screening for cancer and other conditions, applications of clinical decision theory and medical informatics to health policy, technology assessment and the individualization of patient care, cost-effectiveness analysis, clinical cardiology, telemedicine, ethics of various reimbursement models, and efficiency of care delivery.

ROBERT C. SPEAR, Ph.D., is a Professor of Environmental Health Sciences at the University of California, Berkeley. He received an M.S. in mechanical engineering in 1963 from the University of California, Berkeley, and a Ph.D. in control engineering from Cambridge University in Cambridge, England, 5 years later. Dr. Spear's research interests relate principally to the assessment and control of exposures to hazardous agents in both the occupational and community environments. He has an extensive publication record in this field which spans farmworkers' exposures to pesticides to strategies for the characterization and control of the exposure of rural populations to parasites in the developing world. He was appointed Founding Director of the University of California's Center for Occupational and Environmental Health in 1979 and continues to serve in that capacity. He has served on numerous committees advisory to governmental agencies including the National Advisory Committee on Occupational Safety and Health and, currently, the National Institute for Occupational Safety and Health Board of Scientific Counselors.

LESTER N. WRIGHT, M.D., M.P.H., is Deputy Commissioner/Chief Medical Officer responsible for provision of health care to 72,000 inmates in New York State prisons. He has dealt with tuberculosis in primary care in Ethiopia, as tuberculosis control officer for a county public health agency, as a state health officer, and in his current corrections health position in a large state prison system where a multiple drug-resistant tuberculosis outbreak was first identified and the rate of new cases of tuberculosis disease has decreased 83 percent since the peak in 1991. He is certified by the American Board of Preventive Medicine. Dr. Wright spent 7 years working in various parts of Africa including delivery of primary health care and health system development and supervision. He continues to do international consultation in areas such as child survival and prevention of human immunodeficiency virus infection.

Index

S